Handbook of
Behaviour Problems of the
Dog and Cat

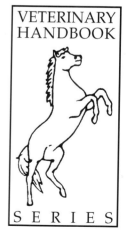

VETERINARY
HANDBOOK

S E R I E S

Handbook of
Behaviour Problems of the Dog and Cat

by

GARY M. LANDSBERG, DVM Dip ACVB

Doncaster Animal Clinic, Thornhill, Ontario, Canada

WAYNE HUNTHAUSEN, DVM

Animal Behavior Consultations, Westwood, Kansas, USA

and

LOWELL ACKERMAN, DVM PhD Dip ACVD

Pet Health Initiative, Scottsdale, Arizona, USA

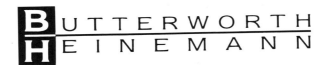

Butterworth-Heinemann
Linacre House, Jordan Hill, Oxford OX2 8DP
225 Wildwood Avenue, Woburn 01801-2041
A division of Reed Educational and Professional Publishing Ltd

 A member of the Reed Elsevier plc group

OXFORD   AUCKLAND   BOSTON
JOHANNESBURG   MELBOURNE   NEW DELHI

First published 1997
Reprinted 1997, 1998 (twice), 1999

British Library Cataloguing in Publication Data
Handbook of behaviour problems of the dog and cat
1 Dogs – Behaviour 2 Cats – Behaviour 3 Dogs – Training
4 Cats – Training 5 Dogs – Psychology 6 Cats –
Psychology I Title Hunthausen, Wayne III Ackerman,
Lowell
636.790887

ISBN 0 7506 3060 4

Library of Congress Cataloguing in Publication Data
Handbook of behaviour problems of the dog and cat/by Gary
M. Landsberg, Wayne Hunthausen and Lowell Ackerman.
p.   cm. – (Veterinary handbook series)
Includes bibliographical references and index.
ISBN 0 7506 3060 4
1 Dogs – Behaviour. 2 Cats – Behaviour. 3 Dogs –
Psychology. 4 Cats – Psychology. 5 Animal behaviour
therapy. I Hunthausen, Wayne. II Ackerman, Lowell.
III Title. IV Series.
SF433.L35   96–15793
636.79089689–dc20   CIP

Disclaimer: Whilst every effort is made by the Publishers to see
that no inaccurate or misleading data, opinion or statement
appear in this book, they wish to make it clear that the data and
opinions appearing in the articles herein are the sole
responsibility of the contributor concerned. Accordingly, the
Publishers and their employees, officers and agents accept no
responsibility or liability whatsoever for the consequences of any
such inaccurate or misleading data, opinion or statement.

Drug and Dosage Selection: The authors have made every
effort to ensure the accuracy of the information herein,
particularly with regard to drug selection and dose. However,
appropriate information sources should be consulted, especially
for new or unfamiliar drugs or procedures. It is the responsibility
of every veterinarian to evaluate the appropriateness of a
particular opinion in the context of actual clinical situations, and
with due consideration to new developments.

Composition by Genesis Typesetting, Rochester
Printed and bound in Great Britain at the Alden Press, Oxford

Contents

Preface

As little as ten years ago, animal behaviour was considered an interesting diversion for veterinarians, but little emphasis was placed on this discipline in veterinary school curricula or continuing education for practitioners. Now, there seems to be a general awakening in the veterinary profession as practitioners realize the importance of this subject to their clients, the well-being of their patients, and the success of their practices.

Clearly, behaviour plays an important role in the life of a pet and its relationship with its owners. As a matter of fact, behaviour problems are one of the more common reasons for abandonment and euthanasia of dogs and cats. North American statistics suggest that more pets are euthanised for behavioural reasons than for all medical reasons combined. Recent studies suggest that those pet owners who receive insufficient advice and guidance on behaviour and training are the most likely to relinquish their pets to shelters. This should be enough of an incentive for veterinarians to incorporate behavioural evaluations and counselling into everyday practice.

This book is designed to provide the veterinarian in general practice with the tools to help owners with concerns they might have about their pets' behaviour. Most importantly, it helps veterinarians incorporate behaviour consultation into their practices in a very meaningful way. Not only does the book introduce topics such as learning theory and behaviour modification techniques but it also covers the diagnostic and therapeutic options for the successful management of behaviour problems. Case examples are used to illustrate real-life clinical situations. To be successful in managing behaviour problems, veterinarians must be more than animal trainers. The proper approach to behavioural problems does not differ significantly from any other medical discipline. One needs to evaluate carefully patient history, perform a thorough physical examination, formulate differential diagnoses, conduct diagnostic testing, initiate treatment options and monitor the patient's responses. Proper diagnosis of the problem and selection of reasonable treatment modalities are solely in the realm of veterinary medicine; let this book serve as your guide.

To all of those who took the time to share with us their thoughts, ideas and observations on behaviour, we wholeheardedly thank you. To our families who saw less of us, to our pets who received fewer walks and less attention, and to our partners and associates in practice who covered for us, you have no idea how much we appreciate your patience and value the support that you gave us while we worked on this project.

Dedication

To my wonderful wife Susan and my adorable children Nadia, Rebecca and David – L. Ackerman.

To the world's greatest wife Susan and children Joanna, Mitchell, and Jordan, our toller Grace, and my partner (in practice) Dr. Steve Waisglass – G. Landsberg.

To my wife, Jan Kyle, my buddies Simon the Standard poodle, Ralphie the Airedale and Russell a most wonderful and talented mutt. – W. Hunthausen.

1

Behaviour Counselling and the Veterinary Practitioner

The Importance of Providing Counselling Services

Pet behaviour problems all too often result in the demise of the pet due to euthanasia or abandonment. The veterinary profession must be a leader in reversing this trend. Although many veterinarians routinely counsel owners (by some estimates accounting for 20% of a veterinarian's time), a comprehensive and standardised approach is sorely needed. It is our intention to provide the foundations for this approach within the pages of this book.

There are many reasons why veterinarians should be enthusiastic about behaviour counselling. In addition to the altruistic reasons of bettering the lives of pets and owners, there are also solid economic reasons for embracing these concepts. Timely behaviour counselling results in fewer behaviour problems so that fewer pets are rejected, abandoned or destroyed. Veterinarians are in the unique position of having repeated contact with most owners during the early, formative months of the pet's life when important information about preventing behaviour problems can be disseminated.

Recent estimates indicate that between 6 and 15 million dogs and cats are euthanised each year in the United States at shelters alone, with less than 5 per cent due to medical reasons. With timely and accurate behaviour counselling, the pet-owner relationship can be greatly improved, fewer pets will meet premature and untimely deaths, and a significant cause of client loss can be eliminated (Sigler, (1991); Arkow, (1994)). To this end, the AVMA has now recognised veterinary behaviour as a board-certified speciality area (i.e. the American College of Veterinary Behaviorists).

Veterinarians also have the medical and pharmacological background that gives them the opportunity to do a more complete job of counselling than behaviourists without a medical background. Behavioural changes can be an important indicator of illness, and many medical conditions cause or contribute to behaviour problems. However, this knowledge alone is insufficient for effective counselling. Veterinarians must learn the basic concepts of normal and abnormal behaviour and the strategies that are most effective for managing behaviour problems.

Behaviour Services that Veterinarians Can Offer Clients

There is a range of services that the veterinarian can offer:

- Preselection consultations
- Preventive behaviour counselling for new pet owners
- Puppy parties and training classes
- Behaviour management products and services
- Surgery
- Basic behaviour counselling
- Medical diagnostics and medical therapy (including pharmacological intervention)
- Advanced behavioural consultations.

Staff Utilisation and Training – The Team Approach

Veterinarians have some valuable allies for pet behavioural counselling. Properly trained veterinary technicians and nurses, assistants and front-office staff can provide owners with a wealth of information and can interface with clients on routine matters. A team approach taken by the veterinary practice instills confidence in owners and increases the probability of owner compliance. When owners receive consistent and timely information over many different office visits, they are more likely to understand the concepts and not to suffer from information overload. Placing a checklist of behaviour topics to discuss during vaccination visits in the file of each new puppy or kitten allows the staff to prioritise the message and to avoid duplication of effort (Figure 2.1). Providing the client with a reading list, utilising handouts, pamphlets and videos, and demonstrating behaviour products and techniques can all help improve the client's understanding and retention of important behavioural concepts.

The key to the team approach is proper education of staff (Fig. 1.1). Office personnel and technical staff should be trained through veterinary instruction and continuing education seminars, and a resource library should be provided. Many veterinary and technician nursing texts contain information on animal behaviour and most major veterinary conferences provide behaviour lectures for both veterinarians and staff. Well-trained staff do a great service but poorly trained or misinformed staff can be devastating to building client confidence and loyalty.

TRAINING AREAS FOR OFFICE STAFF AND TECHNICIANS/NURSES

Normal canine and feline behaviour

Stages of behavioural development

Principles of learning and behaviour modification (including rewards and punishment)

Training techniques

Socialisation

Handling and restraint

Common training and behaviour problems

Recognising abnormal behaviour

Fig. 1.1 Topics to be covered in training for the office team.

Veterinarians will not become experts in behavioural counselling overnight, or even from reading a book or two. Only by putting behavioural concepts into practice will these become second nature (Fig. 1.2). This book addresses the theory of counselling in addition to providing concise and practical information for the busy veterinarian. As with all aspects of medicine, the concepts of behaviour counselling are not static but are constantly evolving. Most major veterinary conferences now provide behaviour seminars and you are advised to attend as many as you are able. It would be advantageous for at least one staff member to belong to the American Veterinary Society of Animal Behaviour which is a professional organisation of veterinarians interested in applied animal behaviour. Newsletters of the society can provide you

---

STAYING UP TO DATE ON BEHAVIOUR COUNSELLING METHODS AND INFORMATION

Residency programme in the veterinary behaviour speciality (in the USA, this involves two years of postgraduate studies under a behaviourist at a veterinary school)

Attending continuing education seminars

Review of literature (veterinary medicine, psychology, ethology, animal behaviour)

Joining veterinary behaviour associations (e.g. American Veterinary Society of Animal Behavior; Companion Animal Behaviour Therapy Study Group)

Subscribe to behaviour newsletters and periodicals

Use computer bulletin boards with an on-line behaviour consultant (e.g. Veterinary Information Network (VIN) via American Online; NOAH via Compuserve)

Fig. 1.2 How to stay up to date on behavioural information.

---

with useful information as well as a forum for information exchange. The Companion Animal Behaviour Therapy Study Group and the European Society for Veterinary Ethology provide similar services for veterinarians in Great Britain and Europe, respectively. A postgraduate certificate in companion animal behaviour counselling will shortly become available in the UK. Addresses for behaviour organisations are listed at the end of this chapter.

There is additional help available for veterinary practitioners with difficult behaviour cases. Specialists in behaviour will accept referral cases and, in most instances, offer advice to veterinarians by telephone. These behaviourists provide an important extension of the veterinarian's own behaviour counselling services.

Providing Behavioural Services in Practice

Providing behavioural services should be an important facet of every veterinary practice. There are several different roles a veterinarian and veterinary clinic can take in this regard. These are highlighted in Fig. 1.3. Each has the effect of promoting healthy behaviours in pets and reinforces the notion that the veterinary practice is a complete care-giver.

A recent study by the American Animal Hospital Association revealed that 78% of pet owners consider their veterinarian to be the first person to contact when seeking help for behavioural problems. As many as 90% of dog owners noted one or more behaviour problems that they would like to improve.

BEHAVIOURAL SERVICES

Approach	Considerations
Preselection consultation	Consult with prospective pet owners to help them select an appropriate pet for their circumstances. Advise the owner about the health, behaviour, and nutritional requirements of their new pet so that the home and family can be prepared in advance
Preventive counselling	Counsel owners how to raise their pet in order to minimise behavioural problems. Use handouts, pamphlets, books, and videos
Puppy parties/training	Encourage owners to participate in puppy programmes to enhance early socialisation and provide training advice. If you have the space and expertise, consider offering classes in the clinic
Behaviour management products	Recommend and supply appropriate training devices (leashes, halters, chew-toys etc.) to prevent or correct undesirable behaviours. If you do not recommend the right products, the owners may make improper decisions
Surgery	Neutering can eliminate unwanted mating as well as preventing both behavioural and medical conditions. Declawing (except in countries where the procedure is illegal or considered unethical) and teeth extraction or dental disarming might be alternatives to consider when euthanasia or relinquishment are likely
Thorough medical history and work-up	Practice good-quality medicine and complete medical assessment on all patients routinely. Perform a medical work-up on every patient that requires a behavioural assessment. Diseases of any organ system can cause or contribute to behavioural problems
Basic behaviour counselling	As puppies and kittens mature, undesirable behaviours may develop. Intervene early and dedicate sufficient time to counselling for each specific behaviour problem. If managed unsuccessfully, consider referral before the behaviour becomes even more ingrained
Advanced behavioural consultations	Make sure you feel competent in performing behaviour counselling for advanced problems, such as aggression or destructive behaviours. If in doubt, contact a behaviour referral centre for advice or refer the case. Inappropriate counselling benefits neither the patient nor the veterinary practice

FIG. 1.3 Types of behavioural service offered by the veterinary practice.

All veterinarians should therefore have enough knowledge of normal and abnormal behaviour to know when and how to give advice, and when and where to refer. When cases are referred to a non-veterinary consultant, the referring veterinarian must take an active role in the diagnostic work-up, as well as any medical, pharmacological, or surgical therapy that might be indicated. Fig. 1.4 lists the most common behaviour problems in dogs.

The veterinarian who wants to provide complete behavioural counselling services must have a good understanding of animal learning, normal behaviour and behaviour modification. Know your limitations and attempt to master one problem area at a time, such as feline housesoiling or canine destructive behaviours. Add additional behavioural problems only after you have mastered your approach to previous ones. For dogs, practitioners could begin by offering behaviour counselling on topics such as puppy training, jumping up, coprophagia, digging, barking, begging, garbage raiding, chewing, play biting, and

MOST COMMON BEHAVIOUR PROBLEMS IN DOGS

According to owners*	Seen at referral practices†
Aggression ✓	Aggression
Barking ✓	Inappropriate elimination
Jumping up	Destructive behaviour
Destructive behaviour ✓	Excitability/unruliness
Begging for food	Barking
Inappropriate elimination ✓	Fears and phobias
Running away	Excessive submission
Fears and phobias	Compulsive and stereotypic behaviours (*see* Chapter 12)
Disobedience	
Excitability/unruliness ✓	
Submission	
Coprophagia	

* Adapted from Beaver (1994)
† Adapted from Landsberg (1991)
✓ Increased risk for relinquishment from Patronek (1996)

FIG. 1.4 Common behaviour problems in dogs according to owners and as seen in referral practices.

housetraining. The common feline problems are litterbox training, plant chewing, jumping on counters, climbing, scratching, and nocturnal activity.

Cases seen at referral behaviour clinics are usually those that are persistent, poorly controlled, disruptive or actually dangerous. The most common problems associated with relinquishment of cats are scratching, inappropriate elimination and aggression (Patronek, 1996). For cats, most referred cases are for elimination problems, aggression, destructiveness, excessive vocalisation, and compulsive disorders. The most common reasons for canine behaviour referrals are listed in Figure 1.4.

Setting up a Consultation Service

It is easier to set up a consultation service if clients are aware of your interest in behaviour. This will happen naturally as you make inquiries about behav-

ioural situations during the course of routine veterinary visits. Discussion of potential problems should not be limited to the initial visit with the client but should take place during each yearly examination. Although all the questions in Figs. 1.5 and 1.6 need not be asked during every visit by the owner and the pet, they will give you some idea of potential areas to explore.

Use routine visits to identify patients in your practice with behavioural problems. There are probably more than you think. If you feel confident counselling them further on specific problems, set up a separate appointment for the problem and allow sufficient time for a thorough consultation. It is a mistake to try to counsel owners during the time allotted for a routine visit and vaccination. Scheduling a separate appointment also shows your concern and interest in working with the problem. The client who agrees to attend a behaviour counselling session is committed to (or at least interested in) correcting the problem at hand.

QUESTIONS FOR DOG OWNERS DURING A VETERINARY VISIT
Regarding basic training and behaviour
Have you and your pet attended any obedience training classes?
Does the pet walk nicely on a leash?
Can you describe the play and exercise that your pet receives – how much and how often?
Does your puppy have any problems that you cannot control?
For adult dogs: Have there been any recent changes in your dog's behaviour?
Note: Before the pet reaches sexual maturity, discuss the advantages of neutering
Regarding housesoiling
For puppies: How is the housetraining going?
For older dogs: Has there been any loss of housetraining skills?
If there have been problems, what has been done so far to correct them?
Regarding aggression
Are there any problems with aggression to people?
Are there any problems with aggression to other animals?
Regarding destructive behaviours
Is there ever any concern about destructive behaviour while you're away?
Is there ever any concern about destructive behaviour while you're at home?

Fig. 1.5 Questions to ask dog owners during the course of a veterinary visit.

QUESTIONS FOR CAT OWNERS DURING A VETERINARY VISIT
Regarding basic training and behaviour
How much play and exercise does your pet routinely get? How often?
Does your cat go outdoors? Any problems?
Does your kitten have any behaviour problems that you cannot control?
For adult cats, have there been any recent changes in your pet's behaviour?
Note: If the owners report problems with excessive scratching, discuss scratching posts and behavioural alternatives as preferable alternatives to declawing. Before the cat reaches sexual maturity, discuss the advantages of neutering
Regarding housesoiling
For kittens: How is the litter box training going?
For cats: Has there been any loss of housetraining skills or urination/defecation in inappropriate locations?
Regarding aggression
Are there any problems with aggression to people?
Are there any problems with aggression to other animals?
Regarding destructive behaviours
Is there ever any concern about destructive behaviour while you're away?
Is there ever any concern about destructive behaviour while you're at home?

Fig. 1.6 Questions to ask cat owners during the course of a veterinary visit.

ADVANTAGES AND DISADVANTAGES OF CONSULTATION LOCATIONS

Location	Advantages	Disadvantages
Clinic visit	See pet and family members	Don't see environmental components
	Distractions can be minimised	Pet's behaviour may be dramatically altered in the clinic
	Can utilise clinic resources (staff, videos, books, handouts)	History and questionnaire will need to be far more comprehensive
House call	Can see environment and problem at first hand	Presence of the veterinarian may alter the behaviour
	Increased investigator awareness of varying home environments	Time-consuming and expensive
		May be interruptions and distractions
		Staff and resources not available
Telephone consultation	Increased accessibility	Cannot observe or examine animal
		Cannot learn as much about owner
		Must rely on verbal history
		No opportunity to demonstrate techniques, products, literature

Fig. 1.7 The advantages and disadvantages of different locations for behavioural consultations.

Also encourage your clients to set up preselection consultations with you before they acquire a new pet. This is an excellent time to offer suggestions before they actually have the animal in their home. The new acquisition should be seen within 48 hours of purchase and given a thorough physical examination; the owners should be educated about behavioural concerns to help prevent problems occurring.

When offering behavioural consultations you should understand that you will get requests for house calls and telephone consultations as well as office visits. Set your criteria beforehand on how you will handle these requests. All have their own benefits and limitations (Fig. 1.7).

Reading List for Pet Owners

Ackerman, L. (1993) *Healthy Dog!* Doral Publishing: Wilsonville, OR, 126pp.

Ackerman, L. (1996) *What Every Dog Owner, Breeder, and Trainer Should Know about Nutrition.* Alpine Publications (in press).

Ackerman, L., Landsberg, G. and Hunthausen, W. (eds) (1996) *Cat Behaviour and Training: Veterinary Advice for Owners.* TFH Publications: Neptune, NJ (available by e-mail at phi@primenet.com).

Ackerman, L., Landsberg, G. and Hunthausen, W. (eds) (1996) *Dog Behavior and Training: Veterinary Advice for Owners.* TFH Publications: Neptune, NJ (available by e-mail at phi@primenet.com).

Anderson, R. K. and Foster, R. E. (1988) *Good Manners For Your Dog.* Ameripet: Center to Study Human-Animal Relationships and Environments: 1666 Coffman #128, St Paul, MN 551081988, 75pp.

Bailey, G. (1994) *The Perfect Puppy: How to Raise a Problem Free Dog.* Hamlyn: London.

Benjamin, C. L.(1985) *Mother Knows Best – The Natural Way to Train Your Dog.* Howell Book House: New York, 256pp.

Benjamin, C. L. (1989) *Dog Problems.* Howell House: New York, 222pp.

Bohnenkamp, G. (1990) *Manners for the Modern Dog.* James and Kenneth Publishers: 2140 Shattuck, #2406, Berkeley, CA,

Bohnenkamp, G. (1991) *From the Cat's Point of View.* Perfect Paws Inc.: PO Box 717 Belmont, CA 94002.

Bohnenkamp, G. (1991) *Help! My Dog has an Attitude.* Perfect Paws Inc.: PO Box 717 Belmont, CA 94002.

Campbell, W. (1992) *Behavior Problems in Dogs*, 2nd edition. American Veterinary Publications, Goleta, CA.

Campbell, W. (1995) *Owners Guide to Better Behavior in Dogs.* Alpina Publications Inc.: Loveland, CO.

Dodman, N. (1996) *The Dog Who Loved too Much.* Bantam: New York.

Dunbar, I. (1987) *Sirius Puppy Training.* (Video). James & Kenneth Publishers: 2140 Shattuck, #2406, Berkeley, CA.

Dunbar, I. (1991) *How to Teach a New Dog Old Tricks.* James & Kenneth Publishers: 2140 Shattuck, #2406, Berkeley, CA.

Dunbar, I. (1992) *Doctor Dunbar's Good Little Dog Book.* Spillers Foods: London.

Dunbar, I. (1995) *A Pre-Puppy Primer.* James & Kenneth Publishers: 2140 Shattuck, #2406, Berkeley, CA.

Fisher, J. (1991) *Why Does my Dog ...?* Howell Book House: New York, 239pp.

Fisher, J. (ed) (1993) *The Behaviour of Dogs and Cats.* Stanley Paul: London, 231pp.

Fogle, B. (1990) *The Dog's Mind.* Viking Penguin Inc.: New York.

Fogle, B. (1992) *The Cat's Mind.* Howell Book House: New York.

Fogle, B. (1993) *101 Questions Your Cat Would Ask its Vet if Your Cat Could Talk.* Michael Joseph Publishers: London.

Fogle, B. (1993) *101 Questions Your Dog Would Ask its Vet if Your Dog Could Talk.* Michael Joseph Publishers: London.

Fogle, B. (1994) *ASPCA Complete Dog Training Manual.* Dorling Kindersley: London, 128pp.

Fox, M. W. (1972) *Understanding your Dog.* St. Martin's Press: New York, NY.

Fox, M. W. (1974) *Understanding your Cat.* Bantam Books: New York, NY.

Heath, S. and Jones, R. (1993) *Why Does My Cat ...?* Souvenir Press: London.

Kilcommons, B. and Wilson, S. (1994) *Child-Proofing Your Dog.* Warner Books: New York.

Marder, A. (1994) *Your Healthy Pet: A Practical Guide to Choosing and Raising Happier, Healthier Dogs and Cats.* Rodale Press: Emmaus, PA, 216pp.

Morris, D. (1986) *Catwatching.* Crown Publishing: New York.

Morris, D. (1986) *Dogwatching.* Crown Publishing: New York.

Mugford, R. (1994) *Never Say No! A Perigree Book.* The Berkley Publishing Group: New York, 207pp.

Neville, P. (1990) *Do Cats Need Shrinks? Cat Behavior Explained.* Contemporary Books: Chicago, IL.

Neville, P. (1992) *Do Dogs Need Shrinks? What to Do When Man's Best Friend Misbehaves.* Citadel Press: Secaucus, NJ.

Neville, P. (1993) *Pet Sex. The Rude Facts of Life for the Family Dog, Cat and Rabbit.* Sidgwick & Jackson: London.

Pryor, K. (1985) *Don't Shoot the Dog.* Bantam Books: New York.

Pryor, K. (1991) *Lads before the Wind.* Sunshine Books: North Bend, WA.

Rafe, S. (1990) *Your New Baby and Bowser.* Denlinger Publications: Fairfax, VA.

Rutherford, C. and Neil, D. H. (1992) *How to Raise a Puppy You Can Live With,* 2nd edition. Alpine Publications: Loveland, CO.

Ryan, T. (1990) *Puppy Primer.* Legacy: Pullman, WA.

Ryan, T. (1994) *The Toolbox for Remodeling Problem Dogs.* Legacy: Pullman, WA, 26pp.

Siegal, M. (1992) *The Cornell Book of Cats.* Villard Books: New York, 435pp.

Tortora, D. (1977) *Help! This Animal is Driving Me Crazy.* Playboy Press: Chicago, IL.

Welcome Home Your New Friend: Your New Cat. [Video]. ImmunoVet: Tampa, FL.

Weston, D. and Ross, E. R. (1990) *Dog Training: The Gentle Modern Method.* Howell Book House: New York.

Weston, D. and Ross, E. R. (1992) *Dog Problems: The Gentle Modern Cure.* Howell Book House: New York.

Wright, J., Lashnits, J. W. (1994) *Is Your Cat Crazy? Solutions from the Casebook of a Cat Therapist.* Simon and Schuster MacMillan Co: New York, NY.

References and Further Reading for Veterinarians

American Veterinary Society of Animal Behavior. (1995) Special Symposium on Animal Behavior. (Available from American Vetinary Society of Animal Behavior).

Anderson, R. K. (1990) Preventing needless death of pets. *Veterinary Forum,* 7 (April), 32–33.

Anderson, R. K., Hart, B. L. and Hart, L. A. (1984) *The Pet Connection: Its Influence on Our Health and Quality of Life.* Center to Study Human-Animal Relationships and Environments: Minneapolis, MN.

Arkow, P. (1994) A new look at overpopulation. *Anthrozoos.* **3**, 202–205.

Askew, H. R. (1994) Animal behavior therapy as a specialty in German veterinary medicine. *Praktische Tierarzt,* **75**(9), 731.

Beaver, B. (1991) *The Veterinarian's Encyclopedia of Animal Behavior.* Iowa State University Press: Ames, IA.

Beaver, B. V. (1992) *Feline Behavior: A Guide for Veterinarians.* W. B. Saunders: Philadelphia, PA.

Beck, A. M., Overall, K. L., McKeown, D. B., *et al.* (1992) *Behavioral Problems in Small Animals.* Ralston Purina Co.: St. Louis, MO.

Blackshaw, J. K. (1994) Management of behavioral problems in cats. *Feline Practice,* **22**(3), 25–28.

Bradshaw, J. W. S. (1992) *The Behaviour of the Domestic Cat.* Redwood Press Ltd, Melksham, UK.

Bradshaw, J. W. S. (1993) *The True Nature of the Cat.* Boxtree: London.

Dunbar, I. (1979) *Dog Behavior: Why Dogs Do What They Do.* TFH Publications Inc.: Neptune, NJ.

Edney, A. T. B. (1986) *Waltham Symposium, No. 8. Canine Development Throughout Life.* British Small Animal Veterinary Association: Cheltenham.

Endenburg, N. and Knool, B. W. (1994) Behavioral, household, and social problems associated with companion animals – Opinions of owners and non-owners. *Veterinary Quarterly,* **16**(2): 130–134.

Evans, J. M. (1985) *The Evans Guide for Counseling Dog Owners.* Howell Book House: New York.

Fox, M. (1965) *Canine Behaviour.* Charles Thories: Springfield, IL.

Fox, M. W. (1978) *The Dog: It's Domestication and Behaviour.* Garland STM Press: New York.

Fox, M. W. (1971) *Integrative Development of Brain and Behavior in the Dog.* University of Chicago Press: Chicago.

Hart, B. L. and Hart, L. A. (1985) *Canine and Feline Behavioral Therapy.* Lea & Febiger: Philadelphia, PA.

Hart B. L. (1985) *The Behavior of Domestic Animals.* W. H. Freeman: New York.

Houpt, K. (1991) *Domestic Animal Behavior*, 2nd edition. Iowa State University Press: Ames, IA.

Hunthausen, W. (1991) It's Time to Offer Behavior Services. *Veterinary Economics*, Nov, 52–57.

Hunthausen, W. (1996) Behavior Problems: Find a long-term solution instead of a quick fix. *Vetinary Economics* (May) 39–40.

Hunthausen, W. and Landsberg, G. M. (1995) *Practitioner's Guide to Behavior Counseling*, AAHA Publications: Denver, CO.

Landsberg, G. (1990) Veterinarians as behavior consultants. *Canadian Veterinary Journal*, **31**, 225–227.

Landsberg, G. (1991) The distribution of canine behavior cases in three behavior referral practices. *Veterinary Medicine*, **86**, 1011–1018.

Luescher, U. A. *et al.* (1995) *How Dogs Learn: The Principles of Learning and Their Practical Application in Dog Training and Behavior Modification.* Professional Animal Behavior Associates: Guelph, Ontario.

McKeown, D. and Luescher, A. (1988) A case for companion animal behavior in the veterinary practice. *Canadian Veterinary Journal*, **29**, 74–75.

Marder, A. and Voith, V. (eds). (1991) Advances in Companion Animal Behavior. *Veterinary Clinics of North America*, W. B. Saunders Co.: Philadelphia, PA, **21**(2).

Mertens, P. A. and Dodman, N. H. (1996) The diagnosis of Behavioral problems in dogs, cats, horses and birds – characteristics of 323 cases (July 1994–June 1995). *Dog Kleintierpraxis*, **41**(3), 197.

Miller, D. D., Staats, S. R., Partlo, C. *et al.* (1996) Factors associated with the decision to surrender a pet to an animal shelter. *J Am Vet Med Assoc*, **209**(4), 738–742.

Mosier, J. E. (1975) Common medical and behavioral problems in cats. *Modern Veterinary Practice*, **56**, 699.

O'Farrell, V. (1986) *Manual of Canine Behaviour.* British Small Animal Veterinary Association: Cheltenham.

O'Farrell, V. (1987) Owner attitudes and dog behaviour problems. *Journal of Small Animal Practice*, **28**(11), 1037–1045.

O'Farrell, V. O. (1989) *Problem Dog: Behaviour and Misbehaviour.* Methuen: London.

O'Farrell, V. O. and Neville, P. (1994) *Manual of Feline Behaviour.* British Small Animal Veterinary Association: Cheltenham.

Overall, K. (1997) *Clinical Behavioral Medicine for Small Animals.* Moseby.

Pageat, P. (1995) Welfare and well-being of pets – an objective evaluation. *Le Point Vétérinaire*, **26**(165), 13–21.

Patronek, G. J., Glickman, L. T. and Moyer, M. R. (1995) Population dynamics and the risk of euthanasia for dogs in an animal shelter. *Anthrozöos*, **8**(1), 31–43.

Patronek, G. J., Glickman, L. T., Beck, A. M. *et al.* (1996) Risk factors for relinquishment of dogs to an animal shelter. *J Am Vet Med Assoc,* **V209**(3), 572–581, 582–588.

Polsky, R. H. (1991) *User's Guide to the Scientific Literature on Dog and Cat Behaviour.* Animal Behaviour Counselling Services, Inc.: Los Angeles, CA.

Robinson, I. (ed.) (1995) *The Waltham Book of Human–Animal Interaction.* Pergamon: Oxford.

Schwartz, S. (1994) *Instructions for Veterinary Clients: Canine and Feline Behavior Problems.* American Veterinary Publications: Goleta, CA.

Scott, J. P. and Fuller, J. L. (1965) *Genetics and the Social Behavior of Dogs.* University of Chicago Press: Chicago, IL.

Serpell, J. (1996) *The Domestic Dog: Its Evolution, Behaviour and Interactions with People.* Cambridge University Press: New York.

Sigler, L. (1991) Pet behavioral problems present opportunities for practitioners. *AAHA Trends*, **4**, 44–45.

Thorne, C. (ed.) (1992). *The Waltham Book of Dog and Cat Behaviour.* Pergamon Press: Oxford, 159pp.

Turner, D. C. and Bateson, P. (1988) *The Domestic Cat: the Biology of its Behavior.* Cambridge University Press: New York.

Voith, V. L. and Borchelt, P. L. (eds). (1982) 'Animal behavior'. *Veterinary Clinics of North America*, W. B. Saunders Co.: Philadelphia, PA, **12**(2).

Watson, N. L. and Weinstein, M. (1993) Pet ownership in relation to depression, anxiety, and anger in working women. *Anthrozöos*, **6**(2), 135–138.

Wills, J. M. and Simpson, K. W. (1994) *The Waltham Book of Clinical Nutrition of the Dog and Cat.* Pergamon: Oxford.

Behavioural Associations and Newsletters

American College of Veterinary Behaviorists: c/o Dr Sharon Crowell-Davis, College of Vetinary Medicine, University of Georgia, Athens, GA, 30602–7382.

American Veterinary Society of Animal Behavior: c/o Dr Laurie Martin, 201 Cedarbrook rd, Naperville, Illinois, 60565.

Animal Behavior Consultant Newsletter: c/o Dr John Wright, P.O. Box 180, NU, Macon, GA 31207, USA.

Animal Behavior Society: S. Foster, Dept of Biology, Clark University, 950 Main St., Worcester, MA, 01610–1477.

Association of Pet Behaviour Counsellors, 257 Royal College Street, London NW1 9LV, UK.

Companion Animal Behavior Therapy Study Group: Mr D. Mills, Secretary, De Montford University, Lincoln, Caythorpe Court, Caythorpe, Nr Grantham, Lincs, NG32 3EP, UK; Newsletter Editor, S.E. Heath, 33 Hayman Road, Brackley, Northants, NN13 6JA, UK.

European Society for Veterinary Clinical Ethology: Dr J. Dehasse, 129 Avenue de la Fauconnerie 92, B-1170 Brussels, Belgium.

International Society for Animal Ethology: Dr S. M. Rutter, ISAE Membership Secretary, Institute of Grassland and Environmental Research, North Wyke, Oke-hampton, Devon, EX20 2SB, UK.

Pet Behavior Rx Newsletter: c/o William Campbell, P.O. Box 1658, Grants Pass, OR 97526, USA.

Veterinary Hospital University of Pennsylvania Newsletter: VHUP, 3850 Spruce St., Philadelphia, PA 19104–6010, USA.

2

Counselling for New Pet Owners

Working with New Puppies and Kittens

Providing timely behavioural advice to new puppy and kitten owners can help prevent undesirable behaviours, as well as help correct existing problems before they become resistant to change. The first veterinary visit is the time to begin reinforcing important concepts and make sure owner and pet are on the right track.

To make matters more expedient during those initial few veterinary visits, it is useful to have a 'new pet checklist' so that points can be addressed in an orderly manner and so important topics don't get missed (Figs. 2.1 and 2.2).

We wish to emphasise again that the veterinarian need not be the only person in the practice qualified to interview the new owners. Properly trained staff can be very effective in this role, and also reinforce the practice's team approach to health care. Depending on the hospital set-up and the amount of training the staff have received, a great deal of behavioural education can and should be handled by trained office staff and technicians. However, it is the veterinarian's responsibility to ensure that the information that the staff are providing is correct and appropriate.

Proper use of hospital staff will give the veterinarian more time to concentrate on important aspects of behaviour and training within the time frame of a typical initial office visit. This is also an important time for the veterinarian to provide a thorough physical

---

NEW PUPPY/KITTEN CHECKLIST

1. **Behavioural advice**
   - Socialisation
   - Housetraining/litterbox training
   - Puppy or kitten proofing
   - Supervision/confinement
   - Chewing
   - Handling
   - Rewards, shaping and training
   - Discipline

2. **Medical advice**
   - Nutrition
   - Vaccinations
   - Spay/Castration
   - Skin and coat care
   - Parasites (internal/external)
   - Dental care
   - Insurance

3. **Educational materials for home use**
   - _____
   - _____
   - _____
   - _____
   - _____

4. **Product advice**
   - Flea/tick control
   - Collars, leashes, halters
   - Permanent identification
   - Shampoos/dips
   - Chew toys
   - Behavioural products

FIG. 2.1 Items for a new checklist. Each should be checked off and dated when discussed, and appropriate entries added to 3.

TOPICS FOR NEW PET OWNERS

Proper socialisation skills

Provide list of appropriate reading material and videos

Puppy- and cat-proofing the home and car (i.e. providing a safe environment)

Supervision/confinement

Housetraining

Crate training

Basic handling techniques

Claw trimming

Basic brushing, coat and home dental care

Exercise, play, and chewing

Nutrition

How to control the unruly puppy/kitten

Proper use of discipline

Appropriate use of rewards

Schedule of medical and dental care

Advantages of spaying/neutering

Products (e.g. collars, leads, harnesses)

Health advice

FIG. 2.2 Topics to discuss with or demonstrate to new pet owners.

examination to detect any medical conditions that might contribute to or exacerbate behaviour problems.

Socialisation is discussed in more detail below but it is mentioned here briefly since it is one of the most important concepts for the veterinarian to relay to the new pet owner. Puppies or kittens removed from the litter at 4 weeks of age or younger may not be able to relate appropriately to members of their own species at a later age. Puppies should stay with their mother and littermates until 6–8 weeks of age so they can develop healthy social skills with other dogs. If puppies are placed in the new home by 6–8 weeks of age, they have approximately 4–6 more weeks of the critical socialis-ation period to begin to develop relationships with people and to habituate with new environments. Puppies at this age are least inhibited so that primary socialisation is readily achieved. Young puppies should be exposed to as many different types of people and circumstances as opportunities allow (Fig. 2.3).

It is equally important for kittens to develop and maintain proper social relationships with other cats. However since the critical socialisation for cats begins to wane by as early as 7 weeks of age, social contact with people and other species must begin before this time. One alternative is to obtain a kitten by 7 weeks of age. Another choice is to ensure that any kitten over 7 weeks of age has been adequately socialised to people.

Take the time during initial visits to address and correct problems early. Ask clients about problems at each visit (Figures 1.5 and 1.6); and do not expect they will volunteer the information. They may not realise that mild behaviour problems can lead to more serious situations as the pet grows. Be especially wary of pets that exhibit excessive growling, aggression, or fear responses. If the pet shows evidence that it may become dangerous to family members, it is incumbent upon the veterinarian to inform the owners fully and give them appropriate options. The pet that is a little too pushy with its new owners needs to begin training immediately so that the owners gain control before the problem gets out of hand.

Explore problems and reinforce information during subsequent visits:

- Housetraining
- Obedience training
- Crying at night; excessive nocturnal activity
- Chewing on furniture
- Play-biting, overexuberant play
- Jumping up, mounting
- Digging, destructiveness, scratching
- Stealing food or household items, garbage raiding
- Eating problems (too much, too little, pica, coprophagia)
- Emerging aggression, protecting food or objects.

When the clients leave the office, it is likely that they have been overwhelmed with medical and behavioural advice and might have trouble digesting and remem-bering it all. So, whenever possible, provide the owner with handout materials and pamphlets that can be taken home. Book and video suggestions may also be appre-ciated. Most pet food companies provide 'puppy packs' or 'kitten kits' that contain free samples and literature, which can be supplemented with your own customised forms. Remember, the new owner often focuses on the new pet during the visit, and may not fully comprehend every message the veterinarian tries to relate.

By 3–4 months of age, puppies are ready for training classes or puppy parties. Although for socialisation and early training it may be advisable to begin these activities as early as 8 or 9 weeks of age, the puppy may not have sufficient immunity from its vaccinations by this time.

STIMULI FOR PUPPIES AND KITTENS	
People	**Environments and stimuli**
Children/babies, Elderly persons, Teenagers	Veterinary clinic
Men with beards	Cars, trucks
People with headgear or glasses	Roadway/pavement (sidewalk)
People in wheelchairs, on skates, on bicycles	Park
People whose appearance differs from family members	Lifts (elevators)
Veterinarians and others in uniform	Crate
	Vacuums, trains, cars, etc.
	Other animals

Fig. 2.3 Examples of stimuli to which puppies and kittens should be exposed.

Pet Selection

One of the most valuable services a veterinarian can perform for clients is to assist them in picking the pet that best suits their home and lifestyle. This is an extremely useful but underutilised facet of veterinary practice. Insufficient effort and forethought into the selection of a pet, and into the preparation for its arrival, are major factors associated with later relinquishment and euthanasia. Many owners spend more time picking a houseplant than they do a pet that will live with them for over a decade.

A selection consultation is the best way to determine the needs of the prospective owner. There are several ways of determining whether the family is suited to pet ownership and, if so, which type of pet would be most compatible. There are several pamphlets (e.g. AVMA's *A Veterinarian's Way of Selecting a Proper Pet*) and questionnaires (e.g. AVMA's *Pet Selection Fact Sheet*) to aid in the process. Most kennel associations and humane societies have also produced useful handouts on the subject. Everyone has a stake in making sure the right pet ends up in the right household.

Some of the decisions may not be as clear-cut as they first appear. By selecting a mixed breed animal from a shelter, an abandoned animal can be saved from death, and the cost is very reasonable. One can even argue that there are genetic advantages to obtaining mixed breed animals. This is often referred to by geneticists as 'hybrid vigour'. However, the best way to predict the behaviour, size, health, coat, and other attributes of an adult dog or cat is to obtain a purebred animal of known parentage. Because there is such wide genetic variation in size, shape, behaviour and health amongst dog breeds, the selection process for purebred dogs is not always a simple task.

Many veterinarians feel uncomfortable discussing pet selection because they themselves do not know much about the process, other than the medical consequences. Acquiring a pet is an emotional experience, and veterinarians would do well to put themselves in the place of clients when considering what recommendations to make. What kind of pet would be best for a young family that has never owned a dog before? How about a family without children whose home is lavishly and expensively decorated? Consider the widow on a pension who loves animals but can't afford to spend much on the purchase and upkeep of a pet. Fig. 2.4 lists the considerations that have to be made during the pet selection consultation.

Because the pet selection consultation is so important, a questionnaire that provides all the necessary information for making an informed recommendation can be very helpful (Fig. 2.5). It should be made clear

FACTORS FOR CONSIDERATION IN PET SELECTION
Type of pet (dog, cat, other)

Breed (purebred versus mixed)
   physical considerations (size, shape, coat)
   heritable medical problems
   behavioural concerns: (breed traits, activity requirements)

Age (puppy or kitten versus adult)
Sex (male versus female; neutered versus intact)
Source (breeder versus shelter versus retail shop)
Expense (high maintenance versus low maintenance)
Ages of family members
Schedules and activities of family
Owners' experience with pets
Home and garden/yard size
Health concerns of family (allergies, AIDS, physical disabilities)

FIG. 2.4 The factors which need to be considered during a pet selection consultation.

TOPICS FOR AN OWNER SELECTION QUESTIONNAIRE	
Topics	**Examples of Pertinent Details**
Family structure	Single; family with children; elderly
Finances	Low-income; moderate; wealthy
Daily schedule	At work all day; travel frequently
Reason for pet ownership	For children; protection; companionship
Household factors	Apartment; no garden or yard; no fencing
Health limitations	Allergies; medical or physical problems
Expected lifestyle changes	New baby expected; moving; schedule changes
Other pets at home	Dogs; cats; birds

FIG. 2.5 Topics that should be included in an owner selection questionnaire.

TEN RULES FOR BUYING A PET: A HANDOUT

1. Be sure a pet fits your present and future lifestyle before you buy one (or accept a free one). That cute little puppy is going to grow. That kitten may use your furniture as a scratching post if not provided with a suitable substitute. Are you planning on moving in the near future and are uncertain whether you could take animals with you? This is no excuse to kill a pet or turn the responsibility over to someone else. Did you know that veterinarians are asked to euthanise more pets for behavioral reasons than for medical reasons. This reflects a failure on the part of owners, not of pets. Pets are demanding of your time and deserve that time when you make the conscious decision to bring one into your home. Be honest with yourself – don't 'give it a try' and see what happens. What happens over 1800 times every hour of every day in the United States alone is that these animals are eventually killed

2. Be sure you can be a responsible pet owner. Although everyone considers themselves responsible, the facts say otherwise. Do you believe cats should always be able to roam outdoors? Wrong! Do you think it is a pity not to have at least one litter from your current pet before it is neutered? Wrong! Is it all right to let your dog out without a leash because it always listens to you? Wrong! Pets need our attention, our protection, and our concern. They are not disposable items when they misbehave, get older, or outlive their entertainment value

3. Be sure you can afford a pet before you get one. Pets have needs and it is short-sighted to think that the purchase price is the last expense other than food. Pets need routine health care, vaccinations, spay/neutering, dentistry, training and licensing. Most would agree however that a pet gives much more than it could ever cost. Should economic constraints arise, there are many public service organizations that will see that you can have your pet neutered at low or no cost. Failure to take advantage of these programmes is a reflection of irresponsibility, not poverty

4. Never buy a pet on impulse. Most puppy/kitten 'mills' thrive on this behaviour. Do you want to rescue that poor puppy from that enclosure? Can't stand to see those kittens kept in that unclean cage? Your intentions may be honorable, but you are directly contributing to more of these animals being produced and sold that way. If you want to break the chain of events that makes this happen, don't buy a pet from these outlets and caution others against it too

5. If you do not need a pet for show purposes, consider adopting an animal that needs a home. Breed rescue organisations do their best to place animals in good homes and they will be familiar with the breed and be able to tell if they have a suitable pet for you. If you don't want a purebred, visit the local shelters. Not all shelters are created equal. Only deal with ones that have the best interests of the animals at heart. Responsible shelters will want to make sure that the animals are going to an appropriate home, that you understand about vaccinations and health care and that you agree to have the animal neutered if it has not yet been done

6. If you do want a show-quality pet or think you may want to breed it someday, deal only with a reputable breeder. Reputable breeders will undoubtedly be affiliated with the appropriate breed clubs, have health care information available for several generations of their animals, and if applicable, have had these animals screened for genetic problems. Call the breed clubs and ask for information and a list of breeders they might recommend in your area. Many good breeders spend more time scrutinising you before they trust you with one of their animals than you'll spend assessing them. A good rule is not to buy any purebred where you can't see at least one of the parents and have access to the medical history and performance record of both

7. If you intend to buy a purebred animal, check with your veterinarian as to the potential hereditary problems in that breed and if they can be determined before purchase. Breeders that are truly interested in the breed will be happy to discuss these concerns with you, and, if possible, will provide proof of being 'clear' or can give a guarantee. The same cannot be said of indiscriminate breeders and many pet shops. What is their policy if your new pet does have a hereditary defect? An exchange-only policy is common for pet-sale outlets but they know that once an animal has been welcomed into a family, most people can't return it. These problems can also happen to reputable breeders occasionally and how they are handled is a mark of just how responsible they are. Always enquire before you buy. *Caveat emptor* – Let the Buyer Beware!

8. Be reasonable when it comes to purchase price. You can buy a pet with 'papers' for $25 or $2500. Either could be disasters. Ask yourself what your money is paying for. Has there been excellent prenatal care for the mother and proper health care for the puppies/kittens or are you paying for freight and cage space for an animal shipped in from a distant location? Were the parents champions (documented), did they hold titles in obedience, and are they 'clear' of heritable disorders? Are the animals kept in clean hygienic quarters and have they been well-socialised? Is the breeder/seller accredited in responsible health care (e.g. Project TEACH)? These are much more important questions than does it have papers, or how much does it cost? Support those breeders that care enough to do the job right and expect to pay more

9. Immediately after acquiring a new pet, make an appointment with your veterinarian and bring along all information you have about its previous health care. It is also wise to bring a stool sample since parasites such as worms are not unusual but will require proper diagnosis and treatment. Puppies and kittens need a series of vaccinations when young and then regular boosters annually. And, make sure you have your new pet neutered or spayed as soon as your veterinarian recommends. Do not wait for the first 'heat' or for a first litter. Did you know that you can significantly diminish the risk of mammary tumours in bitches by spaying them before their first heat? Neutered males are also at reduced risk of experiencing prostate problems later in life

10. If you're truly interested in pets and their welfare, take time to understand the issues and why so many pets are destroyed each year. Give a home to a pet in need. Don't accept a pet that doesn't fit your lifestyle. Don't buy a pet as a whim. Don't support irresponsible pet sales. Don't become a backyard breeder or buy a pet from one. Make sure that your pets have been neutered. And, if you know somebody who doesn't know better, tell them, or give them a copy of this

Fig. 2.6 This is an example of a handout for prospective pet owners – 'Ten Rules for Buying a Pet'. (Modified from Ackermann, 1993.)

to the client, however, that it is not the role of the consultant to choose a particular breed, age, or sex. Rather, the consultant should discuss the advantages as well as any concerns or warnings about each breed, and give suggestions on sex, age and how to choose an individual dog or cat. Fig 2.6 is an example of a handout that has been used for prospective owners.

Breed Considerations

Because there are so many different purebred dogs and cats available, veterinarians should endeavour to narrow the choices down to a few breeds in each class that they know well. If an owner has a query about a breed with which you have less familiarity, be prepared to do the research before you make your recommendations. If you take the time to document pros and cons for each breed as you experience or read about them, eventually you will have an impressive array of facts for the would-be owner. Project TEACH, administered by Pet Health Initiative, Inc, P.O. Box 12093, Scottsdale AZ 85267-2093 (http://www.pet-vet.com) offers educational materials for breeders, veterinarians, shelters, rescue groups and petshop staff, They stress responsible health care of animals being sold to the public, proper genetic screening, socialisation and habituation, parasite control and other important issues. Pet Health Initiative is also in the process of compiling a directory of breed-related medical and behavioural problems and descriptions of all the breeds with which veterinarians may have contact (http://www.pet-vet.com).

Veterinarians should maintain a library of books that provide breed-specific information. They should also encourage owners to read as much about the breed as possible, and to discuss the matter with other informed people, such as breeders, groomers, trainers and kennel clubs. Computerised selection services are also available in some areas.

Even where published breed profiles are accurate, there can be a great deal of variability between different lines, across different geographical areas and amongst individuals within the same litter. Veterinarians, however, should have some idea of the characteristics that are most predictable (e.g. watchdog ability in Rottweilers, vocalisation in Siamese cats, low activity level of Basset Hounds). Other traits, such as tendencies towards destructiveness, housesoiling and affection, may be influenced more by environment than by genetic background. Study the tendencies for which the breed was bred and couple this information with that gleaned from breed profiles. Veterinarians should also be cognisant of potential problems such as tendencies for dominance of the owner, high activity level, fear, sensitivity to pain and noise, and specific conditions such as flank-sucking in Dobermann Pinschers, wool-sucking in Siamese cats and 'spinning' in Bull Terriers.

Pet Age

Puppies are most receptive to socialisation from 3 to 12 weeks of age. It is best for puppies to remain with their mother and littermates until 6–8 weeks and then to be introduced to as many new people and animals as possible in their new home. Kittens are most receptive to socialisation at 2–7 weeks of age. It is important, therefore, that kittens receive adequate contact and exposure to people by 7 weeks. Adult dogs and cats may be insufficiently socialised or improperly trained so that problems may be difficult or impossible to correct. On the other hand, adult pets may be able to handle longer owner departures, may present fewer problems with over-exuberant play, nipping and chewing, and may already be trained.

Pet Gender

Male dogs and cats are slightly larger in stature than females. Male dogs are also somewhat more dominant and more active. Females tend to be easier to train and to housetrain. Castration of dogs reduces sexually dimorphic behaviours (Figure 3.7); male dogs will show decreases in behaviours such as mounting, roaming, urine marking and aggression toward other male dogs. Castration of cats reduces urine odour and decreases sexually dimorphic behaviours such as fighting, spraying and roaming, but has no effect on hunting. Spaying of queens and bitches reduces oestrous behaviour and associated urine spraying. About 10% of spayed female cats and 5% of castrated males continue to spray.

Sources

The best source of a pet is a reputable breeder or a breed rescue service. If dogs are obtained directly from the breeder, the buyer can ensure that the puppies or kittens have been properly cared for and have had sufficient human contact. Ask sources if they are accredited through Project TEACH. Reputable breeders should be happy to provide references (vetinarians, previous buyers).

The buyer should pay close attention to the health and behaviour of both parents since the temperament, size, coat and personality of a puppy or kitten, when grown, will often resemble those of its parents. Purebred dogs and cats that are obtained from pet stores, breeding farms, puppy mills and animal shelters usually have unknown medical and genetic histories. They are highly stressed by weaning, transport, handling and housing and have high levels of exposure to other animals, at a time when their resistance is low or suspect. The risk of respiratory and intestinal diseases is highest in these animals. Saving the life of a pet from a shelter could be seen as a gallant gesture and should be considered, but the owner must be counselled about the potential risks. Families wishing to obtain a cat for rodent control should select a kitten from parents who are known hunters; those who want a social animal should choose a kitten from highly social parents.

The American Kennel Club, Canadian Kennel Club, United Kennel Club and The Kennel Club in the UK publish directories of breed associations and rescue societies. Annual directories, such as *Dogs in USA Annual*, *Cats in US Annual*, *Dogs in Canada Annual*, are available in many countries. Monthly magazines and weekly newspapers aimed at the pet-owning community contain useful information. There may be a local Breeder Referral Service, such as that run by Ralston Purina in Canada, and the local veterinarian may keep a list of reputable breeders.

Temperament Testing

Temperament testing is another useful function that can be performed during the selection process. The value of this type of evaluation is in determining the current temperament and social nature of the animal, not in predicting adult behaviour patterns. Many behaviour and health problems cannot be detected at an early age since they do not emerge until the pet matures. For example, dominance aggression in dogs may not be evident until 2 years of age or older and there is a weak predictive value of testing for social rank at 7 weeks of age. Testing may more accurately predict behaviour in puppies and kittens that have

passed through the primary socialisation period. There are likely traits that are identifiable in young animals but more research is needed before specific recommendations can be made. A specific form of temperament testing used to screen potential guide dogs at 6–8 weeks of age has increased the success of guide dog selection from 30% before tests were initiated, to almost 60% after temperament testing. Testing has also been successfully used to help place shelter dogs in appropriate homes.

Preliminary temperament testing in puppies and kittens can be valuable if one recognises its limitations. Dogs should be observed and evaluated for healthiness, sociability, playfulness and activity level. Puppies with extreme manifestations of undesirable traits such as shyness, overactivity or uncontrollable biting and growling will probably turn out to be unsuitable as a family pet.

A puppy can then be separated from the other dogs and assessed individually. Finally, puppies can be stimulated and assessed by lifting, gently grasping the muzzle, nape of the neck and feet, removing food or a toy from the mouth, and perhaps even nail trimming or light grooming (Fig. 2.7).

A quantitative score can be gained from a puppy aptitude test (PAT) and this is commonly used by breeders and trainers. The test gives a numerical score for different traits, with values representing gradations between the most assertive or aggressive expression of a trait to that representing disinterest, independence or inaction. The traits assessed in the PAT include: social attraction to people, response to restraint, response to social dominance, response to physical control, touch sensitivity, sound sensitivity, stability and energy level. Although the tests do not predict behaviours absolutely, they do fairly well at determining the animal's current temperament and predicting adult behavioural tendencies for puppies at behavioural extremes. The PAT is ideally conducted when puppies are 7–8 weeks old, performed on one puppy at a time, in an environment with few distractions, and by an examiner that the puppy has never met. The test should not be performed within 72 hours of vaccination or surgery.

It may be more difficult to test the temperament of cats, but three common personality types have been identified: sociable, confident and easy going; timid, nervous and unfriendly; and active and aggressive. As many as 15% of cats may not be able to be socialised to people successfully. In general, a healthy, affectionate

TRAITS ASSESSED DURING PUPPY OR KITTEN TESTING	
Behaviour	**Tests**
Fear	Observe facial expressions and body postures during approach and handling by strangers Watch for avoidance Watch for unusual startle responses to loud noises Watch for excessively submissive behaviour
Excitability	Take to a quiet area and observe Attempt to calm; hold in 'sit' or 'down' position for 30 seconds
Resistance to handling	Lift, carry Hold in 'sit' or 'down' position Hold on side or back Gently place the hand around the muzzle Trim claws Brush or comb coat
Sociability	Pick the pet up and stroke it Walk away and call the pet

FIG. 2.7 Some tests that can be used to assess behavioural traits in puppies and kittens.

cat will make the best pet whereas shy, withdrawn, fearful or aggressive cats should be avoided. Cats can therefore be tested in the same three-stage format as dogs. First, they should be observed reacting with littermates and the queen. Are they friendly, shy or aggressive? Secondly, they need to be handled to determine if they tolerate lifting, stroking and brushing with minimal resistance. Thirdly, you should observe how they respond to stimuli such as physical restraint, loud noises or nail trimming. This form of testing is a good (if imprecise) way to identify traits about which the owner should be aware or which might make the pet unsuitable for certain homes.

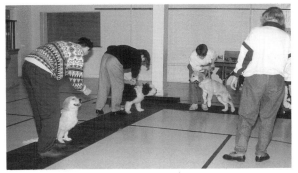

FIG. 2.8 Obedience classes are an excellent way to encourage proper socialisation.

Socialisation and Habituation

Socialisation is the process in which pets develop a relationship with animals of their own species and others (Figs 2.8, 2.9, 2.11). Proper socialisation is one of the most important determinants of how well a pet will do in a home setting. The most critical period for socialisation in puppies is between 3 and 12 weeks of age, while the most receptive period for kittens is from 2 to 7 weeks of age. During these periods, dogs and cats make attachments to their own species, other species and new environments most rapidly. Pets that develop social relationships during these periods are often capable of maintaining these relationships for life. If they have not been properly socialised with people and other pets by the end of this period, they are likely to be fearful, defensive and potentially aggressive when exposed to them at a later age. Although these are

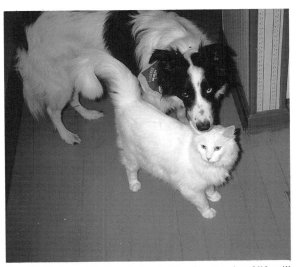

FIG. 2.9 Early socialisation during the first few months of life will help ensure that pets will get along with members of other species when they are adult.

sensitive stages for primary socialisation, continued socialisation is also necessary for these social relationships to be maintained.

For proper social development, handling and enrichment should actually begin shortly after birth. Puppies and kittens that lack sufficient auditory, tactile and visual stimuli may be slower learners, less social and more fearful than properly stimulated littermates. Adequately stimulated puppies and kittens have superior coordination, higher sociability towards people, better problem-solving scores and are less fearful in novel situations. Breeders who isolate puppies or kittens and deprive them of sufficient early handling may produce pets that are overly fearful and lack desirable social behaviour.

Another critical factor in the early development of dogs and cats is the role of the mother. Bitches and queens with good maternal behaviour produce offspring with better digestion, better resistance to disease and better weight gain, which develop and mature faster than puppies born to bitches with poor maternal instincts. Dogs and cats that have been deprived of maternal and peer interactions form poor social bonds later in life. For example, if a puppy or kitten is removed from the litter at birth and hand-reared, it may be unable to mate or care for its own litter later in life. Dominance and submissive signalling and controlled aggression may also not develop normally if there is insufficient early social interaction.

It is generally recommended that puppies remain with their mother and littermates until approximately 7 weeks of age, so they can develop communication skills, develop social skills and have an opportunity to play and interact with other dogs. By 7 weeks of age, puppies are least inhibited and therefore best able to adapt to new experiences. The focus of socialisation should then be shifted toward as many new people and situations as possible (*see* Fig. 2.3). Dogs that have had no social contact with people by 14 weeks of age are unlikely ever to make adequate family pets; they tend to behave more like their wild counterparts.

Cats that have had no social contact with people by 9 weeks of age may never be able to develop a healthy social relationship with humans. For a kitten to be properly socialised to people, other animals and new environments, the kitten should either be removed from the litter and taken into its new home by 7 weeks of age, or the potential owner must ensure that the kitten has had adequate exposure and handling by people before it is obtained.

STEPS TOWARDS NORMAL SOCIAL DEVELOPMENT IN DOGS
Encourage early play and interaction with mother and littermates
Keep puppies with their mothers and littermates for first 6–8 weeks of life
By 8 weeks puppies should be placed in their new homes to ensure adequate socialisation and habituation to people, other pets and new environments
Expose pups to as many different people (age, colour, etc.), animals (dogs, cats, others), locations (parks, other homes, crowded offices, elevators, etc.) and stimuli (e.g. thunder/lightning, gunshots, traffic) as possible during early development. This should be done gradually to avoid overwhelming the puppy
Households with no children (especially potential parents and grandparents), should socialise their puppy with children to minimise the chance of problems when children become part of the family
Continue socialisation even after 14 weeks of age with both people and other animals

Fig. 2.10 Steps to encourage normal social development in dogs.

It is especially important to socialise puppies to non-family members in diverse situations so they will behave appropriately in a variety of settings when they get older (Fig. 2.10). An excellent way for owners to socialise their puppies to new people is to use the concept of 'socialisation biscuits'. The owner should take the puppy into novel situations armed with a box of small, biscuit treats. The puppy should be encouraged to approach everyone it meets along the way (e.g. children, joggers, cyclists, postal delivery people). When the puppy responds appropriately (e.g. responds to the 'sit' command given by the stranger, shows no apprehension), the owner gives the stranger a biscuit treat to give to the puppy. A treat, some play and a few friendly pats are usually all that is required to socialise puppies. The same can be done with the staff in the veterinary clinic and visitors coming to the home. The owner should also be told that properly socialising a puppy does not mean that it won't protect their home and family at a later date. Socialisation should also be done with other animals, but exposure to other dogs should be limited until the vaccination series has been completed. The ideal dog with which to socialise the puppy would be a healthy, fully vaccinated pet that has been recently tested and treated for internal and external parasites and has a social non-aggressive personality.

Socialisation before 14 weeks of age is critical, but continued socialisation after that time is also very important. Obedience classes and puppy parties are an excellent way for the good exposure to continue. Puppy training can begin by 8 weeks of age, but group classes are best avoided until there has been time for adequate response to vaccination. Any behaviour problems that are evident during puppyhood need immediate intervention and counselling.

Puppy Classes

Veterinarians and their staff can play important roles in providing puppy classes for clients. The primary function of the puppy class is socialisation of the puppy to a variety of other dogs and people, while the dog is still young and receptive (Fig. 2.11). They provide an additional opportunity to discuss and demonstrate handling exercises, training, and products that were not adequately discussed during office visits. They also bond clients and patients to the clinic

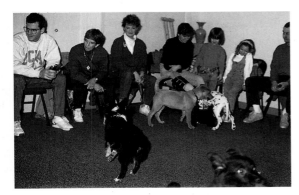

FIG. 2.11 Puppy classes are a great way to provide training and socialisation.

INFORMATION FOR A PUPPY CLASS OR PUPPY PARTY
Socialisation
Establishing leadership
How to teach the puppy to accept handling
How to control unruliness, nipping, mounting, jumping up
How to use punishment and rewards correctly
Housetraining
Prevention of destructive chewing
Basic obedience commands
Basic medical information: parasites, vaccines, nutrition, neutering
Behaviour products and management tools

FIG. 2.12 Information that should be conveyed at puppy classes and puppy parties.

and offer an additional source of revenue. To be successful, the class should have at least four puppies, but fewer than eight per instructor. If there is not space for a formal class, a 1–2-hour social session or 'puppy party' can be scheduled once monthly in the reception area. This provides an excellent opportunity for puppies to socialise and for owners to ask behaviour and health questions (Fig. 2.12).

Exercise and Stimulation

Dogs should be given sufficient exercise to dissipate energy and prevent or greatly reduce behaviour problems. This is especially true of breeds bred for endurance or work (e.g. Siberian Huskies, Labrador Retrievers, German Shepherd Dogs). A 15-minute exercise period once or twice daily may be suitable for most dogs, but working dogs usually need much more. Activities that are more mentally and physically challenging, such as flyball, agility training and pulling carts (off the highway), may be best for these pets. Less active dogs, such as Basset Hounds, may be satisfied with a brief walk and some owner contact. Ultimately, each dog is an individual with its own needs. In general, a dog has had enough exercise if it settles down and rests following its outing. Whereas some owners jog, run or take long walks to satisfy their dog's needs, more sedentary owners can accomplish the same goals by throwing a ball, toy or flying disc for the pet to retrieve. It should be borne in mind that unrestricted exercise is not healthy for all dogs. For example, it has been hypothesised that rapidly growing large-breed dogs should not be strenuously exercised for fear of exacerbating developmental orthopaedic problems such as hip dysplasia.

Play and exercise sessions should be part of the daily routine. It is usually not sufficient to allow the young pet to sit around all week and then take it for a long run at the weekend. Owners should make plans to spend time with their dogs and then honour the commitment – both will benefit. Exercise periods are not only healthy for owner and pet, but are wonderful interactive sessions that help in the bonding process and can also prevent unwanted attention-getting behaviours. When dogs get used to a regular exercise programme, they are less likely to misbehave; they learn to anticipate and wait for scheduled outings. On the other hand, dissatisfying scheduled activity can increase anxiety and may promote unwanted behaviours. Scheduled events encourage the dog to anticipate planned outings and to be calm at other times. For owners unable to exercise or stimulate their pets, there are now videos available that might work at keeping them interested and occupied.

If a kitten's needs for play, exercise and social contact are provided, undesirable behavioural consequences such as excessive nocturnal activity, destructive exploration, scratching, exuberant activity sessions, play aggression and other attention-getting behaviours are less likely to develop. The kitten should be provided with an appropriate scratching post and toys for self play. A play centre with perches, ledges, dangling toys and a variety of surfaces for scratching can be either purchased or constructed. Some cats enjoy investigating and playing in empty cardboard boxes or paper bags.

Since predation is a highly innate behaviour in most cats, play sessions should, at least in part, be designed to provide active chase-and-pounce targets. Battery-operated rolling toys, small plastic balls, walnuts or ping-pong balls will work for some cats. Cat toys that dangle from a door handle or scratching post, and those mounted on springs can also provide good outlets for predatory play. Interactive play is, however, the best outlet for most cats' needs. Interactive cat toys include long wands, ropes or sticks with toys attached to the end that resemble prey. After satisfying these needs for play, attention and exercise during the day and evenings, most cats will sleep through the night. Allowing cats access to the outdoors is generally not essential, provided the owner provides the cat with sufficient outlets for its investigative, predatory and playful instincts.

Some cautions are needed when counselling owners about playing with their pets. Be certain that the toys are not so small or fragile that they can be chewed and swallowed. Be particularly vigilant to keep string and thread away from cats and that all toys are large enough and sturdy enough that they cannot be broken or ingested. Since some dogs have such a strong desire and ability to chew, be certain that all chew and play toys are either safe for chewing and ingestion or large and indestructible enough that they cannot be swallowed. A number of such toys are available from commercial companies (Fig. 2.13). Articles of clothing (such as shoes – Fig. 2.13, or gloves), hands and feet or household items (such as old towels or blankets) should not be used

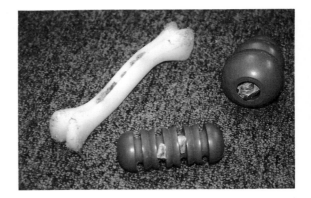

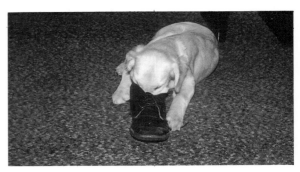

FIG. 2.13 A number of quality chew toys are available (top). Chewing/investigating an old shoe is *not* recommended (bottom).

for play, since some pets will generalise their chewing to possessions that the owner doesn't want damaged. Never allow a pet to initiate play sessions by barking, grasping, pouncing or performing other forms of 'demanding' behaviour, as this may encourage attention-getting or other undesirable behaviours (Fig. 2.14).

BEHAVIOURS REDUCED BY PLAY AND EXERCISE
Destructiveness (chewing, digging, scratching)
Investigative behaviour (garbage raiding, chewing)
Hyperactivity/excitability (exuberant play, nocturnal activity)
Unruliness (knocking over furniture, jumping up)
Predatory and social play – cats (pounce and bite)
Social play – dogs (play biting)
Attention-getting behaviours (barking and whining for attention)

FIG. 2.14 Some examples of behaviours that might be reduced or prevented by adequate play and exercise.

BECOMING A 'PACK LEADER' IN THE HOME

Establish routines with the dog (exercise, feeding)

Initiate obedience training early; attend obedience classes

Before giving the puppy anything of value (e.g. food, patting, walks) have it respond to an obedience command

Save all rewards for training – rewards should be earned

Reward all obedient and subordinate behaviours

Rewards should never be given at the puppy's initiation (barking, pawing, nudging)

Identify and immediately deal with pushy and dominant expressions and displays

Correct inappropriate behaviours as soon as they occur

Handle the pet frequently; reward compliance

Do not play tug-of-war or other boisterous games unless the games are initiated and easily terminated by the owners

FIG. 2.15 Steps to the owner becoming 'pack leader' in the home.

Social Relationships – Dogs

Dogs are pack animals and as such readily establish social relationships with other members with which they live. Although dogs are capable of vocalisation, most of their social communication is accomplished by means of facial expressions, body postures and occasionally by using body contact. This type of communication is innate, shared by virtually all members of the species and is very important in establishing and maintaining the social hierarchy. Within the living group, there is a dominant leader dog (alpha) holding the top position and subordinates holding lower ranking positions in a fairly linear hierarchy. The ability of one dog to become dominant over the others depends on inherited traits, sex, size, hormonal status and the relative dominance of other pack members. The dominant position affords the alpha individual such benefits as better access to food, mates and resting areas. Assertive young dogs will challenge the leader of the pack and, if they are dominant enough, may eventually usurp the role. The same may happen in the home environment with other family pets. Longevity in the household provides a certain degree of authority, but will not deter a domineering newcomer from challenging.

To a certain degree, dogs regard human family members as other members of the pack. If the pet does not respect their leadership, problems can occur. When a pushy puppy does not receive leadership and discipline from the family, it may attempt to climb the dominance hierarchy towards the position of alpha dog. This is an unsuitable position for most family pets, especially when that cute and cuddly puppy

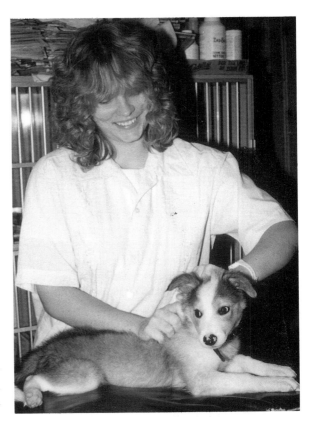

FIG. 2.16 Restraining the exuberant puppy. Being able to handle puppies is an important part of gaining control.

grows to be a disobedient, stubborn or even aggressive adult dog. To prevent this from happening, owners must assert their dominance early, encouraging compliance and obedience from the puppy (Fig. 2.15). This should cover feeding, play and a variety of other behaviour situations. Dogs may be respectful and obedient of some family members but not others, especially children. Accordingly, it is critical that every member of the family gain control over the puppy. Owners must be counselled so that they do not misinterpret control as punishment. Inappropriate punishment does not build respect in dogs any more than it does in children.

Social Relationships – Cats

As individual hunters feeding on small prey, cats are capable of living a rather solitary existence, particularly when food and resources are scarce. Being solitary, however, does not preclude social behaviour. Over the past few years, our knowledge of cat social structure has slowly evolved away from the widespread belief that cats are exclusively a very asocial species. Recently, there have been numerous studies that demonstrate wide diversity in sociability and social structure in cats. The fundamental social unit is a group of females and successive generations of descendants. Relationships between neutered males are more similar to those amongst females than among uncastrated males. Adult males and some females are more solitary and, as such, do not form social groups. There is a great deal of individual variability based on genetic factors, early social interactions during the sensitive period (2 to 7 weeks of age), sexual status and food availability. Encounters between solitary cats are rare while group-living cats display frequent social interactions. Even cats that spend most of their time alone may occasionally be seen in the company of other cats, particularly a mother cat and her kittens.

Social relationships between cats and humans also show widespread diversity. Cats differ greatly in personality and temperament. Again, genetic variability and amount and quality of exposure to humans during the critical socialisation period, are important factors determining how social a cat will be with humans. Some cats are independent, with little desire for contact with humans or other cats. Others maintain social relationships with people or other family pets throughout life. Approximately 15% of cats seem resistant to socialisation with humans. Most cats adapt well to sharing a home or apartment with people, other cats and other pets. On the other hand, it is not unusual for some cats to have difficulty adjusting to changes in the household, particularly the introduction of a new cat.

Handling and Restraint

It is essential that puppies and kittens learn to accept and enjoy all forms of handling from every family member as well as other humans with which they will come into contact. The family should be advised to expose the pet frequently to all types of handling in the context of gentle play and social attention (Fig. 2.16 and 2.17). Handling exercises should include gentle handling of the face, ears, feet, collar, skin and haircoat. Provided there are no signs of anxiety or resistance, the owner should gradually proceed to tooth brushing, grooming, lifting, nail trimming and grasping the muzzle or nape of the neck. The young pet should also be taught to tolerate all approaches and handling by family members while it is eating or playing with a toy. A pet that is not accustomed to being handled may resist or become fearful or aggressive when handled by a groomer, veterinarian, trainer or child.

Any handling that leads to fear, resistance, threats or aggression must immediately be identified and addressed. Training should be undertaken to condition acceptable responses to these forms of handling. Whatever interaction that is upsetting for the pet should be performed in a manner that is so mild and muted that no anxiety is elicited while the handler provides something highly desirable (food, calm talk). The length and intensity of the sessions should gradually increase.

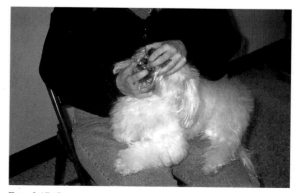

FIG. 2.17 Owners need to accustom the young pet to gentle handling of all parts of its body.

Prevention of Problems

The simplest form of prevention of undesirable behaviours involves separating the pet from the site of the problem, or confining it so that the undesirable behaviour cannot be performed. A common misconception is that confinement is cruel or unfair. On the contrary, leaving a pet unsupervised to investigate, destroy and perhaps get injured is far more inhumane. For kittens, caging may be useful but most kittens can be housed in a 'safe room' with a scratching post and litterbox, provided there are no objects that can be damaged by climbing or chewing. Child locks, secured cupboards and booby traps are useful in designing a cat-proof room.

Although dog-proofing a room might be successful for some dogs, a cage, run or pen is usually the safest and most secure form of canine confinement. Crate training is an excellent way to curb many behaviour problems, including housesoiling, destructiveness, digging, escape behaviour and garbage raiding. As long as a crate is big enough for the pet to stand up and turn around in comfortably, and the dog gets sufficient exercise and attention and is not left in the crate longer than it can control itself, a crate is a safe, secure and humane place to confine a pet when it is unsupervised. When a crate is used as a daily confinement area, its use should be limited for sleeping during the night and for periods not exceeding 4–5 hours during each day. Use of a crate is excessive if the pet is confined all night as well as 8–10 hours each day when the owner is away from home. Also, the crate should not be regarded as a prison cell where a dog is sent if it misbehaves. At each feeding time during the day, the owner should encourage the pet to go into the crate by repeatedly tossing pieces of dry food for the pet to chase into the crate (Fig. 2.18). If the owner says 'Go to your crate' each time the pet runs into the crate, it will eventually be conditioned to run into the crate on command. Toys should also be placed in the crate periodically throughout the day and occasionally a biscuit should be left in the crate so the pet is tempted to go into the crate on its own. This provides plenty of positive associations with the crate. It is ideal to start with short confinement periods and gradually lengthen them. The owner should ignore vocalisations and should not allow the pet out if it is barking or whining. If it needs to be released to eliminate, but continues to vocalise, the owner can try providing a distracting

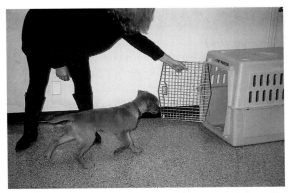

Fig. 2.18 A puppy can be taught to go to its crate on command by tossing dry food and saying 'Go to your crate!'.

noise (whistle, clicker, thump the wall) in an attempt to get the pet to orient towards the sound and be quiet for 10 seconds or more before it is released. However, the crate is simply a tool; it does not replace sound behavioural modification techniques but is a helpful adjunct. Introducing the pet to a confinement pen can be done with the same approach used for crate training. Child gates can also be used to keep the pet confined to a specific area.

Basic Training

There are limits to what should be expected in the training of puppies and kittens. Some animals have natural aptitudes while others are more limited. Learn to work with what you've got. Don't expect a bloodhound to walk perfectly on a leash immediately, because it has been bred to track a scent. The excitable pet will probably train better after it has had the opportunity to play and vent some of that energy. Also be aware that certain medical conditions and a variety of drugs can interfere with the learning process.

All dogs should learn basic obedience command responses such as 'come', 'sit', 'stay' and 'down'. The dog that learns to roll over or play dead may be fun at parties, but the basic skills could mean the difference between life and death. Dogs that will not 'stay' or come when called may end up in front of a car in the road. There are numerous books and videos dealing with training but formal obedience classes are still the best way to learn. This puts the owners under the supervision of a trainer where they are less likely to make fundamental errors. It also affords an opportunity for socialisation with new people and other dogs, an important part of behavioural development. Take the time to visit training classes personally so that you don't inadvertently refer an owner to a trainer who is not reputable.

Dogs can be taught to come, sit and lay down using food lure–reward training. This can even be done during a routine veterinary examination. Standing about 60 cm away from the puppy, a piece of food is held between the thumb and forefinger and extended. As the puppy approaches, its name is called, followed by the command 'come!' (Fig. 2.19). When the puppy reaches the food, it is slowly moved above its head (do not move the food too high over the pet's head or it will jump up instead of sit). As the puppy lifts its head up towards the food, it moves naturally into a sitting position (Fig. 2.20). As it begins to sit, the command 'sit!' is given. Holding the food reward on the ground entices the dog into the 'down' position (Fig. 2.21). Even this basic start helps the owner establish leadership and gain control, and serves as a tool for socialising. It also decreases jumping up and handshyness because the puppy associates greeting with sitting and an outstretched hand with a food reward. Making the dog come and sit before it gets anything also helps define a leadership role for the owner.

Rewards can also be used to train cats, especially young kittens, to perform a variety of tasks and to understand a number of commands. The major difference between dogs and cats is that cats are unlikely to respond to the raised voices, reprimands and physical techniques commonly used (but not always necessary) in dog training. Cats are no more difficult to train than any other animal. All one needs to do is associate a reward with a particular action, and the cat is likely to want to repeat or continue that action. For example, if the cat approaches its scratching post, uses its cat litter, comes to the owner, or sits up on its hindlegs, a desirable reward should be provided and the cat will want to perform the behaviour time and time again. On the other hand, if you call a cat over so that it can be punished for inappropriate scratching or chewing, it is unlikely that your cat will ever respond to your 'Come!' commands. Lure–reward techniques work effectively for most cats. Hold out a piece of food or cat toy, and say 'Come!'. Repeat this exercise a few times and the cat will learn to associate a reward with the 'come'

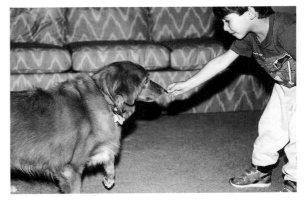

FIG. 2.19 Food lure training is an excellent way to teach a 'come' command. The owner stands about 60 cm from the dog, extends the hand with a food morsel, and says 'Come!'.

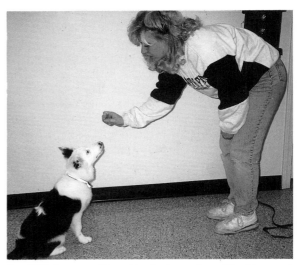

FIG. 2.20 A puppy will quickly sit when a piece of food is moved over the top of its head.

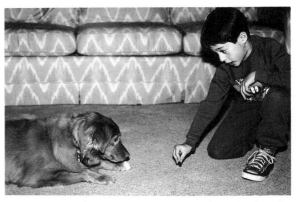

FIG. 2.21 Food lures can also be used to entice a dog into the 'down' position.

command. Hold out a piece of food or toy above the cat's scratching post, and use a different command (e.g. 'scratch') and the cat should soon learn to go to its scratching post on command. Similarly the cat can be taught to sit up and beg, go to its bedroom, or even go to particular people in the home by using the lure–reward technique.

The Role of Punishment and Rewards

The effective use of rewards and punishment is discussed in detail throughout this book as they apply to learning principles and in the correction of undesirable behaviour. Owners must understand that before punishment can be considered, every effort must first be made to provide the pet with appropriate outlets for instinctive and normal behaviours (e.g. chewing, scratching, eliminating, play). The key is to set up the pet to succeed. Prevention, confinement techniques, providing for all of the pet's needs, and constant supervision and guidance are far more productive than attempting only to punish the pet each time an undesirable behaviour is performed. Only after the pet has been encouraged and rewarded to perform appropriately should punishment techniques be considered.

Punishment is intended to reduce the chance that a particular behaviour will be repeated. Animals quickly learn to avoid unpleasant or aversive situations in nature. Similarly, we can teach our pets to avoid certain areas and behaviours with the proper use and application of punishment. **Under no circumstances should the owner ever strike the pet with a hand or anything in a hand.** Owners must understand that if they strike their pet, the consequences can be disastrous. Since the human hand should only be associated with affection, play or rewards, physical punishment (hitting) is never indicated. Physical punishment can lead to handshyness, fear-biting, avoidance of humans, aggression or submissive urination. Remote punishment techniques and booby traps are the preferred forms of punishment since they cause no fear of the owner and they teach the pet to avoid an area or behaviour whether the owner is present or not. In addition, for punishment to be successful, it must be sufficiently aversive to deter the pet immediately, and must be applied immediately and consistently until the behaviour ceases to be performed. Punishment (such as an abrupt, loud noise) is sufficiently aversive if the undesirable behaviour stops immediately, the pet shows a slight startle response without any sign of fear, and will readily come to the owner without any hesitation. **Anything the owner does to stop a behaviour that results in any sign of fear is inappropriate** (For further details see Chapter 3).

References Containing Information on Selection Tests

Bartlett, M. (1987) Follow-up: Puppy aptitude testing. *Pure-bred Dogs/American Kennel Club Gazette*, May, 36–42.

Beaudet, R., Chalifoux, A. and Daillaire, A. (1992) Mise au point d'un test d'évaluation du temperament applicable à la selection de chiens de compagnie. *Proceedings of 6th International Conference*, Animals and Us, Montreal.

Beaudet, R. Chalifoux, A. and Dallaire, A. (1994) Predictive value of activity level and behavioural evaluation on future dominance in puppies. *Appl Anim Behav Sci*, **40**(3–4), 273–284.

Beaudet, R. and Daillaire, A. (1993) Social dominance evaluation: observations on Campbell's test. *Bulletin on Veterinary Ethology*, **1**: 23–29.

Benjamin, C. L. (1990) *The Chosen puppy: How to Select and Raise a Great Puppy from an Animal Shelter.* Howell Book House: New York, NY.

Campbell, W. (1992) *Behavior Problems in Dogs*, 2nd Edn. American Veterinary Publications: Goleta, CA.

Cargill, J. (1994) Temperament tests as puppy selection tools. *Dog World*, April, 40–49.

Carricato, A. M. (1992) *Veterinary Notes for Dog Breeders.* Howell Book House: New York, 230pp.

Dietrich, C. (1984) Temperament evaluation of puppies: use in guide dog selection. In: *The Pet Connection: Its influence on our health and quality of life.* Centre to Study Human–Animal Relationships and Environment: Minneapolis, MN.

Fisher, G. T. and Volhard, W. (1979) Puppy personality profile. *Pure-bred Dogs/American Kennel Club Gazette*, March, 31–42.

Goodloe, L. P. (1996) Issues in description and measurement of temperament in companion dogs. In: *Readings in Companion Animal Behavior*, Voith V. L. and Borchelt P. L. (eds) pp.32–39. Veterinary Learning Systems: Trenton, NJ.

Netto, W. J., van der Borg, J. A. M. and Plant, D. J. U. (1992) Behavioral testing of dogs in animal shelters predict problem behavior. *Proceedings of 6th International Conference*, Animals and Us.

Overall, K. (1994) Temperament testing and training – Do they prevent behavioral problems. *Canine Practice*, **19**(4), 19–21.

References on Breeds and Breed Selection

Ackerman, L., Landsberg, G. and Hunthhausen, W. (Eds) (1996) *Cat Behavior and Training: Veterinary Advice for Owners*, TFH Publications: Neptune, NJ.

Ackerman, L. Landsberg, G. and Hunthausen, W. (Eds). (1996) *Dog Behavior and Training: Veterinary Advice for Owners*, TFH Publications: Neptune, NJ

Alderton, D. (1992) *The Eyewitness Handbook of Cats*, Dorling Kindersley Inc: New York.

American Veterinary Medical Association: *A Veterinarian's Way of Selecting a Proper Pet.* (Pamphlet).

American Kennel Club. (1989) *Complete Dog Book.* Howell House: New York.

Baer, N. and Duno, S. (1995) *Choosing a Dog: Your Guide to Picking the Perfect Breed.* Berkly Publishing: New York.

Beaver, B. V. (1993) Profiles of dogs presented for aggression. *Journal of the American Animal Hospital Association*,29, 564–569.

Borchelt, P. L. (1983) Aggressive behavior of dogs kept as companion animals: classification and influence of sex, reproductive status, and breed. *Appl Anim Ethol*, **10**, 35–43.

Canadian Kennel Club Book of Dogs. (1988) Stoddart: Toronto.

Clark, R. D. (1992) *Medical, Genetic, and Behavioral Aspects of Purebred Cats.* Veterinary Forum Publications: St Simons Island, GA.

Clark, R. D. and Stainer, J. R. (1994) *Medical and Genetic Aspects of Purebred Dogs.* Veterinary Forum Publishing: St Simons Island, GA.

De Prisco, A. and Johnson, J. B. (1990) *The Mini-Atlas of Dog Breeds.* TFH Publications: Neptune, N.J. 48pp.

Gebhardt, R. H. (Consultant editor). (1979) *A Standard Guide to Cat Breeds.* McGraw-Hill

Hart, B. L. and Hart, L. A. (1984) *Selecting the Best Companion Animal: Breed and gender specific behavioral profiles. The Pet Connection – its influence on our health and quality of life.* Center to Study Human–Animal Relationships and Environments: Minneapolis, MN.

Hart, B. L. and Hart, L. A. (1985) Selecting pet dogs on the basis of cluster analysis of breed behavior profiles and gender. *J Am Vet Med Assoc*, **186**(11), 1181–1185.

Hart, B. L. and Hart, L. A. (1988) *The Perfect Puppy.* W. H. Freeman and Co., New York.

Hart, B. L. and Miller, M. F. (1985) Behavioral profiles of dog breeds. *J Am Vet Med Assoc*, **186**(11), 1175–1180.

Howe, J. (1980) *Choosing the Right Dog.* Harper & Row: New York.

Landsberg, G. M. (1991) The distribution of canine behavior cases at 3 referral practices. *Vet Med*, **86**, 1081–1089.

Lowell, M. (1990) *Your Purebred Puppy – A buyer's guide.* Henry Holt: New York.

Palmer, J. (1987) *A Practical Guide to Selecting a Small Dog.* Tetra Press: London 118pp.

Palmer, J. (1987) *A Practical Guide to Selecting a Large Dog.* Tetra Press: London 118pp.

Project Breed: *Breed Rescue Efforts & Education.* (1989) Network for Ani-males & Females, Inc.: Germantown, MD.

Siegal, M. (ed). (1983) *Simon and Schuster's Guide to Cats.* Simon and Schuster: New York.

Siegal, M. and Margolis, M. (1991) *Good Dog, Bad Dog.* Henry Holt: New York.

Tortora, D. (1983) *The Right Dog for You.* Simon & Schuster: New York.

Wilkinson, T. (1985) *Delinquent Dogs.* Quartet Books: London.

Wright, J. C. and Nesselrote, M. S. (1987) Classification of behavior problems in dogs: distribution of age, breed, sex, and reproductive status. *Applied Animal Behavior Science*, **19**, 169–178.

Additional Reading and References

Adams, G. J., Clark, W. T. (1989) The prevalence of behavioural problems in domestic dogs: A survey of 105 dog owners. *Australian Vetinary Practitioner*, **19**, 135–137.

Anderson, R. K. (1990) At What Age Can Dogs Learn? *Veterinary Forum*, August p.32.

Angameier, E. and James, W. T. (1961) The influence of early sensory-social deprivation on the social operant in dogs. *J Genet Psychol* **99**, 153–158.

Askew, H. R. (1994) How scientific is pet behavior therapy. *Praktische Tierarzt*, **75**(6), 539.

Ban, B. (1994) From growl to whimper: the spectrum of canine behavior modification. *J Am Vet Med Ass*, **204**(1), 7–12.

Beaver, B. V. (1994) Owner complaints about canine behavior. *Am Vet Med Assoc*, **204**(12), 1953–1955.

Blackshaw, J. K. (1988) Abnormal behavior in dogs. *Australian Veterinary Journal*, **65**(12), 393–000.

Chapman, B. L. and Voith, V. L. (1990) Behavioral problems in old dogs: 26 cases (1984–1987). *J Am Vet Med Assoc*, **196**, 944–946.

Coppinger, R. and Coppinger, L. (1996) Biologic bases of behaviour of domestic dog breeds. In: *Readings in Companion Animal Behaviour* Voith, V. L. and Borchelt, P. L. (eds) pp.9–17. Veterinary Learning Systems: Trenton, NJ.

Estep, D. O. (1996) The ontogeny of behaviour. In: *Readings in Companion Animal Behavior*, Voith, V. I. and Borchelt, P. L. (eds). pp.19–31. Veterinary Learning Systems, Trenton: NJ.

Feddersenpetersen, D. (1994) Comparative studies of behavioral development of wolves (*Canis lupus*) and domestic dogs (*Canis familiaris*). Domestication traits and selective breeding. *Tierarztliche Umschau*, **49**(9), 527–531.

Feddersenpetersen, D. (1994) Social behavior of wolves and dogs. *Veterinary Quarterly*, **16**(Suppl. 1), S51–S52.

Fox, M. W. (1971) Overview and critique of stages and periods in canine development. *Developmental Psychobiol*, **4**(1), 37.

Fox, M. W. and Stelzner, D. (1966) Behavioral effects of differential early experience in the dog. *Animal Behavior*, **14**, 273–281.

Freedman, D. G. *et al.* (1961) Critical period in the social development of dogs. *Science*, **133**, 1016–1017.

Horwitz, D. F. (1993) Feline socialization: How environment and early learning influence behavior. *Vet Med*, August, 14–16.

Houpt, K. A. (1985) Companion animal behaviour: A review of dog and cat behaviour in the field, the laboratory and the clinic. *Cornell Vet*, **75**, 248–261.

Kerby, G. and Macdonald, D. W. (1988) Cat society and the consequences of colony size. In: D. Turner, P. Bateson (eds) *The Domestic Cat: The Biology of its Behavior.* Cambridge University Press: Cambridge, UK.

Landsberg, G. M. (1993) Confinement Training. *Veterinary Practice Staff*, **5**(3), 19–22.

Mech, L. D. (1981) *The Wolf: The Ecology and Behavior of an Endangered Species.* University of Minnesota Press: MN.

Miller, D. D., Staats, S. R., Partlo, C. *et al.* (1996) Factors associated with the decision to surrender a pet to an animal shelter. *J Am Vet Med Assoc*, **209**(4), 738–742.

Scarlett, J. M., Saidla, J. E. and Pollock, R. V. H. (1994) Source of acquisition as a risk factor for disease and death in pups. *J Am Vet Med Assoc*, **204**(12), 1906–1913.

Scott, J. P. and Fuller, J. L. *Genetics and the Social Behavior of the Dog.* University of Chicago Press: Chicago, IL.

Serpell, J. A. (1987) The influence of inheritance and environment on canine behavior: myth and fact. *J Small Anim Pract*, **28**(11), 949–956.

Stur, I. (1987) Genetic aspects of temperament and behavior in dogs. *J Small Anim Pract*, **28**(11), 957–964.

Vollmer, P. J. (1978) Puppy Rearing. 2: Establishing the leader–follower bond. *Vet Med Small Anim Clin* **73**, 994–000.

Vollmer. P. (1979) Puppy Rearing. 9. Early stimulation. *Vet Med Small Anim Clin*, **74**, 307–311.

Vollmer, P. (1980) Canine Socialization. Part 1. *Vet Med Small Anim Clin*, **75**, 207–211.

Vollmer, P. (1980) Canine Socialization. Part 2. *Vet Med Small Anim Clin*, **75**, 411–412.

Willis, M. B. (1987) Breeding dogs for desirable traits. *J Small Anim Pract*, **28**(11), 965–983.

(For general references on pet care please see Chapter 1).

3

Behaviour Counselling and Behavioural Modification Techniques

Preparation Before the Session

Since behaviour counselling requires a knowledge and understanding of a wide variety of problems, it is seldom practical to perform a behavioural consultation without some advanced preparation. It is therefore, advisable to request that owners fill out a history questionnaire and use this information to research the problem thoroughly before the counselling session. The behaviour data sheet should include references to a variety of factors. The form can be customised using the information provided; alternatively, standardised forms are available in other books. If you feel uncomfortable with your ability to handle some cases, consider referring them, or set up your own telephone consultation with a behaviour referral centre. Regardless of the approach you choose, you will need access to all the information on the behaviour data sheet of your choosing or design (Fig. 3.1).

It is always advisable to counsel and inform clients about simple behavioural concerns during their regular veterinary visits. For more involved problems

BASIC INFORMATION FOR A BEHAVIOUR DATA SHEET	
Client information	Family members – ages – occupations/schedule – special considerations (e.g. special needs, disabilities)
Pet information	Patient profile including neutering and declawing history Source of pet, when obtained, previous owners if known Medical/behavioural information of parents, siblings or littermates General description of pet's temperament Diet, including type of food and frequency, treats/frequency Medical history (medications administered, any recent or pertinent laboratory tests)
Home environment/ lifestyle and daily schedule	Pet's housing, including bedding and where housed day and night Elimination areas, feeding areas, scratching or play areas Play/exercise routines When and how long left alone Time indoors/outdoors Family member and pet responsibilities Other pets in household
Relationships	Other pets in household Family members
Reactions to other people and animals	How does pet react to other animals and people (non-family members) on-property and off-property. Postures, vocalizations, interactions, approach behaviours, fear, aggression
Training	Obedience Crate/cage training Reward use and pet's response (reinforcer assessment) Punishment use and pet's response (punisher assessment)
Response to handling	E.g. bathing, nail trimming, grooming
Primary problem	What is the problem? When began? When does it happen? Where does it occur? Who? Is the problem more likely to occur with specific people or animals? Why? Can the owner identify any events that might have caused or started the problem? Describe circumstances including duration Techniques used thus far and pet's response How serious is the problem? (Are the owners considering euthanasia?)
Additional problems	Are the any behaviour problems that are not part of the principle concern

Fig. 3.1 Basic information for inclusion in a behaviour data sheet.

(e.g. housesoiling, scratching), it is best to schedule a separate appointment. This will allow the practitioner to spend an adequate amount of time discussing the problems rather than hurriedly trying to collect information and give treatment recommendations during a medical visit.

Tackling more difficult problems, such as aggression or complex phobias, is best reserved for behavioural specialists or those veterinarians that have already acquired significant experience in behaviour counselling. Veterinarians should not attempt to counsel cases beyond their abilities. Incomplete, insufficient or inaccurate advice could lead to worsening of the problem, potential liability and loss of confidence from the client.

Scheduling the Behaviour Consultation

A behaviour consultation requires the time and commitment of both veterinarian and client. Rarely is it possible to offer any meaningful behavioural advice for a difficult problem during a 15–20 minute routine office visit. Schedule behaviour consultations accordingly, allowing 1–2 hours for the initial interview. Whenever possible, have all members of the family present.

Fees may be structured in different ways: a set fee might be charged for the visit, no matter how long it takes; an hourly fee might be charged, or an hourly fee with a maximum amount. The average hourly income should approximate at least the amount that would be received if the veterinarian were seeing medical patients during that time. Additional fees should be charged for travel time when the consultation is a house call. Ultimately, the fees that are charged will depend on the demographics of the area and the perceived value of a behaviour consultation for a pet.

Behaviour consultations are like medical consultations; there are rarely any gimmicks that you can offer to fix a long-standing problem. As with any medical case, the veterinarian will be required to diagnose the problem, determine the prognosis, institute or recommend safe and effective correction, and present the treatment plan and all anticipated expenses. The owners then need to decide if such a plan is practical for their home, family and lifestyle, and within their budgets and capabilities. Some owners may decide the problems or expenses in the correction process are greater than they can manage. Those that decide to proceed might want to enlist the aid of a competent trainer or may tackle the problems themselves. It is

critical that the owner understands all the options and alternatives at this time.

The Medical Examination

Prior to performing the actual behavioural consultation, it is critical that a thorough physical examination is done and that underlying medical conditions are ruled out. For example, using behavioural

MEDICAL CAUSES OF ABNORMAL OR UNACCEPTABLE BEHAVIOUR	
Type of medical condition	Example
Congenital/Inherited physiological structural/malformation/ aplasia hypoplasia/dysplasia metabolic/genetic	Narcolepsy; epilepsy Hydrocephalus Cerebellar hypoplasia Lethal acrodermatitis
Infections bacterial viral fungal parasitic protozoal	*Listeria* Rabies; distemper; Feline Immunodeficiency Virus (FIV); Feline Leukemia Virus (FeLV) *Cryptococcus* *Cuterebra*; heartworm *Toxoplasma*
Metabolic hepatic encephalopathy hypoglycaemia storage diseases copper toxicosis multi-system neuronal degeneration	Congenital; acquired Insulinoma; malnutrition Fucosidosis; alpha-mannosidosis As seen in Bedlington Terriers As seen in Cocker Spaniels
Toxic drugs insecticides toxins	Ibuprofen; levamisole; hallucinogens DEET-fenvalerate Lead
Nutritional deficiencies other	Thiamin Adverse food reactions High-protein diet(??)
Neoplasia	Glioma; meningioma Metastatic disease
Immune/Inflammatory inflammatory immune-mediated	Steroid-responsive meningitides Granulomatous meningoencephalitis
Hormonal	Hypo/hyperthyroidism; hyperoestrogenism
Degenerative	Ageing Cognitive dysfunction(??)
Traumatic	Head injury
Vascular	Infarct; haemorrhage
Neural	Psychomotor epilepsy Abnormal neurotransmitter levels (??)
Idiopathic	Rage syndromes(??) Feline interstitial cystitis

Fig. 3.2 Medical causes of abnormal or unacceptable behaviour.

modification for a cat with inappropriate urination is counterproductive if the underlying cause is lower urinary tract disease. When presented with an older pet which suddenly develops behaviour problems, it is important to consider contributing geriatric conditions. A knowledge of medicine is one of the major advantages veterinarians have over many behaviourists and is not something to be minimised. Behavioural counselling is part of comprehensive health care, not a separate entity.

For each behaviour problem it is important to consider all medical and physical conditions or anomalies that might play a role in the development of the problem (Fig. 3.2). Aggression and other alterations in mental state could be due to: primary diseases of the central nervous system such as infections, hyperkinesis or tumours; primary diseases of other organ systems that cause behavioural changes such as thyroid dysfunction or hepatic encephalopathy; or diseases that, in some individuals, may contribute to an aggressive state, such as painful conditions (otitis, arthritis, anal sacculitis) or sensory

dysfunction (loss of vision or hearing). For inappropriate urination problems, it is essential that any medical condition that might lead to polyuria, pollakiuria, dysuria, stranguria or incontinence be ruled out before strictly behavioural causes can be considered.

The Behavioural Consultation

Fig. 3.3 shows the sequence of events from the initial consultation to the treatment plan.

Taking an Accurate History

History taking is the most important diagnostic tool and must be accorded the most time and energy. Taking a verbal history will usually require between 30 and 90 minutes, depending on the complexity of the problem. The behaviour data sheet should be completed for every behaviour consultation and can serve as an outline for the consultation. This becomes part of the permanent medical record.

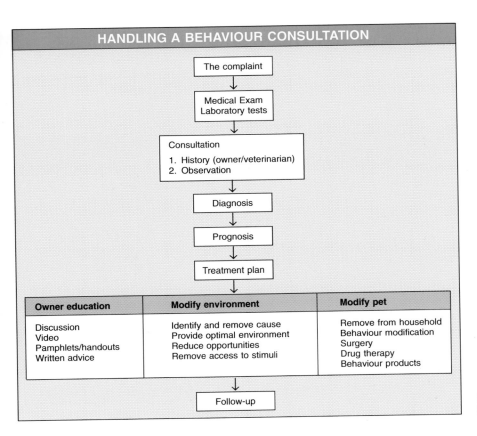

FIG. 3.3 The process of behavioural consultation.

Diagnosis

In most cases, the diagnosis will be made on the basis of the patient history, observation of the pet and physical examination. Diagnostic tests may need to be conducted to rule out organic causes for the problem. Although abnormalities may seldom be found, as medical professionals it is incumbent upon veterinarians to assess all their patients thoroughly for medical problems before rendering a diagnosis, or recommending therapeutic intervention.

When making a behavioural diagnosis, the consultant may have to rely on sketchy information from an emotionally involved owner who may view the pet a bit too anthropomorphically and who may not be present when much of the undesirable behaviour occurs. This can make a firm diagnosis difficult in some cases and impossible in others.

Prognosis

The prognosis is determined based on the diagnosis and is critical for the veterinarian, client and pet. The prognosis given by the veterinarian will often determine if the pet will be treated or removed permanently from the house. Factors that contribute to the ultimate prognosis include the pet itself, the owners, the environment in which the pet lives, the type and extent of the problem, the ability of the consultant to diagnose and communicate with the client, and whether a practical correction programme can conceivably be implemented safely and practically for the problem at hand (Fig. 3.4).

How to Modify and Manage Undesirable Behaviours

The treatment of behavioural problems requires a three-pronged approach. This involves:

- Educating the owner (Figs. 3.3, 3.5)
- Modifying the environment (Fig. 3.6)
- Modifying the pet (Fig. 3.3).

Another important aspect of treatment is **follow-up**. It is essential that the consultant continues to observe each case so that owners can clarify facts or techniques or seek additional advice following the initial consultation, particularly when there are multiple treatment options. When drugs have been discussed or dispensed, regular follow-up is essential. For some cases, additional diagnostic tests and owner information will be required following the initial consultation, so that a formal follow-up telephone call or session may need to be scheduled. Follow-up contacts at 2, 4 and 24 weeks will provide good assessment of progress. At the very least, consultants should monitor and record the outcome of each case 6 months after the initial consultation.

PROGNOSTIC CONSIDERATIONS	
Good Prognosis	**More Guarded or Grave Prognosis**
Problem can readily and accurately be diagnosed	Problem or cause of problem poorly understood
All stimuli can be identified and prevented or controlled	Inability to identify or prevent initiating stimuli
Mild problem of short duration	Severe or advanced problem of long duration High level of intensity or severity High or unpredictable frequency
Low motivation for the behaviour or simple, conditioned behaviour problem	Very strong motivation to perform behaviour Strongly innate factors
Simple, single problem	Complex, multiple problems
Historically, a good prognosis for the diagnosed problem	The type of problem responds poorly to conventional therapy Appropriate correction techniques have been attempted, but were unsuccessful
Degree of danger is low	Marked danger History of severe damage
Commitment and ability of family members is high	Inability or unwillingness of owners to treat Desire of family to remove pet from household
Good understanding and ability to follow necessary correction techniques	Owners cannot comprehend nature of problem or principles of treatment Owners unable to generalise prevention or treatment techniques to similar situations

FIG. 3.4 Factors affecting the prognosis for a behaviour problem.

EXAMPLES OF PROBLEMS AND INFORMATION FOR OWNERS

Problem	Owner Education Required
Dominance aggression	Pack structure; social communication; dominant and subordinate signalling; the dog in the family pack
Canine housesoiling	Better understanding of housetraining; crate training; relationship between eating and eliminating; supervision and confinement
Feline housesoiling	Proper selection, placement and care of litter; odour elimination; supervision and confinement; how to make areas unacceptable for elimination
Feline spraying	The role of neutering; social behaviour of cats; influence of cat density; drug therapy
Unruly dog	Obedience training; halter devices; principles of conditioning
Canine destructive behaviour	Importance of play and exercise; pros and cons of adding a playmate; discussion of appropriate chew toys
Feline play aggression	How to direct play towards moving toys such as a wiggling rope, a fishing toy or a catnip mouse on a rope; adding a second cat

FIG. 3.5 Examples of client education.

Educating the Owner

Educating the owner does not directly influence the pet's behaviour, but the ultimate success of treating the problem is directly related to complete owner comprehension and compliance. Since, in most cases, the behavioural modification will be carried out by family members themselves, the clients must understand their roles and the techniques they will be required to perform (Fig. 3.3).

Providing pets with appropriate outlets for play, exercise, elimination, chewing and digging may be all that is required to solve some problems. Even when the initial cause cannot be determined, providing the owner with the information necessary to work with the problem, may be sufficient to remedy it (Fig. 3.5).

When clients are educated appropriately, they realise more clearly which problems are most likely to be completely eliminated and which are likely to be remedied incompletely. The properly informed client may sometimes prefer to live with the problem rather than institute the necessary steps for corrections, while others may decide that euthanasia is the safest or most appropriate choice for their circumstances.

Changing the Environment

Environmental modification involves manipulating the pet's environment, or placing the pet in a novel situation that is less likely to result in the problem behaviour (Fig. 3.6).

Modifying the Pet (Fig. 3.3)

Removing the pet from the household

Removing the pet from the home remains an option, especially if there is danger posed to family members or if the owners are completely resistant to appropriate behavioural modification techniques. Although removal of the pet may seem like a failure,

WAYS TO MANIPULATE THE ENVIRONMENT

Change	Example
Identify and remove the cause	For urine spraying, reducing the number of cats may eliminate the problem
Provide an environment conducive to the pet's needs	Installing a dog or cat door may successfully manage housesoiling by giving immediate access to the outdoors
Reduce the opportunity to misbehave	Separate the pet from the site of the problem or booby-trap potential problem areas
Set up the environment for success	For feline housesoiling, place the litter tray in the spot of inappropriate elimination. The environment can also be changed by converting a soiled area into one used for feeding, play or sleep. For chewing, provide acceptable and appropriate objects for chewing in an area where the pet investigates and chews
Reduce or prevent access to the stimulus	If neighbourhood or intruding cats are causing urine marking or aggression, modify the environment so that the problem cats can't be seen, heard, or smelled

FIG. 3.6 Manipulating the environment to manage undesirable behaviours.

BEHAVIOURAL BENEFITS OF CASTRATION	
Behaviour	**Effects of Castration**
Undesirable sexual behaviour	Can reduce attraction to females, roaming, mounting and masturbation. Roaming can be reduced in 90% of dogs and sexual mounting of people in 66% of dogs. Roaming in cats can be reduced in over 90% of cases
Marking	Marking with urine is a common territorial behaviour in dogs and cats. Castration reduces marking in about 50% of dogs and 90% of cats
Aggression	Intermale aggression can be reduced in about 60% of dogs and 90% of cats Dominance aggression can sometimes be reduced but behavioural modification is also needed for complete elimination Territorial aggression and predation are not sexually dimorphic and are not influenced by castration

FIG. 3.7 Behavioural benefits of castration.

it is a desirable end if it prevents the animal from hurting members of the household or being inhumanely treated by the owners with inappropriate correction strategies. New owners must, however, be aware of the situation and be in a position to cope.

Changing behaviour through surgery

Castration of male dogs not only helps stem the pet population but also has valuable behavioural and medical benefits. Castration may prevent unacceptable sexual behaviour, reduce aggressiveness, and prevent accidental or indiscriminate breeding. With respect to behaviour, it should be clearly understood that the only behaviours affected by castration would be those that are influenced by male hormones. Thus, castration affects sexually dimorphic behaviours, those seen predominantly in males (Fig. 3.7).

There are also medical benefits of castration. Since castration can help curtail roaming, castrated dogs and cats are less likely to be endangered by viral, bacterial, parasitic or environmental dangers. In dogs, castration is useful in the prevention or treatment of prostatic disease, testicular cancer and in the reduction of perianal tumours.

Other surgical procedures that might also be indicated are olfactory tractotomy for refractory spraying cases, dental disarming, declawing and devocalisation. (Many of these procedures are only considered as a last-resort alternative to euthanasia and in some countries may be unacceptable or illegal.) Surgery or medical therapy might also be necessary when an underlying medical condition (e.g. hyperthyroidism, anal sacculitis) is causing or contributing to the behavioural symptoms.

Modifying the pet with behavioural modification techniques

Behavioural modification is the principle means of correcting or controlling undesirable behaviour. Therefore it is critical for veterinarians to understand the basic principles and definitions of learning and motivation if they intend to perform behavioural counselling in practice. It is also recommended that books on training and behaviour be consulted for more basic instruction on these techniques.

Behavioural Modification Techniques and Terms

Aversion Therapy

Aversion therapy is a procedure for eliminating undesirable behaviour by pairing the unwanted behaviour with a sufficiently unpleasant stimulus. For example, by pairing an aversive stimulus such as bitter taste, a foul odour or irritating noise with the behaviour (e.g. rock-eating, destructive chewing, compulsive licking), the behaviour may be eliminated. In humans, associating shock or a nauseant such as apomorphine with smoking, or a bitter compound with nail biting may successfully stop the undesirable habit. To be successful, the degree of noxiousness or discomfort must outweigh the motivation to perform the behaviour. Taste aversion (*see below*) is a specific form of aversion therapy.

Avoidance and Escape Conditioning

In avoidance conditioning the animal learns to avoid the aversive stimulus, while in escape conditioning the correct response terminates an aversive stimulus. To be effective, the stimulus must be of sufficient intensity to produce the desired response. Timing is the critical element. If the aversive stimulus is applied as soon as the behaviour begins, the pet can learn that escape terminates the stimulus. On the other hand, if the aversive stimulus is immediately preceded by a brief neutral stimulus (e.g. a buzzer), the animal may learn to avoid the neutral stimulus. When a warning stimulus is followed by the aversive event (e.g. shock) and the shock is not presented if the pet responds (e.g. withdraws) this is also known as signalled avoidance. Avoidance learning depends on both classical conditioning of fear (aversive stimulus plus warning stimulus) and negative reinforcement (since the stimulus is terminated by the avoidance response).

Motion detector alarms and noxious tastes and odours can be used to teach animals to escape from particular objects or areas. A dog that jumps off a couch to avoid a shock mat is escaping from the aversive stimulus itself. However, if an unpleasant event (noxious taste, shock, alarm) is paired with a warning stimulus (tag odour, visual cue, audible cue), the pet can learn to avoid objects. For example, by pairing a neutral tone with the shock of electronic fencing or by placing a white pillow case in any area where a shock mat or motion detector is employed, the pet can learn to avoid exposure to the noxious stimulus itself. Similarly, by applying a tag odour such as vinegar or a pet repellent to a more aversive event (cap device, stack of cans, water trap, upside down mouse trap), the pet can quickly be taught to avoid the tag odour itself. It is interesting to note that although early in avoidance training the warning sound or odour may indeed provoke fear, fear diminishes as the avoidance response is learned. Ultimately the pet learns to avoid the stimulus without fear, and the avoidance behaviour is maintained in the absence of the unpleasant stimulus. The dog that retreats at the sight of children may have learned to avoid children from a previous episode of having its ears pulled.

Avoidance conditioning is most likely to be successful when the desired response to the fear evoking stimulus is compatible with the animal's expected defensive or survival reaction (fight, flight or freeze). The response of a dog or cat, for example, is likely to differ from the reaction of a pigeon or a hedgehog. These instinctive responses, which are often referred to as species-specific defensive reactions (SSDRs), are related to the species, the stimulus and the environment. Behaviours that are compatible with the animal's innate defensive reactions are learned most quickly. In practice, most of our applications for avoidance involve training the pet to avoid or retreat from an object (couch, garbage can) or an area of the home (window sill, dining room). However, for some pets in some situations freezing or attacking the fearful stimulus may be a more likely response.

Bridging Stimulus

By pairing a food reward with a cue such as a clicker, whistle or hand clap (see conditioned stimuli below), the cue alone can ultimately be used to bring about a similar motivational state. Next the pet can be taught to expect a delay between the cue and the reward, and this interval can be gradually lengthened. The conditioned cue can then be used as an immediate and powerful reinforcer for training purposes. When the pet performs the appropriate response, the trainer rewards the pet immediately with the 'cue' and the pet approaches the trainer for the food reward. The cue therefore serves as a bridging stimulus – providing the pet with an immediate acknowledgment that an appropriate behaviour has been performed and that a reward will be forthcoming.

Classical Conditioning

This type of learning begins with an unconditioned stimulus (US) that elicits a reflex behaviour called an unconditioned response (UR). A neutral stimulus (NS) that has no influence on the reflex is repeatedly paired with the US until it becomes a conditioned stimulus (CS) that is able to elicit the behaviours by itself. The response to a CS is referred to as a conditioned response (CR).

This type of conditioning is often referred to as Pavlovian conditioning, after the scientist who conditioned dogs to salivate when they heard a bell. Salivation is a reflex response (UR) to the stimulus of food (US). The researcher conditioned the dogs by repeatedly ringing the bell (NS) when the dogs were fed. In time, they began to salivate whenever they heard the bell even when no food was present. At that point, the sound of the bell became a CS which triggered salivation (CR). The experiment is duplicated daily in many households whenever a pet hears the sound of a can opener.

An example of the use of classical conditioning is the formation of a new set of conditioned stimuli (*see below*) by associating neutral stimuli with food. By repeatedly giving food to a dog paired with a specific cue such as a clicker or tone, the cue will eventually become a conditioned stimulus. Similarly by pairing an aversive stimulus with a neutral cue, the neutral cue alone will soon lead to the fear response. This can be of practical and humane importance, since the use of more noxious stimuli such as shock mats or electronic fencing can be greatly reduced by pairing a visual or audible cue with the more unpleasant or uncomfortable stimulus, until the pet learns to avoid the cue alone.

Conditioned Stimuli (Incentive Motivation)

As a result of classical conditioning, specific cues can be used to produce a motivational state (Fig. 3.8). Most animals learn to associate specific cues with highly motivating events such as food or affection. For example, most owners have noted that the pet perks up when it hears the can opener or when a cupboard (where the treats have been kept) is opened. This same process can be used to pair a neutral cue, such as a tone, word, whistle, visual signal or hand-clap with food.

The result is that eventually the cue alone will be able to elicit a motivational response from the pet.

PROPER USE OF CONDITIONED STIMULI

1. The owner selects a cue (whistle, hand-clap, tone) that can be used consistently. Visual cues (e.g. outstretched hand) are also suitable

2. The owner pairs the cue to favoured food rewards, so that each time the reward is given the cue is applied (immediately prior to the food)

3. Within a few sessions, the pet will have paired the cue with the food reward, so that the cue now becomes a conditioned stimulus for response. The cue itself would produce a motivational state which can be used to gain the pet's attention or attract the pet

4. During training, caution must be used since rewards must not be given during the inappropriate behaviour. Therefore the conditioned stimulus should only be used for reinforcement, when the appropriate behaviour is being performed

5. Another use for the conditioned stimulus would be as a bridging stimulus during training (operant or instrumental conditioning)

6. The cue must continue to be paired intermittently with food to prevent extinction and maintain its value as either a conditioned stimulus or as a reinforcer

FIG. 3.8 Steps to the proper use of conditioned stimuli.

This stimulus can be of great practical value in training and counterconditioning applications, since it can serve as an audible (or visual) and immediate means of positive reinforcement. Provided the pet can be interrupted or distracted during exposure training (e.g. for barking, fear aggression), the pet can be immediately rewarded with the conditioned stimulus. If the pet then responds to an appropriate command (e.g. 'sit', 'come'), additional reinforcement (such as food, a toy, affection) could also be given.

Controlled Exposure

When flooding (*see below*) is utilised in behavioural therapy, exposure to the full stimulus may be so traumatic to the pet that effective control and distraction techniques may be impractical and habituation therefore does not occur. A more practical technique is to reduce the stimulus so that fear is minimised to a point where the pet can be controlled safely and effectively. Once habituation to the stimulus occurs, the pet can then be exposed to progressively more intense stimuli at subsequent training sessions. Controlled exposure techniques differ from systematic desensitisation in that the pet is exposed to low or controlled levels of the fear-evoking stimuli rather than levels of stimuli that approach but are below the threshold that would evoke fear (*see systematic desensitisation below*). Inhibitors such as distraction devices (shake can, ultrasonic alarm), control devices (such as head halters or cages) and counterconditioning techniques may all be useful in combination with exposure techniques to ensure that the pet habituates to the stimulus before it is withdrawn or increased.

Counterconditioning

This technique involves conditioning an animal to give a response to a stimulus that is incompatible with the undesirable response. For example, an effective solution for the dog that jumps up on people is to teach it to sit when it greets people. In this way, the learned behaviour interferes competitively with the undesirable behaviour. Similarly, sitting for a food reward is a behaviour that would be incompatible with submissive urination.

Counterconditioning is often used to modify the behaviour of fearful pets. The goal is to replace a fearful response to a specific stimulus with a non-fearful response. This can be done by repeatedly associating a muted presentation of the stimulus with something the animal wants, such as food or play, until the stimulus elicits happy feelings associated with anticipation of food or play instead of fear.

Countercommanding

This is another term sometimes used to describe the situation when a pet is requested to respond to a particular command that is incompatible with the undesirable behaviour.

Drug Desensitisation

When the stimulus cannot be effectively controlled or muted, drugs may be effective for reducing the pet's anxiety, fear or aggressiveness, so that a desensitisation programme can be implemented. (*See Chapter 4 for details.*)

External Inhibition

This occurs when a novel stimulus is presented immediately following the conditioned stimulus so that it subdues the conditioned response. External inhibition can be helpful when counterconditioning an undesirable response of a pet to a certain stimulus. For example, if the goal is to countercondition the pet to be quiet instead of barking (conditioned response) at the doorbell (conditioned stimulus), a high-pitched whistle or shake can can be sounded as soon as the bell rings, but before the barking begins. The barking response will be inhibited as the pet orients to the noise.

Extinction

The withholding of reinforcers leads to the elimination of a behaviour. For example, an owner may inadvertently reward a nuisance behaviour (e.g. whining or begging at the table) by giving the pet a piece of food. If the reward for the soliciting behaviour is taken away (food is no longer given), the behaviour will cease.

The use of extinction may not be sufficient on its own to correct many behaviour problems but it is an important part of the approach. Behaviours that have been rewarded intermittently are much more resistant to extinction. Once extinct, it takes very little

encouragement for the apparently defunct behaviour to resurface.

Extinction Burst

When reinforcement is first removed, the animal may persist and try even harder to achieve the reward before the behaviour is extinguished. Owners must be aware that this increase in behaviour, known as an extinction burst, must also be ignored, or the new and more intense behaviour will be reinforced.

Flooding (Response Prevention)

Flooding involves the continuous exposure of the subject to a stimulus at a level that evokes a response, until the response to the stimulus ceases. Pets that have learned an avoidance response to a fear-evoking stimulus can be retrained to overcome conditioned fears by exposing them to the stimulus so that they cannot escape. To be effective, the animal must be continuously exposed to the stimulus until the fear subsides and the stimulus itself must no longer be associated with fear. If the pet is unable to perform the avoidance response, and the previously fearful stimulus is no longer threatening, the fear response will undergo extinction. If the stimulus is removed before signs of fear abate or if the owner provides patting or attention (in the belief that it might help calm the dog down), fearful behaviour may be reinforced rather than diminished. Similarly, if the pet retreats before the fear abates, the threat will have been removed by the avoidance behaviour (negative reinforcement). Flooding can potentiate problems if used improperly and is most practical for the treatment of mild fears, since full exposure of a pet to a very strong fear-eliciting stimulus may severely traumatise it. Controlled flooding (controlled exposure) techniques, where the pet is exposed to mild, and then to progressively more intense stimuli, may be more useful for overcoming intense fears.

Habituation

Habituation is the process by which animals learn to adapt to novel sounds and experiences, provided they suffer no consequences from such exposure. During habituation, the subject is repeatedly exposed to the stimulus without the presence of negative or positive reinforcers until the response ceases. The animal that is initially anxious during car rides usually settles down after it takes several car rides and realises nothing aversive is going to happen. During the primary socialisation process, it is important to expose young dogs and cats to as many different environments and experiences as possible (e.g. cars, veterinary clinics, stairs) so that they do not become fearful of these situations. Training and behaviour modification must also be performed correctly so that pets don't habituate to certain forms of punishment. When an insufficiently aversive level of punishment is used repeatedly, the pet may learn to ignore the punishment.

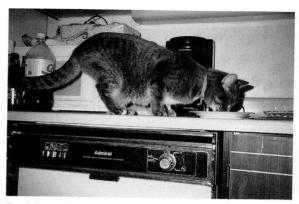

Fig. 3.9 Food left on worktops is a powerful motivator for cats to climb on to those surfaces.

Latent Learning

This type of learning occurs without the presence of purposeful reinforcement and is usually not readily obvious. Latent learning will facilitate the relatively rapid acquirement of accurate performance of a behaviour at a later time when reinforcement is introduced. Rats that are allowed to investigate a maze, but receive no reinforcement, are quicker to learn to run the maze for a food reward than are rats that have had no previous experience with the maze. A dog that is being taught to find an object on command will learn more quickly in an environment that it has previously had the opportunity to explore than in an unfamiliar environment.

Motivation

Motivation is an animal's drive or desire to perform a behaviour. The pet's level of motivation is a key consideration in training and in trying to reduce behaviours through behavioural modification. Motivation is dependent on the degree of deprivation, as well as the attractiveness of the reward. Deprivation of food, for example, leads to the increased drive to attain food. One might say that deprivation of a needed resource leads to arousal, and that the pet is then motivated to perform behaviours to achieve de-arousal or homoeostasis.

When selecting rewards for training and counter-conditioning programmes, the strongest possible motivator (*see reinforcer assessment*) should be used to overcome the pet's desire to perform an alternative behaviour, and to ensure that the pet performs the desired behaviour.

Another practical aspect of behavioural therapy is that the pet's motivation to perform an undesirable behaviour can be reduced to a level where the pet is less likely to perform the undesirable response. Desensitisation and controlled exposure techniques involve the manipulation of stimuli so that the pet's motivation to perform the undesirable behaviour (fear, barking, aggression) is reduced. Then, through the use of counterconditioning techniques and the proper selection of rewards, the pet can be motivated to perform an alternative competing behaviour.

When the pet is highly motivated to perform an undesirable behaviour (Fig. 3.9), stringent control mechanisms and a deterrent of high intensity will likely be required. However, for behaviours that have low levels of motivation (or when the motivation can be reduced by modifying the stimulus or reducing the pet's desire for the stimulus), less intense deterrents and a lower level of control might suffice.

Observational Learning

Observational learning refers to learning that is done passively by watching others. Studies in monkeys, dogs, cats and rats have shown that tasks can be learned more quickly after watching others perform that same task.

Operant Conditioning (Instrumental Conditioning)

This is the type of learning that occurs when the results of a behaviour influence the probability of that behaviour recurring. Giving praise or food for the desired response to an obedience command is a common use of operant conditioning. Although training programmes are designed to provide the pet with reinforcers for appropriate behaviour (and punishment for inappropriate behaviour), a great deal of operant learning occurs independent of owner interactions. Pets that knock over a bin/trash barrel and obtain food or chew on a table leg in the owner's absence will increase the likelihood of these behaviours recurring since they are rewarding to the pet at the time. However, when eliminating on the carpet or raiding the rubbish can results in a severe scolding, the probability of the pet eliminating in front of the owner in the future diminishes.

Overlearning

This involves the continued reinforcement of a behaviour that has already been learned. The consequence of overlearning is an increased resistance to extinction and longer retention of learning once all reinforcement stops. Also, responses are more dependable and consistent in the presence of stressful or distracting stimuli.

Punishment

Punishment involves the application of an aversive stimulus during or immediately (within 1–3 seconds) following a behaviour to decrease the likelihood that that behaviour will be repeated. To be effective, the stimulus must be intense enough to be considered aversive without hurting the animal or causing it to be fearful. Timing and consistency are critical (Fig. 3.10). If punishment is not immediate (and successful) for the behaviour involved, it should not be used at all.

Punishment can be a useful tool in behavioural modification but its inappropriate use can exacerbate the situation and cause other behaviour problems. It is important that the form of punishment be tailored to each pet. If the punishment is too weak, it can lead to habituation as well as not remedying the problem. If too harsh, the punishment can cause additional behavioural problems. Physical punishment should **always** be avoided since it can lead to fear of the owner, handshyness and fear-biting, and could be potentially harmful to the pet.

By initially pairing a highly aversive stimulus (e.g. shake can or horn) with a less aversive 'secondary punishment' (a stern 'No!'), it may be possible to use the command alone for future punishment. The need for repeated, harsh punishment can also be minimised by pairing a neutral stimulus with a sufficiently aversive punishment. For example, a novel odour (e.g. perfume) can be applied to a possession that the dog likes to chew. The next time the dog attempts to chew the possession, he will smell the odour. As he does that, the owner should provide an aversive stimulus (e.g. loud noise, squirt from a watergun, booby trap of cans set to topple). The idea is that the dog will make the connection between the odour and the punishment so that the odour can be used as a deterrent, with no need for actual punishment. Commonly used forms of punishment include direct owner-initiated techniques (e.g. noise, verbal), remote owner-initiated techniques (e.g. sprays of water) and environmental or booby trap techniques (e.g. bitter tastes, bitter smells, motion alarms).

Punisher assessment

Punisher assessment involves predicting which form of punishment will be most practical and

PUNISHMENT FAILURES	
Why Punishment Fails	**Example**
The pet does not understand why it was punished	Punishment is applied too late or inconsistently
The pet is only taught to avoid an area instead of learning to avoid the performance of a behaviour	The pet is punished in some locations where undesirable behaviour occurs but not in others
An alternative, acceptable behaviour was not taught	When the motivation to perform an undesirable behaviour is strong, the pet will continue to perform the behaviour until it is taught the acceptable behaviour
Desirable behaviours inadvertently decrease or undesirable behaviours increase	The pet that is harshly punished for eliminating in the owner's presence indoors may stop eliminating when the owner is present outdoors Punishment may cause fear and avoidance of the owner Punishment may increase fear of the stimulus
The behaviour continues in the owner's absence	The owner punishes an action when supervisory but the behaviour continues without consequence in the owner's absence

FIG. 3.10 Causes of failure when using punishment techniques.

successful for an individual pet. The ultimate success or failure of punishment techniques depends on the individual pet's sensitivity to the punishment, as well as the behaviour for which it is being punished. One might anticipate that any aversive stimulus would be sufficient punishment but this is not true. Many dogs continue to hunt porcupines and skunks even after they have experienced the ill effects of such a meeting.

Punishment techniques

Direct interactive punishment. Direct interactive punishment should only be considered when the pet performs an undesirable act in the presence of the owner. An immediate, startling reprimand or loud noise is often effective and all that is necessary for young or sensitive pets. When the owner is not present to supervise, misbehaviour must be prevented or alternative forms of punishment may need to be considered (e.g. booby traps).

At the first sign that the pet will perform an undesirable behaviour, the owner can try to avert it by redirecting the pet using a command with which it is familiar (such as 'sit', 'come'). Another alternative would be to utilise a form of handling that will successfully interrupt the undesirable behaviour and teach the pet an appropriate response (lifting the puppy, grasping the nape of the neck). Handling should only be utilised if it results in an immediate cessation of the behaviour, without causing undue fear or anxiety, and **should never be used if there is any possibility that the pet may be a danger to the owner or if the sensitivity of the pet suggests that handling may cause fear**. Should a verbal command or a physical exercise be unsuccessful, it must be discontinued immediately. Quicker and more effective control can often be achieved by leaving a long leash attached, and through the use of head halters.

Direct punishment devices are often more practical and effective because they can be more aversive or startling than verbal reprimands, and are less likely to cause fear of the owner. Most emit noises that the pet finds unsettling. Some are audible to people, but many of the new gadgets are in the audible range of pets alone. Punishment is used until the problem behaviour ceases. Then the punishment must be immediately withdrawn. Using a verbal command (such as 'No!' or 'Quit!') at the same time as the primary punishment often results in the command

alone being sufficient punishment in the future (secondary punishment).

Examples of direct punishment devices are: commercial electronic devices that generate an aversive ultrasonic tone that is readily detectable by most dogs and cats but virtually inaudible to humans; commercial electronic devices that generate an aversive tone that is audible to pets and humans; (e.g. rape and pocket alarms; foghorns) bean bag or can (containing pebbles) tossed near the pet; cap gun; shake can containing small pebbles or coins; water gun; and water hose.

Time-out. When the pet first starts to misbehave (e.g. barking), it is given a command (e.g. quiet) and given the opportunity to respond appropriately. If it does, it should be rewarded and praised immediately. If unsuccessful (e.g. the barking continues), the pet is relocated to a confinement area for a period of about 3 minutes. It is only released when it is quiet. To be effective, the isolation room should not be the feeding, sleeping or play area of the pet. A laundry room, basement or bathroom is a good choice. The goal of time-out is for the pet to learn that proper behaviour leads to rewards and misbehaviour leads to temporary isolation and no rewards.

Remote interactive punishment. Remote-control punishment, also known as hidden punishment, is used for misbehaviours that may occur when the owner is not present to supervise. Provided that the pet is properly monitored and effectively punished on each occasion, until it ceases to perform the undesirable behaviour, the pet does not learn that the behaviour can be performed safely in the owner's absence. Peeking around corners, using mirrors, video cameras, or following the situation with an intercom, child monitor or pet monitor (an electronic device that emits a signal when disturbed) will be necessary to ensure that the pet is observed at the instant inappropriate behaviour begins. If punishment can then be meted out while the owner remains out of sight, the pet should associate the punishment with its behaviour rather than with the owner (Fig. 3.11).

Owners can rig up noisemakers, buckets of water, hoses and sprinklers which they can control from out of sight, providing appropriately timed punishment. There are also a number of gadgets which can be activated by remote control to provide aversive stimuli. For example, remote-control switches can be plugged into an outlet and connected to a variety of

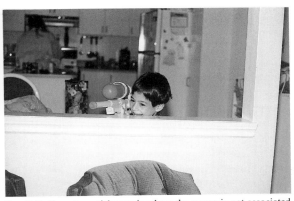

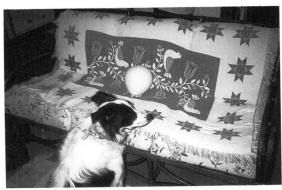

FIG. 3.11 Remote punishment is where the owner is not associated with punishing the behaviour. It is important that the person is not seen.

FIG. 3.12 A balloon can be rigged to pop when the dog attempts to get on to the couch. *Photo courtesy of Dennis Bastian.*

devices including vacuum cleaners, water piks (spray small quantities of water), strobe lights, sirens, alarm clocks, tape recordings of owner saying 'No!' and hair dryers. As soon as the behaviour stops, so should the punishment. Remote-control shock collars work on the same principle. Using a long lead attached to a halter device is another effective way to interrupt or punish undesirable behaviour remotely.

The primary advantage of true remote punishment with the punisher remaining out of sight is that the person is not directly associated with the act of punishment and the risk of the pet becoming fearful of that person is eliminated. This is especially important with cats. Cats are much less likely to tolerate interactive punishment, such as a stern scolding, than are dogs. A cat that is directly punished repeatedly by the owner quickly learns to avoid the person providing the punishment and the relationship deteriorates.

Environmental punishment. Similar to remote-control punishment, environmental punishment works when the owner is not directly in the pet's presence. In contrast, however, environmental punishment does not rely on the owner monitoring the situation. The environment is rigged to provide its own punishment when the pet misbehaves. Booby traps, or home security and child safety alarms can be set to go off when they are 'triggered by misbehaviour'. This can be as simple as perching a bucket of water over a doorway, taping balloons to a couch (Fig. 3.12) or setting a mousetrap rigged to a noisemaker inside a rubbish container. New technology has provided us with other intriguing devices such as mats that provide a very mild electric stimulus, door and window alarms,

receivers that are attached to a punishment device and are triggered when the misbehaviour occurs, and even electronic fencing. The indoor devices are most practical for keeping pets away from furniture, plants, rubbish cans, nappy buckets and the like. Electrically charged mats (which produce a mildly aversive but harmless electrical stimulus) effectively keep cats and small dogs away from areas and are helpful when trying to keep pets off furniture and counters, or out of certain rooms. Motion detectors have been designed for keeping the family pet away from areas indoors (emit an electronic alarm when the pet passes nearby) or for keeping other pets and stray animals away from the property (emit a loud alarm and flashing lights when the animal passes nearby). There are several different devices (collars that emit an aversive sound, citrus spray or shock) that effectively punish dogs with noise each time they bark. Another new device has been designed for owners that are trying to keep one cat out of another cat's bowl. Any cat wearing the special magnetic collar will set off a loud alarm if it tries to eat out of the bowl.

Not all environmental punishments need to be 'new age'. Several 'old time' remedies continue to be effective to keep pets away from certain areas, such as using aversive tastes and smells, two-sided sticky tape, an upside-down plastic carpet runner, or aluminium foil.

Reinforcement – Negative

Negative reinforcement refers to the conditioning of a behaviour through the withdrawal of a stimulus, generally one that is aversive. In practical terms, the pet learns to cease a behaviour or avoid a situation that it finds unpleasant. For example, when a dog has had its tail pulled by young children, it might learn to retreat to its crate for a rest. When outside during a storm, a dog will learn that by seeking shelter under the porch the unpleasant stimulus will be removed (escape behaviour). When the aversive stimulus has been associated with specific cues, the pet may learn an avoidance response so that in time the cues themselves may initiate the avoidance response (avoidance conditioning). Although not recommended, squeezing a dog's or cat's lips until the mouth opens or using a remote-controlled shock collar and terminating the shock at the instant the dog displays the appropriate behaviour are examples of negative reinforcement that have been used in training applications.

Because punishment and negative reinforcement involve aversive stimuli, they are often confused. With punishment, the application of the stimulus during or immediately following the behaviour should lead to a decreased likelihood that the pet will repeat a behaviour. In negative reinforcement the withdrawal of the stimulus increases the chance of a behaviour recurring. Thus, punishment involves the aversive stimulus being applied during or immediately following the behaviour, while negative reinforcement consists of the aversive stimulus preceding the behaviour and being withdrawn when the behaviour occurs.

Reinforcement – Positive

Positive reinforcement involves the application of a positive stimulus immediately following a response that increases the likelihood of the response being repeated. Primary reinforcers are stimuli that satisfy a basic need. For dogs and cats these would include food, water, social interaction, and perhaps chew or play toys. An event or stimulus can become a secondary or conditioned reinforcer if it is paired with other events or stimuli that are already reinforcing. For example, praise (good dog), or events (going for a walk) can become reinforcers if they are paired with primary reinforcers such as a favoured food treat or social play. For rewards to be effective they must be contingent on the behaviour (given only when the desired response is performed). If the reinforcement is also provided non-contingently, the behaviour will be unlikely (or much slower) to change. Timing of reinforcement is also critical. Reinforcement that

occurs immediately after the response promotes the most effective and fastest learning. Therefore when a new response is being developed, immediate reinforcement is essential. Once the response is performed consistently, delayed reinforcement is acceptable. However, if any other response occurs in the intervening period between the desired response and the reward, it will be the intervening response that is rewarded. For example, after elimination in an appropriate outdoor location, the owner that gives a reward as soon as the pet comes back indoors, will be rewarding the pet for coming indoors.

Rather than use punishment techniques to decrease the performance of those behaviours that the owner considers undesirable, it is much more practical and humane to provide pets with desirable outlets for chewing, play, feeding, elimination (etc.), and rewarding the desired response. In this way, little if any, punishment or discipline should ever be required.

Unfortunately, the inappropriate use of reinforcement can also be the cause of many undesirable behaviours. Owners that give any type of attention to nuisance behaviours such as barking, play biting, jumping up or begging, only serve to reinforce these problems. Since the pet's actions are successful at achieving their goal they are constantly being reinforced. Owners who then try to discourage these actions, and only rarely allow them to be performed, provide a variable and intermittent reinforcement schedule, making the undesirable behaviour far more resistant to extinction. The owner that tries to comfort the fearful or aggressive pet by patting, saying 'calm down', or having a heart-to-heart talk with the pet is actually rewarding the fearful or aggressive response. Owners must also be cautioned that mild punishment (stop, get down, light hitting) are unlikely to dissuade the pet, and may inadvertently be rewarding the problem by providing verbal and physical attention. For example, the owner who attempts to dissuade play biting or scratching with a light swat, will usually be unsuccessful and the interactive contact may actually encourage further play. If the physical reprimand is then increased in intensity, the pet could either learn to enjoy rougher and rougher handling, or may desist but become fearful and hand-shy of the owners.

Reinforcement Schedules

Reinforcement delivered after every response is referred to as continuous reinforcement while reinforcement delivered after only some of the responses is referred to as intermittent reinforcement. During initial training a behaviour will be learned most quickly with continuous reinforcement while intermittent and variable reinforcement operates a response that is stronger and more resistant to extinction.

Intermittent reinforcement can be scheduled as either fixed or variable. Either the ratio can be fixed (a response is reinforced after a fixed number of repetitions) or the interval can be fixed (the first response after a fixed interval of time is rewarded). Similarly, the ratio can be variable (a response is rewarded after a variable number of repetitions) or the interval can be variable (the first response after a variable length of time is rewarded).

Performance and responding is higher with variable ratio and intervals compared to fixed ratio and intervals and the learned behaviours are more resistant to extinction. Unfortunately many undesirable behaviours (e.g. begging, jumping up, vocalisation) are rewarded variably and intermittently so that they are highly resistant to extinction.

Reinforcer Assessment

The more valuable the reward, the faster the learning. Since an individual pet's response to any specific reinforcer may vary, it is essential that pet owners determine which rewards (play, toys, food or affection) are most likely to motivate their pet. The effectiveness of the reinforcer can be enhanced by withholding it at all times other than during training. Reinforcers should be used sparingly during training so that shaping can be used for more difficult and complex learned behaviours.

Shaping (Successive Approximation)

Shaping refers to the process whereby pets can be trained to perform increasingly complex tasks by building on their existing knowledge. This is accomplished by gradually withdrawing rewards for general behaviours and progressively rewarding only the behaviours that more closely approximate the desired behaviour. For example, shaping can be used to encourage a dog to bark when someone is at the front door. The initial process involves simply rewarding the dog for barking. Then, rewards are only given when the barking occurs near the front door, and nowhere else. Finally, the barking is only rewarded when someone is actually at the front door.

Systematic Desensitisation

Systematic desensitisation refers to exposing pets repeatedly to stimuli that cause fear, anxiety or aggression in sufficiently small doses so as not to cause the response. The stimuli are then gradually increased at increments that do not lead to a recurrence of the response. The stimuli are repeated so many times with no effect that they become inconsequential.

Systematic desensitisation is often used in conjunction with counterconditioning to facilitate training. For example, a pet may be fearful of thunder but not fearful when a tape recording of thunder is played at low volumes. If the pet listens to the recording and shows no signs of anxiety, it is given a food treat. By gradually increasing the volume over a period of time, the pet can be desensitised systematically to the fear-evoking stimulus and counterconditioned to be in a happy, food-anticipatory state when it hears the sound of thunder. The key is to expose the pet to a level of the stimulus that is below its threshold for anxiety, and then very gradually increase the intensity until it mimics real-life circumstances.

Taste Aversion

Taste aversion is a specific form of aversive conditioning, in which the animal develops an aversion to a particular odour or taste that is associated with illness, following a single taste–illness pairing. Taste aversion is likely to be an innate defence mechanism, so that the animal learns to avoid potentially toxic substances. Taste aversion differs from other forms of aversion therapy or avoidance conditioning in that it generally takes a single event, and the illness may take place a considerable time following the ingestion of the substance. In avoidance conditioning, immediate timing of the aversive stimulus with the unconditioned stimulus, and numerous repetitions may be required before the aversion is conditioned.

Application of Behavioural Modification Techniques

Positive reinforcement, systematic desensitisation, counterconditioning and successive approximation are often used in combination to correct behaviour problems such as fear aggression and phobias. Using food or a toy as a motivator, the pet is first taught to perform a behaviour, such as sit–stay, consistently. (Secondary reinforcers or cues, such as a clicker or tone, may prove particularly helpful for motivating the pet during future training sessions.) Next, the pet is trained to perform the behaviour while exposed to a mild form of the threatening stimulus. Provided the stimulus is beneath the threshold at which the undesirable behaviour is induced, the cues and rewards should motivate the pet sufficiently to perform the desired behaviour and reduce anxious responses to the stimulus. The pet is then gradually exposed to increasing levels of stimuli and rewards are given for successively closer stages to the goal.

Controlled flooding (or exposure) techniques can also be used in conjunction with counterconditioning and positive reinforcement. If the stimuli are very mild, are well controlled and the pet can neither escape nor cause harm or injury, it can quickly be taught that threats will not successfully remove the stimulus and that the stimulus will not harm the pet. A halter and leash or an open mesh cage can work extremely well to control the dog so that it can neither attack nor escape. At each subsequent training session, the pet is exposed to slightly stronger levels of the stimulus.

Controlled flooding techniques and desensitisation are similar in that low levels of the fearful or threatening stimuli are presented at first and gradually increased with each subsequent training session. However, for systematic desensitisation, the pet is exposed to an extremely gradual increase in stimuli with each training session, beginning below the threshold that would stimulate the undesired response. With controlled flooding techniques, the pet is exposed to the stimulus at a level that induces a mild stimulation of the undesired response (but not the full level of the stimulus) until it habituates to the stimulus. The pet must be well controlled so that it can neither escape nor attack, and the stimulus is not removed until the pet responds appropriately. Exposure techniques can be facilitated with counterconditioning, distraction techniques, and the appropriate use of positive and negative reinforcement.

Behaviour Products

Preventive and Training Products

A number of behaviour products have been designed to serve our pet's requirements for play,

chewing and scratching. By discussing and recommending products in practice, we can help the pet owner ensure that proper items are available in the pet's home environment. A demonstration of behaviour products can also be an important and practical way to introduce behavioural concepts and techniques to pet owners. Proper chew and play toys are essential to provide the pet with a sufficiently stimulating environment and reduce the possibility of destructive chewing and furniture scratching. Stain removers and odour eliminators are needed by many dog owners during the early stages of housetraining. Guidance should also be given in the selection of leashes, halters, cat litter and anti-chew sprays.

Products for Correcting Undesirable Behaviour

As problems begin to emerge, there are a number of products that can aid the owner in getting the pet quickly back 'on track'. Some have been designed to ensure better control and faster training, while others have been specifically designed to deter inappropriate behaviour.

There are a variety of products that can be used to deter undesirable behaviour. These products are preferable to physical punishment since they are less likely to lead to fear of the owner. Owners will need to select a product that is practical for the problem at hand, and that is sufficiently aversive to deter the behaviour without causing undue pain or discomfort. For direct punishment or distraction there are ultrasonic and audible devices, water rifles and pocket rape alarms. Since it is imperative that pet owners use these devices **during** the misbehaviour, a pet monitor is another practical training aid. A pet monitor is a device that alerts the owner by producing a signal when a pet is in a particular area. The use of a remote-control device would provide the added advantage of deterring undesirable behaviour remotely so that the pet does not associate the punishment with the owner. Booby traps are often the most practical form of punishment since they train the pet to avoid the site of misbehaviour even in the owner's absence, provided the deterrent is sufficiently aversive to interrupt the behaviour. Although devices that utilise electric shock or discomfort are excessive for most problems, alarms and monitors may not always be sufficiently aversive. Choosing the appropriate device should be based on the application, the pet's level of motivation to

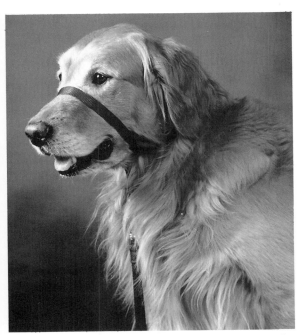

FIG. 3.13 Head halters are an excellent way to maintain effective control. This example is the 'Promise' or 'Gentle Leader' system. Photo courtesy of Dr R.K. Anderson.

By leaving a long leash attached the owner can manage most undesirable behaviours (e.g. jumping up, housesoiling, digging) as far as the leash will allow. Some halters have been designed so that they can be adjusted and left on the dog, while others can only be used when the dog is on a leash. If the owner does not need the control afforded by the head halter but does have a problem with pulling, antipull body harnesses are very effective.

Further Reading on Behaviour Counselling

Beaver, B. V. (1994) *The Veterinarian's Encyclopedia of Animal Behavior*. Iowa State University Press: Ames, IA.

Breazile, J. E. (1987) Physiologic basis and consequences of distress in animals. *Journal of the American Veterinary Medical Association*, **191**(10), 1212–1215.

Chapman, B. (1993) Geriatric behaviour. In: *Animal Behaviour. The T.G. Hungerford Refresher Course for Veterinarians, July 1993*, pp. 133–143. Postgraduate Committee in Veterinary Science, University of Sydney: Sydney, Australia.

Chapman, B. L and Voith, V. L. (1990) Behavioural problems in old dogs: 26 cases (1984–1987). *Journal of the American Veterinary Medical Association*, **196**(6), 944–946.

Chrisman, C. L. (1989) Neurological disorders producing abnormal behavior. In: *Proceedings of the 56th Annual AAHA Meeting*: Denver, CO.

Chrisman, C. L. (1994) Seizures and behavioral abnormalities in dogs and cats with neurological dysfunction. *Veterinary Quarterly*, **16**(Suppl. 1), S28–S29.

Dannerman, P. J. and Chodrow, R. E. (1982) History taking and interviewing techniques. *Veterinary Clinics of North America, Small Animal Practices* **12**(4), 587–592.

Dehasse, J. (1994) Pathological anticipatory defense behavior in dogs. *Veterinary Quarterly*, **16**(Suppl. 1), S49.

Hart, B. L. (1985) Animal behavior and the fever response: theoretical considerations. *Journal of the American Veterinary Medical Association*, **187**(10), 998–1001.

Hart, B. L. (1991) Effects of neutering and spaying on the behavior of dogs and cats: questions and answers about practical concerns. *Journal of the American Veterinary Medical Association*, **198**(7), 1204.

Hart, B. L. and Barrett, R. E. (1973) Effects of castration on fighting, roaming, and urine spraying in adult male cats. *Journal of the American Veterinary Medical Association*, **163**, 290–292.

Heath, S. (1994) Commonly encountered feline behavior problems. *Veterinary Quarterly*, **16**(Suppl. 1), S51.

perform the behaviour, the pet's sensitivity to the product, owner acceptance, cost and the seriousness of the problem.

For barking that cannot be controlled or prevented during the owner's absence, it may be necessary to consider a bark-activated device. If the dog barks in a specific area a door- or cage-mounted device might be successful, but if the dog is not confined an antibark collar would need to be used. Whether antibarking devices are used or not, control of problem barking will be most successful when the stimuli and motivation for barking are elucidated and controlled.

One of the most effective means of controlling unruly, disobedient and 'headstrong' dogs are halter systems (Fig. 3.13). With a halter, the owner gains control naturally through pressure exerted behind the neck and around the muzzle. Since the head halter is attached around the muzzle, it does not choke, and can be used effectively to control barking, chewing, coprophagia and even some forms of aggression. Control is gained through negative reinforcement and rewards, and not through punishment, fear or anxiety. As soon as the misbehaviour ceases the owner merely releases the leash and rewards the dog for calmness.

Hewson, C. J. and Luescher, U. A. (1996) Compulsive disorders in dogs. In: *Readings in Companion Animal Behavior*. Voith, V. L. and Barchelt, P. L. (eds) pp. 153–158. Veterinary Learning Systems: Trenton, NJ.

Hopkins, S. G., Schubert, T. and Hart, B. L. (1976) Castration of adult male dogs: effects on roaming, aggression, urine marking, and mounting. *Journal of the American Veterinary Medical Association*, **168**, 1108–1110.

Hornhfeldt, C. S. (1994) *Nepeta cataria* (catnip) 'poisoning' in cats. *Veterinary Practice Staff*, **6**(5), 1,7.

Hunthausen, W. (1994) Collecting the history of a pet with a behavior problem. *Veterinary Medicine*, **89**(10), 954–959.

Hunthausen, W. (1994) Identifying and treating behavior problems in geriatric dogs. *Veterinary Medicine*, **89**(9), 688–700.

Jaggy, A., Oliver, J. E., Ferguson, D. C. *et al.* (1994) Neurological manifestations of hypothyroidism – a retrospective study of 29 dogs. *Journal of Veterinary Internal Medicine*, **8**(5), 328–336.

Kohlke, H. U. and Kohlke, K. (1994) Animal behavior therapy – Characteristics and specific problems from the psychological point of view. *Kleintierpraxis*, **39**(3), 175–180.

Knol, B. W. (1994) Social problem behavior in dogs – Etiology and pathogenesis. *Veterinary Quarterly*, **16**(Suppl. 1), S50.

Krawiec, D. R. (1988) Urinary incontinence in dogs and cats. *Modern Veterinary Practice*, **69**(1), 17–23.

Landsberg, G. (1994) Products for preventing or controlling undesirable behavior. *Veterinary Medicine*, **89**(10), 970.

Lieberman, D. A. (1993) *Learning, Behavior and Cognition*, 2nd edition. Brooks/Cole Publishing Co.: Pacific Grove, CA: 134–143, 227–233, 315–357.

Luescher, U. A. (1993) Hyperkinesis in dogs: six case reports. *Canadian Veterinary Journal*, **34**, 368–370.

Mook, D. G. (1987) *Motivation. The Organization of Action*. W.W. Norton and Co: New York, 226–239.

Nolan, K. (1994) Flea collars may cause erratic behavior. *Irish Veterinary Journal*, **47**(5), 230.

O'Farrell, V. and Neville, P. (1994) *Manual of Feline Behaviour*. British Small Animal Veterinary Association: Cheltenham.

Overall, K. L. (1994) Management-related problems in feline behavior. *Feline Practice*, **22**(1), 13–15.

Overall, K. L. (1994) Stereotypic and ritualistic behaviors. *Proceedings of the North American Veterinary Conference*, 55–57.

Owren, T. and Matre, P. J. (1994) Somatic problems as a risk factor for behavior problems in dogs. *Veterinary Quarterly*, **16**(Suppl. 1), S50.

Polsky, R. H. (1993) Does thyroid dysfunction cause behavioral problems? *Canine Practice*, **18**(4), 8–11.

Polsky, R. H. (1994) The steps in solving behavior problems. *Veterinary Medicine*, **89**(6), 504–507.

Rapaport, J. L. (1989) *The Boy Who Couldn't Stop Washing*. E.P. Dutton: New York.

Reisner, I. (1991) The pathophysiologic basis of behavior problems. *Veterinary Clinics of North America, Small Animal Practice*, **21**, 207–224.

Reisner, I. R., Erb, H. N. and Houpt, K. A. (1994) Risk factors for behavior-related euthanasia among dominant-aggressive dogs: 110 cases (1989–1992). *Journal of the American Veterinary Medical Association*, **205**(6), 855–863.

Salmeri, K. R., Bloomberg, M. S., Scruggs, S. L. and Shille, V. (1991) Gonadectomy in immature dogs: Effects on skeletal, physical, and behavioral development. *Journal of the American Veterinary Medical Association*, **198**(7), 1193.

Seksel, K. (1993) Feline elimination problems. In: *Animal Behaviour. Proceedings of the T.J. Hungerford Refresher Course for Veterinarians, July 1993*, pp. 147–153. Postgraduate Committee in Veterinary Science, University of Sydney: Sydney, Australia.

Towell, T. L. and Shell, L. G. (1996) Endocrinopathies that affect the central nervous system of cats and dogs. In: *Readings in Companions Animal Behaviour* Voith, V. L. and Berchelt, P. L. (eds) 116–121. Veterinary Learning Systems: Trenton, NJ.

Voith, V. (1979) Multiple approaches to treating behaviour problems. *Modern Veterinary Practice*, **60**, 651–654.

Voith, V. L. (1996) Interview forms. In: *Readings in Companion Animal Behavior* Voith, V. L. and Borchelt, P. L. (eds) Vetinary Leaving Systems: Trenton, NJ.

Voith, V. L. and Borchelt, P. L. (1985) History taking and interviewing. *Compendium of Continuing Education for the Practicing Veterinarian*, **7**(5), 433.

Voith, V. L. and Borchelt, P. L. (1996) (Update by Debra F. Horwitz.) History-taking and interviewing. In: *Readings in Companion Animal Behavior* Voith, V. L. and Borchelt, P. L. (eds). Vetinary Leaving Systems: Trenton, NJ.

Further Reading – Behavioural Modification Techniques and Terms

Adler, L. and Adler, H. (1977) Ontogeny of observational learning in the dog (*Canis familiaris*). *Developmental Psychobiology*, **10**, 267–272.

Askew, H. R. (1993) Use of punishment in animal behavioral therapy. *Praktische Tierarzt*, **74**(10), 905–909.

Beaver, B. V. (1981) Modifying a cat's behavior. *Veterinary Medicine Small Animal Clinic*, **76**, 1281–1283.

Borchelt, P. L. and Voith, V. L. (1985) Punishment. *Compendium of Continuing Education for the Practicing Veterinarian*, **7**, 780–788.

Borchelt, P. L. and Voith, V. L. (1996) Punishment. In: *Readings in Companion Animal Behavior*. Voith, V. L. and Borchelt, P. L. pp. 72–80. Vetinary Learning Systems: Trenton, NJ.

Crowell-Davis, S. L. (1990) Negative reinforcement is not punishment – Help clients know the difference. *Veterinary Forum*, March, 18.

Gustavson, C. R. (1996) Taste aversion conditioning vs. conditioning using aversive peripheral stimuli. In: *Readings in Companion Animal Behavior*. Voith, V. L. and Borchelt, P. L. (eds) pp. 56–67. Veterinary Learning Systems: Trenton, NJ.

Hart, B. L. (1985) *The Behavior of Domestic Animals*. W. H. Freeman & Co.: New York.

Hart, B. and Hart, L. (1985) *Canine and Feline Behavioral Therapy*. Lea & Febiger: Philadelphia, PA.

Hengst, A. (1994) Animal behavior therapy. *Praktische Tierarzt*, **75**(12), 1138.

Houpt, K. (1991) *Domestic Animal Behavior*. Iowa State University Press: Ames, IA.

Keller, F. S. and Schoenfeld, W. (1968) *Principles of Psychology*. Appleton-Century-Crofts: New York.

Kirkpatrick, M. and Rosenthal, G. G. (1994) Animal behavior – Symmetry without fear. *Nature*, **372**(6502), 134–135.

Marder, A. and Reid, P. (1996) Treating canine behavior problems: Behavior modification, obedience and agil-ity training. In: *Readings in Companion Animal Behavior*. Voith, V. L. and Borchelt, P. L. pp. 62–71. Veterinary Learning Systems: Trenton, NJ.

Nobbe, D. E., Niebuhr, B. R., Levinson, M. and Tiller, J. E. (1978) Use of time-out as punishment for aggressive behaviour. *Canine Practice*, **5**, 12–18.

Overall, K. L. (1993) Treating canine aggression. *Canine Practice*, **18**(6), 24–28.

Owren, T. (1987) Training dogs based on behavioural methods. *Journal of Small Animal Practice*, **28**(11), 1009–1029.

Reid, P. and Marder, A. (1996) Learning. In: *Readings in Companion Animal Behavior*. Voith, V. L. and Borch-elt, P. L. (eds) pp. 62–71. Vetinary Learning Systems: Trenton, NJ.

Spreat, S. and Spreat, S. R. (1982) Learning principles. *Veterinary Clinics of North America*, **12**, 593–606.

Thorndike, E. L. (1911) *Animal Intelligence: Experimental studies*. Macmillan Co.: New York.

Thorpe, W. H. (1963) *Learning and Instinct in Animals*. Harvard University Press: Cambridge, MA.

Voith, V. L. (1979) Learning principles and behavioral problems. *Modern Veterinary Practice*, **60**, 553–555.

4

Drugs Used in Behavioural Therapy

Introduction

The timely and appropriate use of drugs may allow the pet owner an opportunity to resolve the pet's behaviour problem successfully, or modify its behaviour sufficiently to allow the pet to remain in the home. Failure to identify and suggest potentially helpful pharmacological agents may mean the difference between a safe and healthy pet–owner relationship, and the pet's demise.

Drug prescription must proceed in agreement with local regulations and licensing requirements. In the UK, for example, the drug of first choice should be one that is licensed for the species being treated, provided there is a suitable choice available. The second choice of drug to consider should be one which has been licensed in another animal species. The third choice should be one which has been licensed for use in man and the final choice, when the other three choices are not possible, would be a drug that is available (perhaps on trial or through another country), that is as yet an unlicensed drug.

Although some of the old favourites (relatively speaking), such as acepromazine and the progestins, are still in frequent use, newer drugs that are non-addictive, relatively free of potential organ toxicity and cause minimal sedation are now available. Many of these so-called 'smart drugs', exert their effects on the specific behaviours with little or no alteration of other behaviours. Most of these medications have been used widely in humans but have not been approved for use in animals.

Drug dosage information is provided in the *Appendix* at the end of this book.

There are three types of situation where drug therapy might be indicated. The most common use is as an adjunct to behaviour therapy. The treatment of separation anxiety, fears and phobias, and aggression are examples of where a drug may help to facilitate the initiation of behaviour therapy. Choosing an appropriate drug may provide an opportunity to resolve the problem in a quicker or safer manner by providing some initial control. However, without concurrent behavioural modification, the problem is likely to recur when the drug is removed. Pharmacological desensitisation of the pet is a technique that can be applied when the stimulus cannot be effectively controlled or reduced, or when there are multiple stimuli that lead to fear or aggression. The drug should be given at sufficient dosage so that the pet can be safely exposed to the stimulus and taught to perform the desired response (counterconditioning). In other words, the pet's response to the stimulus (rather than the stimulus itself) is modified. Whenever possible, drug-aided desensitisation should be combined with other behavioural modification techniques such as systematic desensitisation, controlled flooding and counterconditioning, so that behavioural techniques, rather than the drug itself, are the principal methods of altering behaviour.

A second indication for drug use is when a behaviour problem is unlikely to be corrected by behavioural modification techniques alone. This might be the case for problems such as urine marking, and compulsive disorders such as acral lick dermatitis (granuloma) or tail chasing. Not only might these behavioural problems require drugs to help control the condition, but it may never be possible to withdraw the drugs without recurrence of the condition.

A third indication for drug use is when a medical condition is the cause of a behaviour problem. For some behaviour problems with underlying medical conditions (e.g. cystitis, epilepsy, hepatic encephalopathy, hyperthyroidism, hypothyroidism), drugs may be a critical part of therapy.

Since most drugs used in canine and feline behaviour therapy are not licensed for use in pets, they should be used cautiously.

In the US, the owner should sign a release where appropriate, advising that the drug is considered

PRETREATMENT CONSIDERATIONS

1. Complete medical work-up
2. Accurate behavioural diagnosis
3. Institution of an appropriate behavioural programme
4. Individuality in response to psychoactive drugs
5. Side effects
6. Cost

FIG. 4.1 Considerations prior to drug treatment for behaviour problems.

investigational and that its use is 'extra-label' with respect to the manufacturer's recommendations. Owners should monitor their pets for a reduction in severity, frequency or intensity of the targeted behaviours. Adverse or unexpected effects should be reported immediately. Veterinary literature should be regularly reviewed for reports of adverse effects or changes in dosage recommendations. Although potential adverse reactions in humans cannot necessarily be extrapolated to animals, it is also advisable to consult the human literature and manufacturers data, to determine areas of potential concern. Blood and urine tests should be considered before any behavioural drug is dispensed to rule out underlying medical problems and establish a baseline against which future tests can be measured. Testing (based on the pet's health and the potential side effects of the drug) should be repeated at regular intervals.

Drug selection requires an accurate diagnosis of the behaviour problem and a comprehensive knowledge of which drug or drugs would be the safest and most effective for resolving the problem at hand (Fig. 4.1). The pet's age, sex and health, the cost of medication, and owner compliance and ability to administer the medication are also important aspects of drug selection. When there is more than one potentially effective treatment regimen, the safest course of action should be followed. Accurate doses have not yet been established for many of the drugs used in pet behavioural therapy so that, in some cases, wide dosage ranges can be found in the veterinary literature.

When treatment fails or untoward side effects are identified, it should first be determined whether a dosage adjustment is practical and whether longer duration of therapy might be indicated. Alternative regimens, which might be potentially more harmful to the pet, must be weighed against all other options.

Neurotransmitters

In order to make an intelligent decision when choosing a psychoactive drug for behavioural therapy, it is important to have an understanding of central nervous system (CNS) neurotransmitter activity. Neurotransmitters are responsible for the transmission of impulses from one neuron to another or to a non-neuronal cell. Neurotransmission can be increased or decreased to accommodate any physiological situation. Alterations in the levels of neurotransmitters can be responsible for neurological and behavioural disorders and these alterations can sometimes be modified by the administration of certain drugs. While drugs can be used to manage disease conditions they can also result in aberrations of neurotransmitters causing adverse effects.

Following stimulation of the presynaptic neuron, neurotransmitters are released from the terminal endings and act on the postsynaptic cell (Fig. 4.2). They are then inactivated by enzymes in the interneural space or attach to re-uptake receptor sites on the presynaptic neuron where they re-enter the neuron from which they were released. Re-uptake blockage therefore prolongs the effect of the neurotransmitter and this is the basis for the action of many of our psychoactive drugs.

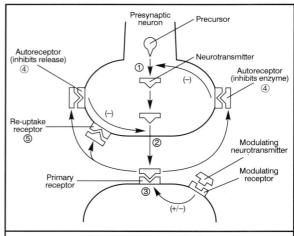

Stages of Neurotransmission

1. Synthesis of neurotransmitter in the prejunctional neuron
2. Release of neurotransmitter in response to an action potential
3. Interaction of neurotransmitter with the receptor
4. Auto-regulation
5. Re-uptake

FIG. 4.2 The stages of neurotransmission and receptor sites.

All neurotransmitters interact with receptors on the postjunctional cell. These receptors can have either excitatory or inhibitory effects. In addition, receptors that are stimulated continuously by neurotransmitters or drugs (agonists) can become hyposensitive or 'down-regulated', whereas receptors that are not stimulated by their neurotransmitters or are blocked by drugs (antagonists) can become hypersensitive or 'up-regulated'. The result is a decrease or increase in the physiological response of the effector cell.

Amino Acids

Amino acids are the most prevalent of the CNS neurotransmitters. They are involved in rapid point-to-point communication. Glycine, glutamate and aspartate are three of the most important of the 20 amino acids that function as neurotransmitters. Glutamate is the primary excitatory messenger in the brain. Gamma-amino butyric acid (GABA) is synthesised from glutamate and is the most prevalent inhibitory neurotransmitter (*see below*).

Acetylcholine

Acetylcholine is synthesised from choline and is generally an excitatory neurotransmitter. It is the only major neurotransmitter not derived directly from an amino acid. In vertebrates, acetylcholine is the neurotransmitter at all neuromuscular junctions and is involved in preganglionic to postganglionic neurotransmission for both the sympathetic and parasympathetic nervous systems (nicotonic synapses). Acetylcholine is also the postganglionic neurotransmitter of the parasympathetic nervous system (muscarinic synapses). Muscarinic stimulation leads to a decrease in heart rate and cardiac output and arteriole vasodilation, and an active digestive system. It is present in subcortical structures above the brainstem, especially in the area of the lower part of the basal ganglia named the nucleus basalis of Meynert. It plays an important role in memory; degeneration of acetylcholine function is seen in Alzheimer's disease.

Acetylcholine action is rapidly terminated by the enzyme acetylcholinesterase. Levels are regulated by the enzyme choline acetyltransferase and by choline uptake. Atropine blocks muscarinic synapses and therefore the effect of the parasympathetic system at the target organs while curare blocks nicotonic synapses, thereby paralysing skeletal muscles. Acetylcholinesterase inhibitors, such as some organophosphate compounds, potentiate the effects of cholinergic activity, while atropine acts as an antidote by blocking cholinergic receptors in the brain.

Monoamines

This neurotransmitter group is divided into two classes, catecholamines and indoleamines. The **catecholamines** noradrenaline (norepinephrine), adrenaline (epinephrine) and dopamine are all synthesised from the same amino acid, tyrosine, and share a common chemical structure. The **indoleamines** serotonin (5-hydroxytryptamine) and melatonin are synthesised from tryptophan. The cell bodies for the neurons that produce these neurotransmitters are present in small groups or nuclei located in a relatively small area of the brainstem. The distribution of axons from these nuclei has a rather diffuse disposition affecting a large number of cells in various areas of the brain. Catecholamines are the neurotransmitters associated with the arousal of the autonomic nervous system. During stressful or fearful moments, the catecholamines dopamine and noradrenaline are released, resulting in CNS stimulation and anxiety. The locus ceruleus in the pons is the principal noradrenergic nucleus. In monkeys, stimulation of the locus ceruleus leads to the fear response while the drug clonidine or lesions of the locus ceruleus nucleus decrease fear. Chronic stress might lead to exhaustion and depletion of noradrenaline and dopamine and resultant depression. Almost all classes of psychotropic drugs interact in one way or another with catecholamine-containing neurons.

Dopamine

Dopamine is a neurotransmitter that is synthesised from tyrosine by dopaminergic neurons. Tyrosine is converted to levodopa and then dopamine and stored in prejunctional vesicles. After release, dopamine interacts with dopaminergic receptors. This is followed by re-uptake by the prejunctional neuron. Levels are held constant by changes in tyrosine hydroxylase activity. Dopamine is inactivated by the enzymes monoamine oxidase (MAO), primarily MAO B and by catechol-O-methyltransferase (COMT). Dopamine depletion may lead to behavioural changes such as depression, extrapyramidal signs, Huntington's chorea in humans and Parkinsonian-like tremors, and may be a contributory factor in certain forms of pituitary-dependent hyperadrenocorticism. The selective MAO B inhibitor, L-deprenyl, may therefore be useful in the treatment of some of these conditions. A relative increase in brain dopamine levels may be associated with certain stereotypic and compulsive disorders.

Noradrenaline (Norepinephrine)

Noradrenaline is a neurotransmitter that is synthesised from tyrosine in noradrenergic neurons. Following synthesis, dopamine is further hydroxylated to form noradrenaline. Noradrenaline is stored in prejunctional vesicles and, when released, interacts with noradrenergic receptors. The effects of noradrenaline are primarily terminated by re-uptake at the prejunctional neuron, similar to dopamine. Noradrenaline is also broken down by monoamine oxidase A (MAO A) and by catechol-O-methyltransferase (COMT). Drugs that inhibit noradrenaline uptake, such as tricyclic antidepressants and drugs that inhibit MAO, increase noradrenaline availability and have been used to treat depression in humans.

Adrenaline (Epinephrine)

In response to noradrenaline release, adrenaline is secreted from the adrenal gland and together they cause sympathetic effects, e.g. pupillary dilation, piloerection, tachycardia. There are both alpha and beta adrenergic receptors. Activation of alpha receptors leads to vasoconstriction, increased cardiac contractile forces, iris dilation, intestinal relaxation, pilomotor contraction, contraction of the intestinal and bladder sphincters, and inhibition of the parasympathetic nervous system. Stimulation of beta-one (β_1) receptors leads to an increase in cardiac output while β_2 receptor stimulation causes vasodilation, intestinal relaxation, uterine relaxation and dilation of coronary vessels as well as bronchodilation. Drugs that block beta receptors, such as propranolol, may therefore block some of the physiological signs associated with fear. Nicergoline is a competitive antagonist to alpha-adrenoreceptors that has recently been marketed for the treatment of a variety of behaviour problems. The benefits proposed by the manufacturer include increased cerebral blood flow and neuroprotection.

Serotonin

Serotonin (5-hydroxytryptamine) is synthesised from tryptophan by serotonergic neurons and is found mainly in cells in the midline raphe. Its molecular structure is very similar to the psychedelic agent, lysergic acid diethylamide (LSD). It plays a major role in the sleep–wake cycle, mood and emotion, and in other functions mediated by the limbic system.

Levels are controlled by cellular uptake of tryptophan and the action of tryptophan hydroxylase which is involved in the rate-limiting step in serotonin synthesis. Inactivation is by re-uptake or by breakdown by MAO. An increase in serotonin may be associated with an activation of the pituitary adrenal axis. A decrease in serotonin may lead to depression, increased anxiety, aggression and decreased food intake. In humans, altered serotonergic system function is associated with hyperaggressive states, schizophrenia, affective illness, major depressive illness and suicidal behaviour. Increasing or normalising serotonin levels may be useful in the treatment of depression in people, compulsive and stereotypic disorders, and some forms of aggression and anxiety. Specific serotonin re-uptake inhibitors and tricyclic antidepressants increase serotonin availability by decreasing re-uptake, and MAO inhibitors increase serotonin by decreasing serotonin breakdown. Serotonin agonists have been shown in rat studies to reduce offensive aggression, without blocking defensive aggression.

Gamma-Aminobutyric Acid

Gamma-aminobutyric acid (GABA) causes mostly inhibitory effects and is synthesised from glutamic acid. After it interacts with its receptor, there is active re-uptake by the prejunctional neuron. GABA is metabolised by GABA transferase (GABA T). Seizure activity and Parkinson's disease may be associated with GABA decreases or disorders, so that GABA agonists such as benzodiazepines can be useful in the treatment of these conditions. GABA agonists may also be helpful in the treatment of anxiety disorders. GABA T inhibitors, such as sodium valproate, have also been used in the treatment of epilepsy.

Vasopressin

Vasopressin, in addition to its effects as an antidiuretic hormone, is a neurotransmitter that affects a variety of functions including cardiovascular regulation, antipyresis, learning and memory, and arousal. In hamster and rat studies, injections of vasopressin in multiple CNS sites leads to offensive aggression, while vasopressin receptor antagonists inhibit aggression. It has been hypothesised that, at least in the hamster, vasopressin promotes aggression and dominant behaviour, that is normally restrained by serotonin. A similar reciprocal relationship between vasopressin and serotonin may also exist in humans, so that in some personality disorders associated with aggression there may be elevated vasopressin, which may be inhibited by serotonin.

Neuropeptides

This group of short-chained amino acids includes endorphins, substance P and substance K. They mainly function as modulators of other neurotransmitters, evoking facilitation or inhibition of neurotransmitter activity at the postneuron receptor site. Central nervous system endorphin release has been implicated in some compulsive disorders involving stereotypic behaviour, although the role is still not too well understood.

Other Neurotransmitters

There are numerous other neurotransmitters (e.g. encephalins, histamine, nitric acid), but further discussion is beyond the scope of this text.

Monoamine Oxidase

Monoamine oxidase is an enyzme that metabolises noradrenaline, dopamine and serotonin. MAO inhibitors (e.g. phenelzine, isocarboxazid, tranylcypromine) inhibit both MAO A and MAO B and are irreversible in their actions. They thus cause elevations of the neurotransmitters, and are therefore used in the treatment of depression and phobic states in humans.

HUMAN CONDITIONS WITH DEFECTS IN NEUROTRANSMISSION	
Condition	**Proposed Neurotransmitter Involvement**
Anxiety	Associated with reduced action of GABA. Benzodiazepines increase GABA binding and the inhibitory action reduces anxiety
Depression	Associated with reduced norepinephrine and serotonin levels, combined with increased number of beta adrenergic and serotonergic receptors. Antidepressants may work by increasing neurotransmitter levels, inhibiting monoamine oxidase or inhibiting the re-uptake system
Mania	Associated with increased noradrenaline, decreased serotonin and a decreased number of adrenergic receptors. Lithium increases noradrenaline uptake
Parkinson's disease	Associated with loss of specific brain cells, loss of dopaminergic function, depleted GABA and an overactive cholinergic system. L-DOPA increases dopamine levels, bromocriptine stimulates dopamine receptors, and anticholinergic drugs counteract the overactivity of the cholinergic system
Schizophrenia	Possibly associated with overactivity of the dopaminergic system. Antipsychotic drugs block dopamine receptors and reduce dopaminergic overactivity

FIG. 4.3 Some human conditions associated with defects in neurotransmission.

DRUGS THAT AFFECT NEUROTRANSMITTERS		
Neurotransmitter	**Drugs that Increase Effects**	**Drugs that Decrease Effects**
Acetylcholine	Carbachol, neostigmine, cholinesterase inhibitors, arecoline (muscarinic), black widow spider venom	Atropine, botulinum toxin, curare (blocks nicotinic synapses)
Dopamine	L-DOPA, amphetamine, apomorphine, bromocriptine, L-deprenyl, MAO inhibitors	Neuroleptics (e.g. chlorpromazine), lithium
GABA	Benzodiazepines, sodium valproate	Tetanus toxin, picrotoxin
Noradrenaline	Alpha adrenergics (ephedrine, phenylpropanolamine), amphetamine, MAO inhibitors	Metyrosine, reserpine, lithium, beta blockers (pindolol, propranolol), clonidine
Serotonin	Tryptophan, fluoxetine, clomipramine, sumatriptin, MAO inhibitors, eltoprazine, buspirone	Cyproheptadine, methysergide, nicergoline

FIG. 4.4 Examples of drugs that affect neurotransmitters.

They are prescribed cautiously in human medicine because they have a number of side effects and, under certain circumstances, can cause hypertensive crises. (For details, see MAO inhibitors in drug therapy, below.) More selective reversible inhibitors of MAO such as moclobemide, which only inhibits MAO A, or deprenyl that inhibits only MAO B, may be safer alternatives.

Receptor Pharmacology

The role of neurotransmitters in behavioural problems in pets is at present in its infancy. What is known is that neurotransmitter imbalance is contributory to a number of human maladies (Fig. 4.3), and that the use of many of the same drugs used in human psychiatric medicine have been used with similar affects on animal behaviour. It is thus likely that neurotransmitters play a role in some behavioural problems in animals. It is also likely that drugs used in pets may help control behavioural problems due to their effects on individual neurotransmitters.

Some drugs have rather general effects on the behaviour of an individual (e.g. phenothiazines, anticonvulsants, antihistamines), while others are more selective in their results (e.g. tricyclic antidepressants, fluoxetine). Use of drugs in the latter category can be advantageous in that desirable behaviours, like play and social interaction, are less likely to be sacrificed for the benefit of altering a single undesirable behaviour such as fear or aggression.

A drug is able to act in a selective manner when it has a specific effect on a distinct group of cells. This occurs when the drug's chemical configuration allows for a unique fit with a distinct neurotransmitter receptor macromolecule on the surface of the effector cell. A number of distinct neurotransmitter receptor sites exist on the surfaces of pre- and postsynaptic cells. Activation of these sites can result in a wide variety of cellular responses. Any of these receptor sites provides a potential location for drug interaction.

The **primary receptor** sites on the postsynaptic cell interact with the neurotransmitter from the presynaptic neuron, resulting in major biological changes within the postsynaptic cell. Activation of these sites may influence a variety of physiological activities including ion movement across the cell membrane, changes in cell membrane potential and activation of intracellular enzymes. Drugs that have molecular conformations that are similar to that of the primary neurotransmitter can attach to the receptor sites and either mimic neurotransmitter activity or block normal neurotransmitter activity, depending on the specific character of the molecule.

After detaching from postsynaptic receptor sites, the neurotransmitter molecules are either enzymatically degraded or diffuse to **re-uptake receptor** sites on the presynaptic neuron, where they attach and are transferred into the cell. In addition to decreasing the neurotransmitter's interneural concentration by physically removing molecules from the interneural space, re-uptake indirectly results in a decrease in interneural concentration by increasing the intracellular storage pool. This occurs because an intracellular feedback system inhibits neurotransmitter synthesis as the concentration of neurotransmitter increases within the neuron. Thus, the re-uptake receptor site provides an excellent target for drug action by effectively increasing the amount of neurotransmitter available to interact with the postsynaptic cell.

The influence of the primary neurotransmitter on the effector cell may be modulated by secondary neurotransmitters, such as polypeptides, as they interact at separate **modulator receptor** sites on the postsynaptic cell membrane. Attachment of modulatory neurotransmitters at these sites can result in the inhibition or facilitation of the effect of a primary neurotransmitter on the postsynaptic cell. Drugs with a correct fit can also work at these sites to regulate neurotransmitter effect.

Other locations on the presynaptic neuron where drugs can modulate neurotransmitter activity are the **autoreceptor** sites. Activation of these sites following attachment of neurotransmitter molecules diffusing through the intercellular space provides negative feedback probably by having an inhibitory influence on neurotransmitter synthesis and release. Inhibition of neurotransmitter synthesis occurs due to decreased activation of the synthesising enzyme from its inactive to active form or by directly downgrading the enzyme's activity. Autoreceptor activation can also have an inhibitory effect by directly decreasing the amount of neurotransmitter that is released from the presynaptic cell. This is an effective feedback system that results in less synthesis and release as extracellular neurotransmitter concentration increases. Pharmacological blockage or desensitisation at these sites results

SITES OF MODULATION OF NEUROTRANSMITTERS		
At the Presynaptic Neuron	**Interneural Cleft**	**At the Postsynaptic Neuron**
Synthesis	Catabolic enzymes	Primary receptor sites
Storage		Modulator receptor sites
Release		
Re-uptake receptor sites		
Autoreceptor sites		
Catabolic enzymes		

FIG. 4.5 Potential sites of pharmacological modulation of CNS neurotransmitters.

in less inhibition and increased synthesis and release of neurotransmitter molecules. It is interesting to note that when a strong serotonergic re-uptake blocker, such as fluoxetine, is given, the initial increase in serotonin results in activation of inhibitory autoreceptors that initially counterbalances the drug's effects. With time, however, the overstimulated autoreceptors become hyposensitised and inhibition of serotonin synthesis and release wanes. This is the likely reason for the delayed effect of fluoxetine and other re-uptake blockers.

Another way that a drug might increase the interneural concentration of a transmitter is by having an inhibitory effect on enzymes involved in the catabolism of that neurotransmitter. An example of a drug that works in this way is an MAO inhibitor which inhibits the enzyme that metabolises mono-amine transmitters.

Psychoactive Drugs and their Activity

Neuroleptics

Neuroleptics are commonly used in veterinary medicine as tranquillisers. They decrease motor function at the level of the basal ganglia in the brain and may reduce aggression through their action as dopamine antagonists. Phenothiazine tranquillisers such as acepromazine are non-specific in their effects. Since they decrease motor function, cause a reduced awareness of external stimuli and are effective antiemetics, they may be useful for motion sickness and anxiety associated with travelling, for some forms of aggression and anxiety, and when a decrease in exploratory or investigative behaviours is desired. However, their primary value is for restraint and sedation. Tranquillised pets should be cautiously assessed as phenothiazines have a variable effect on

aggression, and some patients may be more reactive to noises and may easily startle.

Low levels of neuroleptics such as chlorpromazine or thoridiazine may be effective at reducing anxiety associated with specific situations and, in people, are less likely to generate drug dependency. Benzodiazepines are preferable to neuroleptics for treatment of anxiety because of the potential for extrapyramidal signs with neuroleptics.

Potential side effects of phenothiazines include hypotension, decreased seizure threshold, bradycardia, ataxia, and extrapyramidal signs such as muscle tremors, muscle spasms, muscle discomfort and motor restlessness.

Promazine is one of the most hypotensive phenothiazines. Caution should be taken in patients with liver disease because of slow hepatic clearance, and in epileptic patients, since seizure activity may be potentiated. Higher-potency neuroleptics, such as perphenazine, might be considered for the treatment of fear-based conditions such as separation anxiety and thunderstorm phobias, since they are less sedating, less anticholinergic and may cause fewer extrapyramidal effects. High-potency neuroleptics, such as the dopamine receptor antagonist haloperidol, are amongst the least hypotensive, least sedating and least anticholinergic of the neuroleptics, but are also non-specific. They are used in the acute treatment of psychotic and aggressive states in people, and may be of some use in compulsive and aggressive states in dogs, but their doses and effects have not been fully established. They are more likely to produce extrapyramidal signs than the low-potency neuroleptics. Droperidol is approved in veterinary medicine in combination with fentanyl (dogs only). Potential adverse effects include bradycardia, salivation, defecation, respiratory depression and startling to loud noises. On occasion it has been reported to produce behavioural changes, such as aggression, following its use. Pimozide has been used to augment anti-depressant therapy in the treatment of obsessive–compulsive disorders in people. It may produce extrapyramidal signs and should not be used in patients with cardiovascular disease or respiratory diseases. Clozapine, a tricyclic antipsychotic, is unlikely to produce extrapyramidal symptoms and has been shown to be effective against aggression in experimental animals. Because of the significant risk of agranulocytosis in people, human patients must have a white cell and differential count prior to therapy and should be monitored weekly throughout the course of therapy. It should be used with caution in patients with underlying cardiovascular disease.

Phenothiazines may be combined with anxiolytics such as benzodiazepines but their cumulative effects are additive so that profound sedation may result. Since both tricyclic antidepressants and phenothiazines are anticholinergic, there may be an intensification of both sedative and anticholinergic effects if these drugs are used together.

Benzodiazepines

Benzodiazepines can be considered for the treatment of any condition that may have a fear or anxiety component, including fear aggression and some forms of feline inappropriate elimination. They potentiate the effects of (GABA), an inhibitory neurotransmitter. Like phenothiazines, benzodiazepines lack behavioural specificity. In general they cause decreased anxiety, hyperphagia, muscle relaxation, decreased locomotor activity and varying degrees of sedation. They also act as anticonvulsants.

Studies of animal models of anxiety have shown that locomotion, feeding and drinking behaviours that had been suppressed by fear, were increased with benzodiazepine administration. This may therefore mean that a pet which is suppressed, anorexic, withdrawn or non-aggressive due to fear may begin to eat and become more active and aggressive with benzodiazepine therapy. Diazepam is the benzodiazepine of choice for most forms of anxiety in cats, but because of its short half-life in dogs (2.5 hours compared with 5.5 hours in cats), as well as the short half-life of its active metabolite nordiazepam (3 hours in dogs compared with 21 hours in cats) it has limited value. Clorazepate may therefore be more suited for use in dogs, because of its longer half-life. In cats,

diazepam has been used successfully for spraying, anxiety-motivated inappropriate elimination, fears and anxieties (including fear aggression). It has also been used successfully to stimulate the appetite, to control seizures and to treat feline hyperaesthesia. Diazepam may also decrease predation through its inhibitory effect on acetylcholine. In humans, low-potency longer-acting and more-sedating benzodiazepines such as diazepam are more commonly used for generalised anxiety, since they are less likely to produce a rebound effect between doses as might occur with the high-potency shorter-acting benzodiazepines such as alprazolam.

Alprazolam is a short-acting high-potency benzodiazepine. In people it is one of the more useful benzodiazepines for the treatment of panic situations and agoraphobia, and may be useful in some cases of depression. Because of its short duration of action and high potency, it is most useful for acute fears. In pets, it has been used successfully for some forms of fear or anxiety-related aggression, for pets that wake up anxious at night, and in refractory cases of feline inappropriate elimination. At low doses, it may successfully reduce fear and aggression with less effects on motor function than diazepam. High-potency longer-acting benzodiazepines such as clonazepam are also less sedating than diazepam. In addition to its use as an anticonvulsant, clonazepam may be useful in the treatment of panic and obsessive–compulsive disorders in people, because of its longer duration of action, less frequent dosing and faster onset of action. Oxazepam is an effective appetite stimulant for cats and provides a longer duration of action than diazepam. In people oxazepam is a favoured benzodiazepine in the elderly and in patients with impaired hepatic function. Lorazepam provides more sustained release in people but has a slower onset of action. It has been used for the control of acute aggression in people. Since diazepam has such a short half-life in dogs (2.5 hours) it may be a useful adjunct to desensitisation programmes for fears and fear aggression, and may be useful for departure anxiety and noise phobias of short duration. In general, however, clorazepate, clonazepam, oxazepam or lorazepam might be preferable when a longer duration of action is required. Chlordiazepoxide combined with clinidium may be effective for stress-induced colitis.

Another group of benzodiazepines, the hypnotics, exert their effects on sleep. In people, their primary use is for the treatment of insomnia. Flurazepam and triazolam fall into this category. Flurazepam has rapid absorption, a long half-life and may sedate during the next day (in people), while triazolam has slower absorption and a very short half-life. When used for pets that wake during the night, flurazepam may be preferable if pets wake too early on triazolam or alprazolam. Triazolam has been reported to be effective in some cases of aggression in cats.

In addition to sedation and hyperphagia, benzodiazepines may cause a paradoxical increase in aggression or excitement (which generally resolves within a few days). Long-term use may lead to dependence. Therefore, all benzodiazepines, particularly those of high potency, should be withdrawn slowly (e.g. 10% per week). This is especially true in patients that have been administered benzodiazepines for the control of seizures, as status epilepticus may be precipitated if the drug is not tapered slowly. Behaviour problems may recur when the drug is withdrawn. In one study, 91% of cases of inappropriate urination in cats recurred when the drug was discontinued. As mentioned, since fear may be a factor inhibiting aggression, pets on benzodiazepines may become more aggressive. Since some benzodiazepines have been associated with hepatic failure, liver function should be assessed prior to therapy and pets should be monitored closely throughout the course of therapy. Rare cases of fulminant hepatic failure, within 3 to 5 days of onset of diazepam therapy have been recently reported. Baseline screening with close attention to ALT and reassessment 3 to 5 days after onset of therapy is recommended. Benzodiazepines may interfere with learning and can therefore affect the outcome of training programmes.

Benzodiazepines are commonly used to complement behavioural modification techniques such as desensitisation, controlled flooding and conditioning techniques. In general, short-acting high-potency benzodiazepines such as alprazolam are preferred for acute fear situations such as those associated with a visit to the veterinarian, car travel or a temporary visitor to the home. Longer-acting lower-potency and more-sedating benzodiazepines, such as diazepam in cats, are preferred for generalised fearful situations. Although drugs such as tricyclic antidepressants may be more appropriate for chronic anxiety situations, such as separation anxiety, shorter-acting drugs that do not require several weeks to reach a therapeutic state, such as benzodiazepines, may be better suited to anxieties of shorter duration such as a boarding situation, or for a few days after a move or other changes in the household.

Benzodiazepines have been combined with tricyclic antidepressants or fluoxetine in people for panic attacks, obsessive–compulsive disorders, and as an adjunct to antipsychotic therapy with phenothiazines or lithium. Benzodiazepines such as alprazolam or clonazepam have been used in combination with propranolol in people for treating social phobias (e.g. stage fright), and in panic disorders that have not responded to other forms of drug therapy. Combination therapy of benzodiazepines plus tricyclic antidepressants, propranolol or phenothiazines have also been used occasionally in veterinary medicine.

Beta-blockers

Since fear leads to the release of the neurotransmitter noradrenaline, beta-blockers such as propranolol have been used successfully to treat some forms of anxiety, and have been shown to suppress the offensive aggression of mice towards intruders. By blocking beta adrenergic activity, the physical symptoms of anxiety (muscle tremors, tachycardia, palpitations, sweating, trembling, gastrointestinal upset) are decreased. Although they are seldom effective for generalised anxiety or panic situations, beta-blockers have been used successfully in people with situational or social anxiety (e.g. stage fright), sometimes referred to as 'fight or flight' situations. One of the primary mechanisms for their calming effect is that they reduce the somatic components of anxiety. Without these signals of fear the fear response is diminished. Propranolol may also act to inhibit aggression by elevating serotonin at the synaptic level.

Propranolol has been used in conjunction with benzodiazepines in people for social fears and phobias and in panic disorders that have not improved with benzodiazepines or antidepressants. It has also been combined with tricyclic antidepressants in dogs for refractory cases of separation anxiety, with phenobarbital in cases of separation anxiety in which there appears to be a fear component, and with buspirone or benzodiazepines for some fears and phobias. Beta-blockers are contraindicated in pets with bradycardia, hypotension or bronchospasm. Since pindolol has more effect on serotonin receptors it may have a central effect on aggression. Potential side effects of pindolol are panting, increased anxiety and urinary incontinence.

Other Anxiolytics:

Buspirone, an azapirone, is a selective anxiolytic that produces minimal side effects. It is a serotonin receptor agonist (serving to enhance the neurotransmission of serotonin) as well as both a dopamine receptor agonist and antagonist. It has been shown to be a relatively successful drug in controlling feline urine spraying. In one study, it was found to be effective in reducing feline urine marking in over 50% of the cases. The drug may be effective in the reduction of fearful conditions as well as the treatment of aggressive and compulsive disorders. Buspirone produces no significant sedation or muscle relaxation and does not impair motor function, so that it is a good first choice for mild chronic fears and anxieties. Since it does not lead to dependence, it is more likely that a pet can be withdrawn from buspirone (compared to a benzodiazepine) without recurrence of the problem. As with other anxiolytics, treatment with buspirone can lead to an increase in aggression, as the inhibitory effects of fear are removed. It does not cause sedation, and it may cause restlessness in some people. When buspirone is effective, its major drawback is its expense in comparison with the benzodiazepines and propranolol. Buspirone may take 2–4 weeks to reach full effect as an anxiolytic, so that it is not effective in the short-term therapy of acute anxieties. For feline spraying behaviour, however, effects are generally seen within 1–2 weeks.

Buspirone does not interact with other sedatives so that it may be useful in combination with beta-blockers, sedatives, antidepressants such as clomipramine and fluoxetine or even benzodiazepines when additional anxiolytic effects are desired.

Meprobamate was a favoured antianxiety drug in the 1950s but has been since replaced by more specific anxiolytics such as benzodiazepines and buspirone. It produces marked CNS depression and muscle relaxation, and at higher doses may impair learning. It may be useful in reducing aggression and anxiety, particularly when therapy with other anxiolytics produces excessive agitation or when more profound sedation is required. It is also useful in the treatment of insomnia in people. In addition to excessive drowsiness and ataxia, meprobamate can cause hypotension and drug dependence.

Antihistamines

Antihistamines are useful for the treatment of pruritus, self-trauma and anxiety. Those antihistamines which have sedative CNS effects (hydroxyzine, chlorpheniramine, diphenhydramine, trimeprazine) may also be useful in situations of mild anxiety or overactivity. Anxiety associated with car rides, excessive vocalisation and night-time activity are conditions that may respond to antihistamine therapy. They also may be useful as a postoperative sedative, and for anxiety associated with pruritus. Since these antihistamines are anticholinergic, pet owners should be warned that they may cause a dry mouth and constipation, and are contraindicated in patients with glaucoma, urine retention or hyperthyroidism. Cyproheptadine, an antihistamine with antiserotonergic effects, may also be an effective appetite stimulant in cats and dogs.

Serenics

Serotonin agonists, such as eltoprazine, reduce offensive aggression, while leaving defensive aggression, social and exploratory behaviours intact. Eltoprazine is currently under investigation for the treatment of offensive aggression.

Hormonal Therapy

Synthetic progestins have been used for many years to treat feline inappropriate urination and some forms of anxiety and aggression. They are anti-androgenic, and cause non-specific depression of the CNS and an increase in appetite. However, because of their effects on the endocrine system, numerous unacceptable side effects may result. High doses or long-term use may lead to diabetes mellitus, adrenocortical suppression, bone marrow suppression, acromegaly, endometrial hyperplasia, pyometra, and mammary hyperplasia and carcinomas. Behavioural use of progestins should be avoided in intact females and, whenever possible, other drugs should be used first. When all else fails, progestins may be an effective treatment for controlling aggression (e.g. dominance aggression in dogs, territorial aggression in cats), and for cases of feline spraying and anxiety-motivated inappropriate urination that are refractory to antianxiety agents. Progestins may also be the drug of choice for sexually dimorphic behaviours that do not respond to castration or when castration is contraindicated.

Diethylstilboestrol is used for the treatment of oestrogen-responsive incontinence in spayed female dogs by increasing sphincter tone. Oestrogens, however, can be toxic to the bone marrow and cause blood dyscrasias so that the lowest effective dose should be utilised and complete blood counts should be monitored regularly. Phenylpropanolamine therapy (*see below*) may also be effective and may be associated with fewer adverse or undesirable effects.

Incontinence in neutered male dogs has been successfully treated with repository parenteral treatment of testosterone propionate, since most oral testosterone is rapidly broken down by the liver. The prostate should be regularly assessed in dogs undergoing testosterone therapy. Potential side effects are the development, aggravation or recurrence of sexually dimorphic male behaviours.

Alpha Adrenergics

Alpha adrenergics (sympathetic agonists) decrease incontinence by increasing urethral sphincter tone in cases of urethral incompetence. Ephedrine or phenylpropanolamine may be successful, although phenylpropanolamine is used more frequently since it is generally more effective and has fewer cardiovascular side effects. Once the pet regains urethral competence, the amount and frequency of administration should be decreased gradually to the lowest effective dose. Some pets become refractory to long-term use so that increased doses may ultimately be required. Side effects include bronchodilation, restlessness, hypertension, excitability, anxiety, panting, anorexia, irritability, tremors and cardiac arrhythmias. These drugs are contraindicated in patients with glaucoma, prostatic hypertrophy, hyperthyroidism, diabetes mellitus, cardiovascular disorders or hypertension. Phenylpropanolamine can be found in human medications such as decongestants and diet pills. Side effects may also therefore be associated with other ingredients found in the compound. Drugs with anticholinergic effects such as the tricyclic antidepressant imipramine may also be effective in the treatment of urethral incompetence.

Alpha-Adrenergic Antagonists

Alpha-adrenergic antagonists inhibit peripheral vasoconstriction. A product called nicergoline (Fitergol: Rhône Mérieux) has been released in the UK with claims of acting as a neuroprotective agent and increasing cerebral blood flow. It is recommended for dogs with age-related behavioral changes, decreased vigor, sleep disorders and psychomotor disturbances. Independent clinical studies are not yet available. The product comes as a freeze-dried tablet; because of this format, the tablet cannot be broken for dosing small dogs. The company provides instructions for converting the product into a solution for dosing very small animals. Each tablet contains 5 mg nicergoline and the manufacturer recommends 0.25–0.50 mg/kg/day each morning for 30 days.

Opiate Antagonists And Agonists

Opiate peptides are released during stress and conflict. They activate the dopamine system, which may in turn lead to compulsive or stereotypic behaviours. Endogenous opioids may also induce analgesia, reducing the pain that might otherwise inhibit self-mutilation. Thus, opiate (endorphin) receptor blockers may be effective in reducing some compulsive stereotypic behaviours, especially those of recent origin. The resultant increase in pain perception may further reduce selfmutilation. Narcotic antagonists have been variably effective in the treatment of a number of compulsive and stereotypic disorders, such as self-mutilation, acral lick dermatitis, tail chasing and flank-sucking in Doberman Pinschers. Naltrexone can be given orally, but most other opiate antagonists or mixed agonist-antagonists are only available in injectable form. A trial with naltrexone would indicate its effectiveness, however the drug may not be practical for long-term therapy because of its expense.

It has also been found that supplying an exogenous source of opioids, such as hydrocodone, may be successful in the treatment of some self-mutilatory behaviours such as acral lick dermatitis.

Ergot Alkaloids

These are dopamine agonists which activate dopamine receptors in the brain and inhibit prolactin from the anterior pituitary. Although bromocriptine, an injectable drug, is no longer available, preliminary studies by Dr Kersti Seksel in Australia revealed that urine spraying decreased in 85% of 27 males and 40% of 5 females improved after therapy. The drug was administered subcutaneously at 2–4 mg per cat and repeated after 2–4 weeks. No long-term side effects were seen. Side effects included increased affection, prolapsed nictitating membranes and inappetance for 24–48 hours. Oral tablets are available but exact dose rates have not been determined. It is thought that steady state plasma levels are reached in 10 days and that the medication should be given twice daily for 4–8 weeks.

In humans the drug may cause dizziness, hypotension and nausea (so it should be taken with food), and transient elevations in alanine aminotransferase (ALT), creatinine phosphokinase (CPK), blood urea nitrogen (BUN), aspartate aminotransferase (AST) and serum alkaline phosphatase (SAP). Bromocriptine may also be useful in the treatment of false pregnancy in dogs and in occasional cases of pituitary-dependent hyperadrenocorticism. Vomiting, diarrhoea, hypotension (especially with the first dose) and behaviour changes such as sedation and fatigue have been observed in dogs.

Anticonvulsants

The most commonly used anticonvulsant in veterinary medicine is phenobarbital. It has few applications for clinical veterinary behaviour unless an epileptic component to the behaviour problem (psychomotor epilepsy) is suspected. Spinning in bull terriers, hyperaesthesia syndrome in cats and sporadic behaviour changes with no obvious stimuli (e.g. so-called 'rage' syndromes) may be responsive to anticonvulsants. Phenobarbital may also be useful for mild cases of overactivity and excessive vocalisation. It may be useful in combination with other drugs such as clomipramine or propranolol for conditions such as separation anxiety and some forms of aggression. Reported side effects of phenobarbital and propranolol combinations include increased thirst and night wetting in spayed bitches. Phenobarbital may reduce the effects of beta-blockers while antihistamines and phenothiazines may potentiate the sedative effects of phenobarbital. During initiation of therapy, ataxia and sedation may be noticed, which generally resolve with continued treatment. Lipaemia and hepatotoxicity may develop with long-term use.

Clonazepam (previously discussed under benzodiazepines) and carbamazepine are two other anticonvulsants that may have behavioural applications in veterinary medicine. Carbamazepine is a tricyclic compound, similar in structure to imipramine, and as such may be useful in the treatment of compulsive disorders and aggression due to anxiety or frustration. In addition to the treatment of seizures in people, it is also useful in the treatment of depression, mania and for some explosive aggressive states, particularly those that might be associated with temporal lobe epilepsy or other organic diseases. In animals, carbamazepine is slightly sedating, mildly anticholinergic and does not cause significant muscle relaxation. In cats, carbamazepine has been found to reduce some forms of fear-induced aggression, and may make individual cats more affectionate towards people. However, as with other drugs that reduce the inhibitory effects of fear, aggression towards other cats within the home is a potential adverse effect. In cases where psychomotor epilepsy might be a component of the problem, a trial with an anticonvulsant such as carbamazepine might also be warranted. The drug is monitored in people by maintaining therapeutic plasma ranges of 4–10 μg/ml. Both in people and in feline case studies, clinical response may be achieved with lower levels. Since the drug induces its own metabolism, reduction in blood levels may occur after a month of therapy. Side effects in people include ataxia, clonic/tonic convulsions, gastrointestinal upset and locomotor difficulties. The drug is contraindicated in patients with known renal, hepatic, cardiovascular or haematological disorders, and should not be used in pets kept for reproductive purposes.

Antipsychotics

Antipsychotics such as lithium chloride are used in the treatment of manic depression and explosive behaviour disorders in people. An ECG, blood profile, urinalysis and thyroid level should be assessed prior to treatment. Lithium inhibits the release of dopamine and adrenaline and enhances serotonin release. It may also cause a mild increase in noradrenaline levels. Lithium has been utilised for some forms of unpredictable severe aggression in dogs, but it is highly toxic and has a narrow window of efficacy. It therefore requires careful monitoring. Therapeutic blood levels should be in the range of 0.8–1.2 mEq/litre. Lithium may be useful in combination with benzodiazepines or tricyclic antidepressants when these drugs alone have been unsuccessful in the treatment of stereotypic or compulsive behaviours. Potential side effects in humans include arrhythmias, dizziness, gastrointestinal disturbances, nephrogenic diabetes insipidus, hypothyroidism, hyperparathyroidism, tremors, leucocytosis and hypercalcaemia.

MAO Inhibitors

Most MAO inhibitors non-selectively inhibit both MAO A and B, and have few animal applications. MAOs increase the breakdown of the monoamines dopamine, adrenaline, noradrenaline and serotonin. Therefore, MAO inhibitors prevent this breakdown and stimulate mood elevation. In humans, MAO inhibitors are used as antidepressants and in the treatment of some panic and phobic states. They may also be effective in some phobic and anxiety conditions in animals. They are less anticholinergic and less sedating than tricyclic antidepressants (TCA), but have the potential for greater side effects and may interact with a number of foods and drugs to precipitate a hypertensive crisis. These crises may be precipitated when individuals take other drugs with sympathomimetic properties, or eat or drink items that are rich in tyramine, such as cheeses and wine. Tyramine is normally inactivated by MAO in the gut. However, when non-selective irreversible MAO inhibitors are administered, tyramine may not be inactivated. This may lead to an increase in noradrenaline release leading to vasoconstriction and an increase in blood pressure. MAO inhibitors should not be taken concurrently and tyramine-containing compounds (e.g. cheese) must be avoided or decreased during MAO therapy. Adverse reactions include CNS stimulation, hepatoxicity, dizziness, hypertension or hypotension, dry mouth, blurred vision, and constipation. Newer selective reversible inhibitors of MAO A are far less likely to precipitate a hypertensive crisis and may therefore be a safer and more practical treatment option.

The drug L-deprenyl (selegiline) is the only MAO inhibitor which is selective for monoamine oxidase type B. It also increases dopamine levels by inhibiting dopamine re-uptake and by increasing phenylethylamine levels (which is a facilitator of dopamine activity). L-deprenyl may also enhance the release of norepinephrine and serotonin. Deprenyl also activates superoxide dismutase and catalase, two enzymes which are responsible for removing free radicals. Because free radicals cause cell injury and may contribute to brain pathology and signs of ageing, it has been hypothesised that L-deprenyl decreases nerve damage and degeneration. Recent studies in several laboratories have confirmed that L-deprenyl also exhibits 'rescue' of CNS and peripheral neurons damaged by trauma or neurotoxins.

Decreased dopamine levels may also lead to muscle tremors (as in Parkinson's disease in humans), reduced muscle movements on walking, memory loss and disorientation. Preliminary studies indicate that deprenyl may improve cognitive function in ageing dogs, and may be useful in the treatment of disrupted sleep–wake cycles, indifference to the environment, decreased responsiveness to commands, decreased attentiveness and activity, weakness or stiffness, and geriatric-onset housesoiling with no concurrent organic disease.

L-Deprenyl is also effective in the treatment of some forms of pituitary dependent hyperadrenocorticism (PDH) which may result from hypothalamic dopamine depletion. Dopamine inhibits the release of adrenocorticotropic hormone (ACTH), so that lack of dopamine would lead to oversecretion of ACTH. Administration of L-deprenyl may promote normalisation of dopamine levels, thus ameliorating clinical signs and returning balance of the hypothalamic–pituitary–adrenal (HPA) axis. L-deprenyl may also be effective in suppressing cataplexy in cases of canine narcolepsy. Few adverse effects (none serious) have been reported in dogs to date so that it is likely that the drug is extremely safe. Clinical trials involving elderly pet dogs are underway in several countries for use of L-deprenyl to treat PDH and to treat cognitive dysfunction. At the time of writing, l-Deprenyl is licensed in Canada and the United States (Anipryl) for the treatment of pituitary dependent hyperadrenocorticism, and is now also licensed in Canada for the treatment of cognitive dysfunction.

Since increases in dopamine levels cause CNS stimulation and an increased onset of stereotypic behaviours, it is likely the drug would be contraindicated for the treatment of pets (particularly young pets) with normal or increased activity levels and in most stereotypic behaviours. In healthy laboratory dogs, spontaneous behaviour was unaffected by once daily oral doses below 3 mg/kg, while at higher doses there was stereotypical responding characterised by increased locomotion and decreased exploratory behaviour (sniffing). These behavioural effects were thought to be due to increased levels of phenyl-ethylamine resulting from inhibition of MAO B and/or dopaminergic enhancement by L-amphetamine metabolites of L-deprenyl. It is important to note that the amphetamine that is a metabolite of L-deprenyl is L-amphetamine and not D-amphetamine (which is a much more potent inducer of stereotypy).

Catnip

Catnip or catmint produces an apparent euphoric or hallucinogenic reaction in some cats. The active ingredient, nepetalactone, exerts its influence on the CNS through the olfactory bulb. When cats sniff even a small amount of catnip they may begin to head-shake, lick, chew or rub up against the catnip, and then begin to twitch, salivate and roll on the ground. The response is transient, lasting for up to 15 minutes. Approximately 50–75% of cats respond to catnip odour. Since catnip is so appealing to most cats it can provide a useful reward for training and for encouraging approach and play, and may also be useful in counterconditioning programmes.

Antidepressants

Included in this category are the tricyclic anti-depressants (TCAs) such as clomipramine, amitripty-line, carbamazepine (previously discussed under anticonvulsants), doxepin, imipramine and protripty-line and the selective serotonin re-uptake inhibitors (SSRIs) such as fluoxetine and sertraline. Their primary function is as a stimulating or mood-elevating drug for the depressed human patient. In humans they are also used to treat narcolepsy, bedwetting, obsessive–compulsive disorders and agoraphobia, to reduce chronic and recurrent fears and anxieties, and to decrease volatile and impulsive forms of aggression. Increased irritability and hostil-ity may, in part, be due to reduced central serotonin functioning. In pets, antidepressants have been used successfully to treat a variety of conditions including compulsive disorders, urine marking and some types of aggressive behaviour. Antidepressants may also be successful in the treatment of chronic or recurrent fears and anxieties, but are seldom effective for acute anxieties (unless they are combined with other drugs such as beta-blockers and benzodiazepines) since they may take several weeks to reach therapeutic levels.

Depending on the antidepressant selected, there may be inhibition of noradrenaline re-uptake, serotonin re-uptake or both. In general, blocking noradrenaline reuptake should have an activating effect, while blocking serotonin re-uptake should have a sedating or calming effect. Antidepressants also produce varying degrees of sedation depending on the degree of anticholinergic and antihistaminic effects they pro-duce. Doxepin and amitriptyline produce the strongest antihistaminic effects so that they may be particularly useful when sedative or antipruritic effects are desired. Clomipramine, fluoxetine, paroxetine, fluvoxamine and sertraline are serotonin re-uptake inhibitors with little effect on the noradrenergic system, so that they are the first choice when serotonergic effects are desired, without concurrent stimulation. However clomipramine is metabolised to chlordesipramine, which inhibits noradrenaline uptake. Antidepressants that inhibit noradrenaline uptake and have less effect on serotonin re-uptake, such as desipramine and protriptyline, generally produce a more rapid response and might be better for pets that would benefit from mild stimulation. The anticholinergic and alpha-adrenergic effects of imipramine, clomipramine and amitriptyline may also be useful in the treatment of some forms of incontinence.

Antidepressants may have a number of applications in pet behaviour therapy. For generalised and recurrent fears and anxieties, antidepressants such as fluoxetine and clomipramine may be preferable to the anxiolytics since they are non-addicting, less sedating, and are unlikely to affect learning or training. In humans, antidepressants such as imipramine are used for the treatment of panic attacks, agoraphobia, and separation anxiety and school phobias in children. Although TCAs may be effective at reducing panic, benzodiaze-pines such as alprazolam (short-acting) or clonazepam (long-acting) may also be needed to control the anxiety, particularly in acute situations. Since ami-triptyline blocks both the re-uptake of serotonin and catecholamines, and is moderately sedating, it may be particularly useful in situations where a calming effect and mood elevation are desired, such as in cases of separation anxiety and anxiety-related feline urine marking. Clomipramine and imipramine might be useful in the therapy of separation anxiety in dogs, while clomipramine might be considered in refractory cases of urine marking in cats.

Serotonin re-uptake inhibitors may be particularly effective in the treatment of compulsive and stereotypic behaviour problems. Anxiety, stress or conflict can lead to displacement behaviours depending on the genetic make-up of the pet. In time, these behaviours may become stereotyped and compulsive. They may continue to be performed even in the absence of the stressors in non-related situations during which the pet is even minimally aroused. In dogs, stone-chewing and other picas, blanket-sucking, circling, tail chasing, fly snapping, acral lick dermatitis and other forms of self-mutilation may all be compulsive behaviours. In cats, overgrooming, self-mutilation, tail chasing, paw shaking, wool-sucking and perhaps hyperaesthesia may be manifestations of compulsive disorders. Clomipramine and fluoxetine are the drugs of choice for treatment of these behaviours in people and are effective in approximately 50% of all cases. Treatment will require several weeks to several months before dramatic improvement is likely to be seen particularly in self-mutilatory behaviours such as acral lick dermatitis. Doxepin, because of its strong antihistaminic effects and amitriptyline, because of its combined antihistaminic, serotonergic and sedative effects, may also be useful in the treatment of self-mutilatory behaviours.

Antidepressants such as clomipramine and carbamazepine have also been used to treat behaviours that might have underlying pathology. Spinning in Bull Terriers, hyperaesthesia in cats and some forms of aggression, where the arousal seems to be excessive and the stimuli are vague or non-existent, may be responsive to antidepressant therapy. Carbamazepine has been used to treat organic brain disorders and temporal lobe epilepsy leading to violent outbursts of aggression in people. Similar conditions in dogs (mental lapse aggression, rage syndrome) and cats may possibly benefit from therapy with tricyclic antidepressants.

Serotonin re-uptake inhibitors such as clomipramine, paroxetine, amitriptyline and fluoxetine may have a mood-stabilising effect in some cases of affective aggression in dogs and cats. Aggression associated with high levels of arousal (territorial, fear and redirected aggression) in cats, and some forms of fear and dominance aggression in dogs have responded favourably to therapy with these drugs. Since acetyl-choline is a principal mediating neurotransmitter in predatory aggression, anticholinergic TCAs may be of some benefit in moderating or reducing predation.

Selection of the appropriate antidepressant requires an understanding of the behaviour problem at hand, the neurotransmitters that might mediate the behaviour, and the effect that each antidepressant has on the histaminic, serotonergic, noradrenergic, cholinergic, dopaminergic and alpha-adrenergic receptors. When CNS pathology or temporal lope epilepsy is a possibility, carbamazepine or clomipramine might be indicated. For compulsive disorders, serotonergic antidepressants should be selected, while antidepressants that sedate may be most useful when a quieting effect is indicated (such as in the initial treatment of separation anxiety). Of course, potential adverse effects, contraindications and cost also play an important role in selection. Drugs that reduce dopamine levels may also play a more valuable role in reducing compulsive and stereotypic behaviours but may be more prone to producing extrapyramidal effects.

Antidepressants may produce a general calming effect and may be successful at reducing panic states in humans. However, anxiolytics such as alprazolam, clonazepam or buspirone may also need to be added to reduce anxiety. These drugs and propranolol may also be useful should acutely stressful or fearful situations arise while the pet is undergoing antidepressant therapy. Concurrent therapy with benzodiazepines may be of particular importance during the initial stages of antidepressant therapy since antidepressants take several weeks to be effective and may produce a transient restlessness and increase in anxiety (*see below*). Antidepressants have been combined with pimozide or lithium in humans for refractory obsessive–compulsive disorders.

Serotonergic antidepressants may take up to 14 days to take full effect, and therefore cannot be used on an 'as needed' basis. Due to uptake inhibition, serotonin quickly begins to accumulate in the synaptic cleft; however, serotonin autoreceptors lead to a concurrent reduction in firing of serotonin neurons. Over the longer term (up to 14 days), these receptors become desensitised and serotonin neurons resume their normal firing. Fluoxetine has a plasma half-life of approximately 1 day in dogs (compared to approximately 2 days in man), while its active metabolite norfluoxetine has a plasma half-life of approximately 5 days in dogs and 9 days in humans.

EFFECTS OF TCAs IN PEOPLE		
Most anticholinergic amitriptyline/protriptyline	**Moderately anticholinergic** doxepin/imipramine/clomipramine	**Least anticholinergic** doxepin/imipramine/clomipramine
Most hypotensive doxepin/clomipramine/amitriptyline/imipramine	**Moderately hypotensive** protriptyline/desipramine	**Least hypotensive** fluoxetine
Most sedating doxepin/clomipramine/amitriptyline	**Moderately sedating** imipramine	**Least sedating** desipramine/protriptyline/fluoxetine
Most antihistaminic doxepin/amitriptyline	**Moderately antihistaminic** imipramine/protriptyline	**Least antihistaminic** clomipramine/fluoxetine
Most serotonergic fluoxetine/clomipramine	**Moderately serotonergic** imipramine/protriptyline/amitriptyline	**Least serotonergic** desipramine/doxepin
Most noradrenergic desipramine/protriptyline	**Moderately noradrenergic** imipramine/amitriptyline	**Least noradrenergic** fluoxetine
Most antidopaminergic? clomipramine/protriptyline	**Moderately antidopaminergic?** amitriptyline/doxepin	**Least antidopaminergic?** fluoxetine/imipramine

Fig. 4.6 Comparison of the effects of tricyclic antidepressants (TCAs) in humans.

Paroxetine and Fluvoxamine have shorter half lives in humans (20 hours and 15 hours respectively, and no active metabolites). Sertraline has a half life of 25 hours in man, but only 5 hours in dogs.

Antidepressants that increase serotonin may cause a serotonin syndrome in people (restlessness, diarrhoea, nausea, insomnia and abdominal cramps). However these side effects are less common with SSRIs than other serotonergic drugs because, although they accumulate in the synaptic cleft and thereby increase serotonergic neurotransmission, the increased activation of presynaptic autoreceptors leads to decreased firing of serotonin neurons. The net effect is an increase in serotonin availability but the magnitude of the increase is limited by the decrease in serotonin release.

In humans, side effects of tricyclic antidepressants include insomnia, anorexia, diurnal mood variation, and anticholinergic effects such as dry mouth, constipation, urine retention and dry eyes; however, after several weeks the effects of these begin to taper off. Antidepressants that stimulate the dopaminergic or noradrenergic systems may cause an initial increase in restlessness, irritability, anxiety or even aggression, which might resolve in a few weeks when the neurotransmitter levels stabilise. Antidepressants that activate noradrenergic systems have the potential for causing tremors and, in rare cases, an increase in aggression. Tricyclic antidepressants may also cause tachycardia, arrhythmias and hypotension, may potentiate seizures, may interfere with thyroid medications, and are contraindicated in patients with cardiovascular problems. Antidepressants that are hypotensive and those that may predispose the pet to cardiac arrhythmias or tachycardia should be started at low doses and gradually increased to optimum or maximum doses over several weeks. Antidepressants also produce variable anticholinergic effects: dry mouth, constipation, urine retention, inappetance, dry eyes, glaucoma and hypotension (Fig. 4.6). Antidepressants that block dopamine receptors (such as clomipramine) might on rare occasions be associated with extrapyramidal signs.

CNS Stimulants

Stimulants have a paradoxical calming affect on hyperkinetic dogs, but are contraindicated in dogs that are displaying overactivity or aggression from other causes. Most cases of hyperactivity are not due to any physiological disorders. In humans attention deficit disorders (ADD) may or may not be associated with hyperactivity (ADHD). Hyperkinetic dogs have been reported to exhibit overactivity (barking, chewing, pacing), tachycardia, panting, salivation, lack of trainability, aggression, and failure to calm down in neutral environments. However it has recently been speculated that dogs without hyperactivity that show signs of repetitive behaviours, increased aggressiveness or anxiety, poor learning or inattentiveness and perhaps GI signs, might also 'suffer' from ADD. The diagnosis can be made by administering 0.2–0.5 mg/kg dextroamphetamine orally and then observing the dog every 30 minutes for 1 to 2 hours to determine if the dog's respiratory or heart rate decreases or the dog becomes calmer. Alternatively methylphenidate can be prescribed for 3 days after which the target behaviours (repetitive, aggression, anxiety, overactivity, learning ability) can be assessed to determine if there has been any measurable improvement. Although the drug can often be discontinued after retraining, it may be needed throughout life in others. CNS stimulants may be indicated for narcolepsy and other conditions associated with underactivity as well as drug- or anaesthesia-induced respiratory depression (e.g. doxapram hydrochloride).

Further Reading

Allen, D. G., Pringle, J. K., Smith, D. A., Conlon, P. D. and Burgmann, P. M. (1993) *Handbook of Veterinary Drugs*. J.B. Lippincott: Philadelphia, PA.

Beaver, B. V. (1994) *The Veterinarian's Encyclopedia of Animal Behavior*. Iowa State University Press: Ames, IA.

Brignac, M. M. (1992) Hydrocodone treatment of acral lick dermatitis. *Proceedings of the 2nd World Congress of Veterinary Dermatology, Montreal 1992*.

Bruyette, D., Ruehl, W. W. and Smidberg, T. L. (1995) Canine pituitary-dependent hyperadrenocorticism: a spontaneous animal model for neurodegenerative disorders and their treatment with L-deprenyl. *Progress in Brain Research*, **106**, 207–215.

Burghardt, W., Jr. (1991) Using drugs to control behavior problems in pets. *Veterinary Medicine*, **86**(11), 106–109.

Burghardt, W. (1996) Repetitive and self traumatic behaviors. *Presentation to the American Veterinary Society of Animal Behavior Specialty Meeting AAHA, San Antonio*.

Center S. A., Elston, T. H., Rowland, P. H. *et al.* (1995) Heptatoxicity associated with oral diazepam in 12 cats. *Proc ACVIM*, **13**, 10009.

Center, S. A., Elston, T. H., Rowland, P. H. *et al.* (1996) Fulminant hepatic failure associated with oral administration of diazepam in 11 cats. *J Am Vet Med Assoc*, **209**(3), 618–625.

Cooper, J. R., Bloom, F. E. and Roth, R. H. (1991) *The Biochemical Basis of Neuropharmacology*. Oxford University Press: Oxford.

Cooper, S. J. and Hendrie, C. A. (1994) *Ethology and Psychopharmacology*. John Wiley and Sons: Chichester.

Dodman, N. (1994) Pharmacologic approaches to problem behavior. *Presentation to the American Veterinary Medical Association Annual Conference, San Francisco*.

Dodman, N. H. (1995) Pharmacological treatment of behavioral problems in cats. *Veterinary Forum*, April, 62–71.

Dodman, N. H. and Shuster, L. (1994) Pharmacologic approaches to managing behavior problems in small animals. *Veterinary Medicine*, **12**, 960–969.

Fuller, R. W. (1994) Uptake inhibitors increase extracellular serotonin concentration measured by brain microdialysis. *Life Sciences*, **55**(3), 163–167.

Goldberger, E. and Rapaport, J. L. (1991) Canine acral lick dermatitis: response to the antiobsessional drug clomipramime. *Journal of the American Animal Hospital Association*, (27), 179–182.

Goodman, A. G., Rall, T. W., Nies, A. S. and Taylor, P. (1990) *Goodman and Gilman's The Pharmacologic Basis of Therapeutics*, 8th edn. Pergamon: New York.

Hart, B. L. (1985) Behavioral indications for phenothiazine and benzodiazepine tranquilizers in dogs. *Journal of the American Veterinary Medicine Association*, **186**(11), 1175–1180.

Hart, B. L., Eckstein, R. A., Powell, K. L. and Dodman, N. H. (1993) Effectiveness of buspirone on urine spraying and inappropriate urination in cats. *Journal of the American Veterinary Medicine Association*, **203**(2), 254–258.

Hewson, C. J. and Luescher, U. A. (1996) Compulsive disorders in dogs. In: *Readings in Companion Animal Behavior*. Voith, V. L. and Barchelt, P. L. (eds) Veterinary Learning System: Trenton, NJ.

Hornfeldt, C. S. (1994) *Nepeta cataria* (catnip) 'poisoning' in cats. *Veterinary Practice Staff*, **6**(5), 1,7.

Houpt, K. A. (1993) Drugs used for behavior problems. In: *Animal Behavior. The T.G. Hungerford Refresher Course for Veterinarians, July 1993*, pp. 51–59. Postgraduate Committee in Veterinary Science, University of Sydney: Australia

Krawiec, D. R. (1988) Urinary incontinence in dogs and cats. *Modern Veterinary Practice*, **69**(1), 17–23.

Leonard, B. E. (1992) *Fundamentals of Psychopharmacology*. John Wiley and Sons: West Sussex, UK.

Levy, J. K., Cullen, J. M., Bunch, S. E., Weston, H. L., Bristol, S. M. and Elston, T. H. (1994) Adverse reaction to diazepam in cats. Letters to the editor. *Journal of the American Veterinary Medicine Association*, **205**, 155–156.

Luescher, U. A. (1993) Hyperkinesis in dogs: six case reports. *Canadian Veterinary Journal*, **34**, 368–370.

Marder, A. R. (1991). Psychotropic drugs and behavioral therapy. *Veterinary Clinics of North America, Small Animal Practice*, **21**(2), 329.

Maxmen, J. S. (1994) *Psychotropic Drugs: Fast Facts*. W.W. Norton & Co.: New York.

Melman, S. A. (1995) Use of Prozac in animals for selected dermatological and behavioral conditions. *Veterinary Forum*, August, 19–27.

Milgram, N. W., Ivy, G. O., Head, E., Murphy, M. P. *et al.* (1993) The effect of L-deprenyl on behavior, cognitive function, and biogenic amines in the dog. *Neurochemical Research*, **18**(12), 1211–1219.

O'Farrell, V. and Neville, P. (1994). *Manual of Feline Behaviour*. British Small Animal Veterinary Association Publications: Cheltenham.

Overall, K. L. (1992) Practical pharmacological approaches to behavior problems. In: *Behavioral Problems in Small Animals. Purina Specialty Review.* Ralston Purina Co.: St Louis, MO.

Peterson, M. E. and Kintzer, P. P. (1994) Medical treatment of pituitary-dependent hyperadrenocorticism in dogs. *Seminars in Veterinary Medicine and Surgery (Small Animal)*, **9**(3), 127–131.

Plumb, D. C. (1995) *Veterinary Drug Handbook,* 2nd edn. Pharma Vet Publishing: White Bear Lake, MN.

Reisner, I. R. (1994) Use of lithium for treatment of canine dominance – related aggression. *Applied Animal Behavioral Science*, **39**: 183.

Restak, R. M. (1994) *Receptors.* Bantam Books: New York.

Ruehl, W. W., Bruyette, D.S., DePaoli, A., Cotman, C.W., Head, E., Milgram, N.W. and Cummings, B.J. (1995) Canine cognitive dysfunction as a model for human age-related cognitive decline, dementia and Alzheimer's disease: clinical presentation, cognitive testing, pathology and response to L-deprenyl therapy. *Progress in Brain Research*, **106**, 217–225.

Ruehl, W. W., DePaoli, A. C. and Bruyette, D. S. (1994) L-deprenyl for the treatment of behavioral and cognitive problems in dogs: preliminary report of an open label trial. *Applied Animal Behavior Science*, **39**, 191.

Schwartz, S. (1994) Carabamazepine in the control of aggressive behavior in cats. *Journal of the American Animal Hospital Association*, **30**, 515–519.

Shanley, K. and Overall, K. (1995) Rational selection of antidepressants for behavioral conditions. *Veterinary Forum*, **12**, 30–34.

Tatton, W. G. and Greenwood, C. E. (1991) Rescue of dying neurons: a new action for deprenyl in MPTP Parkinsonian. *Journal of Neuroscience Research*, **30**, 666–672.

Wiener, J. M. (1966) *Diagnosis and Psychophramacology of Childhood and Adolescent Disorders,* 2nd edn. John Wiley and Sons: New York.

Voith, V. L. (1979) Multiple approaches to treating behaviour problems. *Modern Veterinary Practice*, **60**, 651–654.

Voith, V. L. (1982) Possible pharmacological approaches to treating behavioural problems in animals. In: *Proceedings of the First Nordic Symposium on Small Animal Veterinary Medicine.* Pergamon: Oxford, 227–234.

Wiener, J. M. (1996) *Diagnosis and Psychopharmacology of Childhood and Adolescent Disorders*, 2nd edn. John Wiley and Sons: New York.

White, S. D. (1990) Naltrexone for treatment of acral lick dermatitis in dogs. *Journal of the American Veterinary Medical Association*, **190**, 1073–1076.

Zito, J. M. (ed.) (1994) *Psychotherapeutic Drug Manual*, 3rd edn. John Wiley and Sons: New York.

5

Unruly Behaviours

Jumping Up on People

Dogs can be a real nuisance when they jump up on people. Sometimes they do this when they first meet someone, sometimes when they want to play, and sometimes for no discernible reason. The common denominator is that the behaviour persists because of inconsistencies among family members in trying to deal with the situation. In order to prevent or correct this nuisance behaviour, it is very important that everyone in the household follows the same basic rules in training.

Diagnosis and Prognosis

The diagnosis is evident from observing the dog jumping up on the owners. Veterinary staff are also not immune from the advances of these sociable (but poorly controlled) dogs. However, with behavioural modification therapy, there is an excellent prognosis for complete correction of the problem.

Management

The successful management of dogs that jump up is a balance of rewards and punishments. The owner

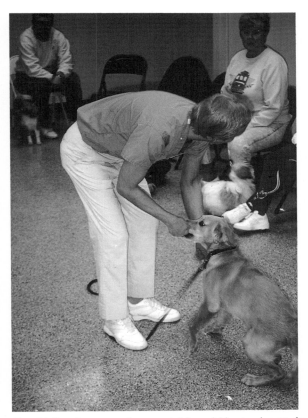 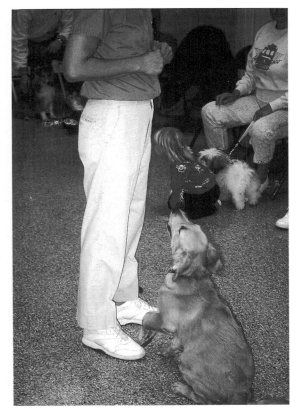

FIG. 5.1 Jumping up can be corrected by quickly stepping on the dog's leash to stop the behaviour and then asking it to sit for a reward.

should keep greetings very low-key to prevent the pet from becoming highly aroused, excited and more likely to jump up. The dog should be lightly and calmly praised when it approaches and does not jump up. Under no circumstances should it be praised for jumping up and the owner should not indulge the dog in games that involve jumping up. When the dog does jump up it can be punished (not physically) with a stern reprimand and an aversive stimulus such as a noisemaker. The audible stimulus (verbal or noise-maker) must be strong enough, relative to the pet's temperament, to stop the behaviour immediately without eliciting any signs of fear. Punishment that is not sufficiently aversive is likely to reward the behaviour by providing attention, while punishment that is overly harsh may cause undue fear or anxiety. The punishment that is used should immediately interrupt the behaviour, thereby providing a window of opportunity in which the owner can command and encourage the dog to greet in a sitting position (Figs. 5.1 and 5.2). The appropriate behaviour, sitting, is then rewarded. Once the dog is effectively controlled and trained, obedience commands and rewards should be successful in counterconditioning the pet to perform an appropriate competing behaviour such as sitting at greeting.

Prevention

Jumping up can be prevented effectively by encouraging owners to practise basic obedience techniques. Dogs jump up because owners have not learned to be consistent in applying appropriate correction measures, or do not reinforce proper greetings, or inadvertently reward the problem behaviour and thereby reinforce it.

MANAGEMENT FOR THE DOG THAT JUMPS UP	
Method	**Comments**
Avoid eliciting the behaviour	Keep greetings very low-key
Ignore the behaviour	Behaviours that are not rewarded will become extinct with time, but only if the owner has enough patience. One of the problems with this approach is that, initially, the behaviour often gets worse before it decreases as the pet tries harder to elicit a response from the owner
Rewards	The dog should be lightly and calmly praised when it approaches and does not jump up. Praise must immediately cease if the dog attempts to jump up
Reward motivation	Strong motivators such as food or toys can be used to motivate the dog to perform an appropriate alternative behaviour such as 'sit' or 'down'
Punishment	Stern verbal reprimands such as 'No!', accompanied by an aversive stimulus (e.g. noisemaker, water), should be sufficient. This should be repeated until the behaviour ceases. Punishment must be sufficiently aversive to deter the behaviour without eliciting any sign of fear. If punishment is the only treatment used, it is not uncommon for the dog to habituate to the aversive stimulus
Negative reinforcement	An aversive device (horn, ultrasonic) is applied until the pet jumps down and the aversion is immediately withdrawn
Distraction	Choose a device or sound that will interrupt the behaviour in order to get the pet's attention (ultrasonic device, whistle). The dog can then be commanded to perform an appropriate acceptable (non-jumping) behaviour
Obedience training	An owner with good control and a well-trained dog may be able to correct the behaviour with an appropriate obedience command and reward. (*See counterconditioning, below*)
Counterconditioning	A behaviour is taught that is incompatible with jumping up. For example, the dog can be taught to sit upon meeting someone, in exchange for food, a toy, or social reward. Make it maintain that position for a few seconds at first, and gradually shape the behaviour so that the dog sits for 10 seconds or longer before giving the reward (e.g. 'Good boy'). Timing is important because you do not want to reinforce a chain of behaviours in which the dog first jumps up and then sits so it can be rewarded
Control devices (head halter and leash)	For owners that have difficulty gaining verbal control, a head halter and long leash can be left attached to the dog and the leash used either in a direct manner to train the 'sit' command or from a distance (remote training) to deter the jumping behaviour
Surgery	Neutering has little or no effect on this behaviour unless it is associated with male mounting behaviour
Drugs	There are no indications for using drugs with this behaviour problem

Fig. 5.2 Management of the dog that jumps up.

Owners should follow these basic rules:

- Attend obedience classes and learn proper use of training collars and halters
- Call the dog, give a 'sit' command, and reward the proper behaviour
- Never reward pets when they jump up by giving them food, walks, or attention
- Reward the pet each time it approaches and does not jump up
- Immediately reprimand the pet when it jumps up, with a verbal 'No!'
- Make sure all family members and visitors abide by the same rules.

Case Example

Lucy, an 8-month-old spayed female Irish Setter, would jump on the owners and most visitors when they came into the home. The owners had attempted to reprimand Lucy verbally and when that was unsuccessful, they attempted to knee Lucy in the chest. Despite these and even more physical techniques (e.g. toe pinching) the problem only seemed to escalate.

Lucy enjoyed greeting people and, as a young puppy, had been intermittently rewarded by the owners and some visitors with patting or attention during greetings. As Lucy grew, the owners attempted to punish the pet verbally and then physically but as the 'punishment' gradually escalated, Lucy habituated to the reprimands and physical contact. In fact, through 'punishment' the owners were inadvertently rewarding the behaviour because Lucy enjoyed rough handling (play) and attention.

The owners were instructed to work on reward-motivated training techniques during non-greeting times. They were taught how to train Lucy to sit instantaneously on command and remain sitting for 10 seconds or longer. Since Lucy enjoyed playing with her ball, it was used as a reward for training. The owners then attempted to use counterconditioning techniques (having Lucy sit and then receive ball playing as a reward) whenever anyone entered the home. When the owners entered the home, if Lucy did not immediately respond to a 'sit' or 'down' command, they were to ignore Lucy completely (no eye contact and as little physical contact as possible). These techniques were moderately successful but Lucy did not always respond to commands when

visitors entered the home, because some continued to give her attention when she greeted them. The owner then left a 10-foot leash and head halter attached to the dog so that when visitors arrived a quick pull on the leash could be used to interrupt the behaviour. In a short time, Lucy learned to greet owners and strangers in a sitting position and on those occasions when Lucy did begin to jump up, a verbal 'Down!' command would get an immediate response.

This type of approach works very nicely with most dogs. By spending a little extra time at greetings, though, the owner can increase the speed of resolution of the problem. After the pet has been corrected or rewarded for the initial greeting, the person should leave and re-enter multiple times in order to reward a number of correct responses in succession. This will result in more rapid learning.

Stealing, Raiding Rubbish, and Jumping on Furniture or Worktops

Stealing, raiding rubbish (garbage), jumping onto furniture or worktops, or getting into any room or area that the owner considers out of bounds may be considered quite different behaviours, but there are many similarities when it comes to cause and treatment. Pets indulge in these behaviours because of their inquisitive and investigative natures and because they are self-gratifying (the pet may obtain food or a desired rest station). In addition, despite owner attempts at punishment, most pets are not aware that they have done anything unacceptable. Owners are often certain that their pets know they have done wrong when they are caught but, in most cases, this logic is seriously flawed.

Diagnosis and Prognosis

The diagnosis is made based on the owner's observation that the dog or cat performs the activities. Many owners report that the dog or cat knows it is misbehaving because it looks guilty or runs away when the owner approaches or is heard coming home. In these cases, the pet has learned that there are unpleasant consequences for being on the furniture or worktop, or in the rubbish, when the owner approaches. It has also learned that there are no unpleasant (only pleasant) consequences when going onto the furniture or worktop or into the rubbish in the owner's absence. Fortunately, with behavioural modification, the prognosis for correction is good.

Management

Teaching the desired behaviour is the first course of action. The pet should receive a food treat or lavish social reward for chewing on its own toys. Also be certain that the pet has been provided with adequate play, exercise and attention to meet its requirements. Preventing access to problem areas and safeguarding valuables by keeping them in pet-proof (or child-proof) containers or cupboards may be practical for some households. For pets that steal items, raid rubbish or chew the owner's possessions, the most practical deterrents are taste aversion and booby-traps. Taste aversion is the next course of action. This is best done by coating two or three of the owner's possessions that are being chewed with something that is bitter or hot to the taste. Commercial antichew products or a coating of oil of eucalyptus, oil of citronella, menthol or cayenne pepper mixed with water may be successful. Products such as tabasco sauce may also be effective but, for some pets, may enhance chewing as the pet develops a 'taste' for the product.

When the problem is not related to chewing, taste deterrents will not be successful and most pet repellents are not sufficiently aversive to keep pets away from furniture, worktops or other 'out-of-bounds' areas. Some garden centre products that use nasal irritants (or 'sneezing powder') may prove to be practical. Another technique that might be effective is to teach the pet to develop an aversion to a particular odour by spraying a very small amount of the product (e.g. an aerosol repellent or unscented underarm deodorant) across (not into) the pet's nose. Paired with the quickly advancing can and the sharp hiss, the odour may then be sufficient to deter the pet's approaches when sprayed on other items.

Booby-traps, such as a stack of empty cans or a bucket of water that is set to topple when disturbed, balloons set adjacent to mousetraps or tacks so that they pop on contact, electronic motion detectors, alarm mats, shock mats, and indoor electronic fencing, may be necessary or appropriate to keep pets away from selected objects or areas. Remote punishment techniques are also effective provided the pet is constantly monitored. Prevention, however, is by far the best approach when these problems continue to

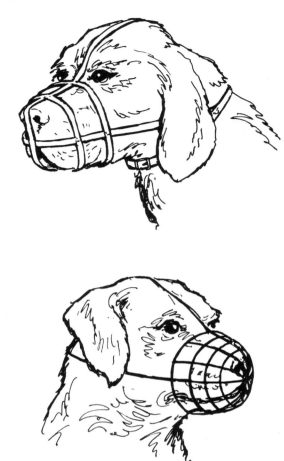

FIG. 5.3 Basket-type muzzles can be used with exposure techniques, handling of dominant aggressive dogs, or temporary control of destructive behaviour.

occur in the owner's absence. A temporary solution for some dogs that steal food or raid the rubbish is to apply a basket-type muzzle for short periods of time when the owner cannot supervise (Fig. 5.3). For those dogs that raid rubbish or steal items in the owner's presence, an increased level of control and training is necessary. A remote leash left attached to a head halter can be an excellent means of interrupting and gaining control over these behaviours.

Prevention

Encourage proper habits initially by making sure the pet has enough of its own toys to meet its need for

GUIDELINES FOR CORRECTING CHEWING AND 'STEALING'	
Step	**Comments**
Ensure adequate play, exercise and attention	Provide an adequate number of play and exercise periods to provide for the pet's needs
Control and supervision	Train and provide sufficient supervision to ensure that problem behaviours do not occur in the owner's presence (remote punishment or remote leash might be helpful)
Prevent access to potential targets and areas	Child locks, locking or child-proof containers, barricades, or partial confinement may be useful
Enhance acceptable toys and reward desired behaviour	During this whole process, smear something the pet likes (e.g. cheese, peanut butter) on the pet's favourite toys. For cats, catnip treats and moving toys (toys that dangle or roll) may increase appeal. Every time the pet chews on an acceptable object, it should receive a social or food reward
Use aversive tastes	Apply the aversive-tasting materials to two or three household items. Be certain that initial applications are strongly aversive by applying a thick coating. Products that have a 'tag' odour can help deter pets from chewing other items that are coated with the same products. Odourless products may be more useful when it is necessary to teach pets universally to avoid chewing on certain types of objects or areas (e.g. coprophagia, chewing houseplants)
Ensure aversiveness of product	Observe the pet's response to the product to be sure that it deters the behaviour effectively. Owners can potentially have a disaster on their hands if the pet is left alone with objects that have been coated with a substance that it actually likes rather than finds aversive
Relocate items	Each day, move the coated items to different locations in the home
Alternate items	Once a week, change the items that have been coated for other possessions that are of different shapes and textures
Continue the process	The goal is to shift preference from household possessions to the pet's own toys. If the exercise has been run properly, after a few weeks the pet should conclude that all household possessions taste bad (no matter where they are found or what their shape) and all toys taste good
Consider booby-traps if taste aversion therapy fails	If taste aversion is not successful, booby-traps can be used to alert owners when the unruly behaviour is occurring so it can be corrected instantaneously. Booby-traps can also be used to keep pets away from rubbish bins, stairs, food cupboards, plants, and worktops. (For more information, see the section on booby-trapping.)

FIG. 5.4 Guidelines for correction of dogs and cats that chew or take items that are not their own.

play. Do not give discarded clothing to pets (e.g. old shoes) to use as playthings it only makes it more difficult to distinguish between household possessions and chew toys. If a pet is found chewing on a household item, it should be verbally corrected (not hit), the possession retrieved, and a more suitable chew toy provided. Reward pets when they make proper use of their own toys.

Be consistent! Do not allow the pet into a particular room or area at some times and then expect it to stay away from these areas at others.

Supervise or confine! Be aware of the investigatory, exploratory, and feeding desires of pets. This means that if there is an area that it is likely to investigate, raid, or chew in, be certain that the pet is properly supervised so that it can be interrupted and corrected as the problem begins. At all other times, the pet should be denied access to the problem areas by closing off doors to these areas, using child locks or child-proof containers, confining it to a dog-proof room, run or cage, or booby-trapping the problem

areas (*see above*). Remote training (with a halter and 10-foot leash) may also be a useful way to keep the pet away from furniture, rubbish bins, and rooms that are 'out-of-bounds' (Fig. 5.4).

Case Examples

Case Example 1

Gilligan, a 2-year-old male Standard Poodle, could not be 'trusted' by the owners whenever he was out of the owners' sight. His exploratory, playful and destructive nature had persisted into adulthood, and whenever he was left alone or unsupervised he would go into rooms where he was not allowed, steal food off tables or out of cupboards, raid rubbish bins for items that could be eaten or chewed, and climb on to furniture where he would often chew on the upholstery. Gilligan enjoyed playing with the owners and other dogs outdoors and was kept confined to his owners' half-acre property with an electronic fencing unit. The owners had attempted to confine Gilligan to a cage but this resulted in extreme anxiety on Gilligan's part (howling, salivating, chewing at the bars), and he was capable of escaping from or damaging most cages.

Because of Gilligan's size and the anxiety associated with being caged, confinement techniques were not practical in this case. Many of the potential problem areas could be closed off but a few of the rooms had no doors and no physical means of denying entry.

Gilligan's highly energetic and exploratory nature was dealt with by increasing exercise and providing more attention, by playing chase and fetch games and taking longer walks before each departure. Gilligan enjoyed playing with other dogs, so he was also given the opportunity to play with two of the neighbours' dogs every morning before the owners departed for their daily activities. Although obtaining a second compatible, playful dog for the household may have helped in this situation, the owners had no interest in possibly adding to their problems with another dog. When the owners departed, all bedrooms, the study, and the basement were closed off and the only remaining rooms that Gilligan had access to were the living room, dining room, and kitchen. Child locks were placed on the kitchen cupboards so that these could not be raided and all rubbish was placed in the garage before the owners departed. Three or four toys with treats (meat, peanut butter) hidden inside, and a few small bowls of food (with a hidden treat of meat or cheese inside) were provided each time the owner had to leave home. Gilligan's problems were dramatically decreased but his explorations into the living room and dining room occasionally led to damage or destruction. Since motion detectors and other forms of booby-trap had not been successful, the owner installed additional wiring for the electronic fencing unit which was run along the basement ceiling directly below the entrance to the dining room and living room. Gilligan quickly learned to stay away from these rooms when wearing the receiver collar.

Case Example 2

Samantha, a 4-year-old spayed female cat, lived in a one-bedroom apartment with her 23-year-old owner. Because of her owner's concerns about cleanliness and health, Samantha was not allowed on the kitchen worktops or tables. When the owner was present, the cat had been taught to stay away from the tables and counters with a water rifle, but whenever the owner went out of the room or out of the apartment, Samantha continued to climb on the worktops and table. The owner had tested this by leaving some food on the counter, which Samantha quickly ate when the owner left the room. Remote punishment techniques with the water sprayer had not been successful (presumably because the owner did a poor job of hiding out of sight and Samantha was able to determine when the owner was watching). The owner was not willing to confine Samantha to the bathroom, bedroom or a crate.

Samantha continued to climb onto the tables and worktops as part of her daily exploratory and play behaviours and because food, leftovers or tasty spills could occasionally be found in these areas (not to mention the test foods that the owners had purposely provided) that would intermittently reward her 'travels'. The first step was to provide Samantha with a play centre which consisted of scratching surfaces, a few cubby holes for hiding and a number of ledges and platforms for climbing and perching. On these platforms and dangling from the ledges were toys and small morsels of food and treats. Samantha soon began to explore and investigate the play centre regularly but continued occasionally to wander across the table and worktops. The owner purchased an electronic mat which was used to keep the cat away from the worktop when she was out, and a piece of plastic carpet runner (nubs up) was draped across the table except at meal times. The cat was never seen on the work surfaces or table top again.

Pulling/Forging Ahead and Lunging on Lead

Many dogs have habits of lunging ahead on their leash and pulling their owners along during a walk. These behaviours are unsafe for the dog and not a pleasurable experience for the owner. Both will enjoy the walk more if the dog correctly maintains its position next to the owner during the walk.

Diagnosis and Prognosis

The diagnosis is made based on history. The dog controls the owner during the walk, not the other way around. In many cases, the dog persists even if the owner uses a choke collar, but without correct technique. Fortunately, there is a good prognosis for correction of the problem.

Management

Lunging and pulling on the leash are much easier to prevent than to treat but can be managed effectively with some behavioural modification and the use of some equipment. Obedience classes are very useful, because one of the first lessons learned is the heel command. A slip training collar or head halter and the guidance of a good trainer will quickly put the pet under control so that it can be taught how to walk on the lead without constantly pulling. Training involves a light 'pop' of the leash or abruptly changing direction, to get the pet's attention and stop the pulling. This permits the owner to use social attention or food lures to condition the pet to walk alongside without pulling.

It should be apparent very quickly whether training and traditional collars will be effective. For those dogs that cannot be controlled effectively by the owners during walks, a useful diagnostic technique may be to determine the success a competent trainer has with the same dog. If the trainer is immediately successful, a more intensive training programme and a thorough discussion of the techniques for gaining control are necessary. For refractory cases or when the owner needs to gain immediate control, head halters provide the control necessary to prevent lunging but also allow the owner to restrain the dog properly and retrain it to perform to the 'heel' command. Other

harness-like devices deter or prevent pulling and lunging by means of straps that apply pressure to the axillary areas, but don't improve the owner's overall control of the dog. Distraction devices (e.g. ultrasonic and audible trainers) and conditioned cues (clickers) may also be helpful for getting the dog's attention during a retraining programme.

Prevention

Lunging and pulling on the lead is effectively prevented by teaching the 'heel' command to dogs when they are young or when they first learn to walk on a lead. Training collars are very useful for this purpose.

Case Example

Fester, a 4-year-old 50 kg male entire Rottweiler, could not be physically restrained by his 50 kg female owner in the presence of male dogs. Fester threatened and lunged at other male dogs and would probably have attacked if not physically restrained. The husband, who weighed 85 kg and had taken Fester to obedience classes as a puppy, could physically restrain Fester on walks and could usually get him to respond to a 'heel' command with a strong tug on the choke collar and harsh verbal corrections. Fester had been fitted with a prong collar which was of no benefit for the female owner. The prong collar helped the male owner gain better control over Fester but Fester's aggression towards other male dogs had further escalated. Although the prong collar provided the male owner with a more intense means of suppressing Fester's aggression, it only served to fuel his aggression towards other dogs since Fester would now associate pain and increased fear and anxiety with the approach of other dogs. The only real control the male owner had was through physical suppression and this was impractical and unsuccessful for the smaller female owner.

Fester was first retrained to the 'heel' command using a head halter and reward training by the female owner. The owners were advised to have Fester neutered as this might help reduce his aggression to other male dogs, but the owners preferred to defer this until all other aspects of training had been put into place. Once Fester could successfully 'heel' for both owners in dog-free environments, he was gradually reintroduced to other dogs, beginning first with

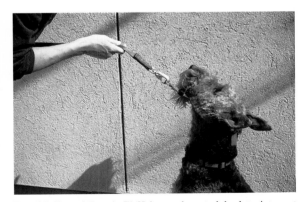

FIG. 5.5 Use of Promise™ Halter and control lead to interrupt undesirable behaviour (e.g. jumping up, barking, nipping, chewing, coprophagia) and ensure appropriate behaviour (e.g. sit, quiet).

female dogs, then neutered males and the occasional male dog which was housed or tied up on his own property. The halter provided exceptional control and Fester could be kept at the heel except when an unexpected male dog approached. Neutering and continued use of the head halter led to much greater improvement so that within 6 months, the female owner reported that virtually all walks were enjoyable and problem-free.

Feline Nocturnal Activity and Exuberant Play

Cats are nocturnal by nature and this can cause problems in a household. Not only can they provide unwanted attention to their owners during sleep, but they can also run through the house at night, during exuberant play sessions. Owners might complain of lack of sleep, or damage done to the house at night while they were sleeping. Owners may even report that the cat or kitten contacts them physically during the night, perhaps by trying to sleep on their face or nibbling their toes. Although many of these problems are more frequent at night, it is not unusual for exuberant play and jumping on or pouncing at owners to occur at any time during the day or night.

Diagnosis and Prognosis

The diagnosis is made based on the history provided by the owner. The complaint is one of feline over activity during the night that is not well tolerated by the owner. The prognosis for successfully stopping the behaviour is fair, but the prognosis for acceptable resolution of the problem is good. Exuberant play and chasing and pouncing behaviours have a much better prognosis in a young playful kitten and are more of a concern if they persist into adulthood.

Management

Most of the annoying behaviours mentioned above are more common in kittens and the behaviours decrease significantly when they reach 12–18 months of age. However, for some cats that are eternally 'young at heart', the behaviour can continue throughout adulthood.

The cat may sleep better through the night if it is given more attention, activity and play in the early evening, before the family retires for the night. Cat play is best directed at moving objects so that toys thrown or dragged along by the owners, and those that can be batted along the ground or dangled from cat perches or door handles work best. Restricting the areas accessible to the cat can also be helpful. This might involve closing the bedroom door, or confining the cat to another room or a crate.

When the problem persists, punishment techniques may be necessary. Water sprayers, ultrasonic devices or compressed air may deter night-time play; booby-traps can be used to keep cats away from particular areas. Cats that exhibit exuberant play can be directed into a special play room until their activity diminishes, and cats that seem to enjoy pounce and play games may do better with a second cat in the home (provided it is also young, hearty and playful).

Prevention

Since cats enjoy play and are somewhat nocturnal in their habits, providing appropriate play in the day and during the evenings can help get the cat into a more diurnal schedule. Providing interactive games and appealing play toys is very important in meeting the cat's social and play requirements. For cats that get too rough or energetic in play, it may be necessary to set limits by stopping any game or activity when the cat gets too boisterous. A spray of water, compressed air, loud horn or locking the cat into a separate room until it calms down, are all ways of ensuring that the owner controls the situation. A second playful kitten can prove to be the best play partner for a young, growing and boisterous kitten.

Case Example

Ralphy Boy, a 9-month-old neutered male domestic shorthair cat, lived in an apartment with a couple in their late 60s. Ralphy was a gregarious kitten who liked to initiate play by jumping onto the owners' laps or shoulders. However, the major problem was that Ralphy loved to chase across the bedroom furniture and bedcovers at about 2 o'clock every morning. The owners had recently had Ralphy neutered which had had no effect on this behaviour, and had taken to locking Ralphy out of the bedroom at night where he would howl and run around knocking items off the table tops and work surfaces.

The owners were providing little if any interactive play, so that Ralphy boy slept throughout the evening and was up and raring to go at night. The owners had no control over Ralphy so that he was allowed to play, eat and be patted whenever he desired. The owners began gaining more control by providing no further rewards of any kind (food, play, or affection) except on the owner's initiation. The cat quickly learned the 'Come!' command which the cat always had to respond to before rewards were given. Ralphy was also taught to sit on his owner's lap and be stroked for several minutes before each feeding or play session. Interactive cat wands for chasing and a cat play centre with dangling toys were placed in the den, and play sessions were planned each evening. From 7 to 11 p.m. Ralphy was provided with numerous play sessions and a catnip treat so that he had little chance to sleep. A feeding session was added at 11 p.m. and Ralphy was confined to the den each night. The situation improved dramatically but Ralphy continued to wake and vocalise on some nights. A playful 6-month-old neutered male kitten was obtained from a local shelter. Although Ralphy Boy and his new friend 'Norton' occasionally woke and played at nights there was no further vocalisation and the cats caused no problems for their owners as they were housed in the den at nights.

Excessive Barking

Barking is a normal and natural means of canine communication. The primary reasons for barking are an innate need to stave off conflict, innate desires for food or social contact, and anxiety or conflict behaviours. Barking is then further motivated when reinforcement of any type is associated with it. This is frequently the case when owners accede to their dogs' desires by providing food, play or some other form of attention. Reinforcement may be inadvertent, such as when the owner attempts to stop the barking or calm the pet down by providing treats or by any verbal or physical attention. Attempts at punishment, especially light scoldings, may also serve to reward the behaviour if they are not sufficiently aversive. Barking is also reinforced when the threat (e.g. a stranger approaching) is successfully removed (stranger retreats) or the conflict is successfully resolved by the barking.

Diagnosis and Prognosis

The diagnosis for any barking case is based upon the history of the problem, especially those situations in which the problem occurs. The owner's response to the barking and the dog's response to the owner's attempts at 'correction' are also critical issues in both the diagnosis and the prognosis. By the time the case is presented to the practitioner, the barking may have multiple contributing factors, and there may in fact be more than one type of barking occurring. Barking can be quite difficult to correct since it is a highly innate behaviour in some dogs, and often occurs in the owner's absence. Barking that occurs in the owner's presence and problems in which the stimuli can be controlled should have a much better prognosis.

Vocalisation may be categorised:

- territorial/protective/alerting
- conflict/anxiety-induced
- stereotypic compulsive
- attention-getting
- play/social
- separation/distress-induced

Management

Behavioural modification is based on the following (Fig. 5.6):

1. Identify/eliminate the cause
2. Control or avoid stimuli that elicits barking
3. Reward/quiet training (*see below*)
4. Remove reinforcing factors
5. Exposure/counterconditioning to stimuli
6. Punishment (e.g. bark-activated devices)

While most barking problems can be interrupted by training the dog to be quiet on command, these techniques are unlikely to be effective when the dog barks in the owner's absence. Depending on the dog's level of motivation and the intensity of the stimulus, many of these owner-absent problems can be reduced by the use of bark-activated deterrents. (The management of separation anxiety is discussed in chapter 7). Those products that are designed to sit on counters or attach to walls or cages may be effective for dogs that bark in specific areas (e.g. water-spray bark devices, bark-activated alarms). Bark-activated collars are particularly useful for the pet that is not restricted to

MANAGING THE DOG THAT BARKS	
Step	**Comments**
Identify and remove or limit stimuli for barking	Whenever possible, remove stimuli that lead to barking or modify the stimulus (e.g. change the doorbell). Controlling and muting the stimulus is also an important aspect of desensitisation techniques
Remove reinforcers for barking	Identify reinforcers for the behaviour and ensure that they do not continue (e.g. treats, attention, mild punishment, release from confinement). When the reinforcement is the retreat or withdrawal of the stimulus, use control and exposure techniques
Train quiet command	(See Prevention below)
Behavioural modification (desensitisation and counterconditioning)	To accomplish exposure or desensitisation training, the owner must first have good control of the dog. Obedience reward training techniques and the use of head halter devices should be used to ensure control. Once control is achieved, the dog should be exposed to controlled or muted levels of the stimulus. Initially the stimuli might be recordings of the stimuli (e.g. knocking on a door or the sound of a doorbell) or single controllable stimuli such as a car door shutting or a family member knocking on the door. The key to exposure is that the dog cannot escape, the stimulus does not retreat and the barking can be controlled with either the training/reward method and/or the head halter device. The level of stimulus is gradually increased with each subsequent training session
Devices For barking in the owner's presence:	Owner-activated punishment • alarms (ultrasonic, foghorns, rape alarms) • water (watergun, hose, sprinkler system)
For barking in the owner's absence:	Bark-activated area devices (for room, run, cage, etc.) • bark-activated water sprayers or bark-activated audible alarms Bark-activated collars • citronella-emitting collars • ultrasonic and audible collars • shock collars
For separation anxiety	Treatment for separation anxiety – drug therapy
For compulsive behaviour	Treat as for compulsive behaviour – drug therapy
For inadequate stimulation	More exercise, obedience training, more social contact with the owner, teach a game (fetch)
Surgery	Devocalisation unacceptable in some countries may result in an unacceptable muffled vocalisation the formation of scar tissue may result in a recurrence of barking

FIG. 5.6 Management of excessive barking.

specific areas. In one study by Dr.'s Juarbe Diaz and Houpt, barking was decreased in 88.9 per cent of cases with the citronella spray collar, but only 50 per cent of cases with an electronic bark-activated collar. In an unpublished study of 62 dogs in two veterinary hospitals (personal communication, Patrick Melese, Gary Landsberg) approximately 70 per cent of dogs stopped barking and another 20 per cent were decreased with the citronella spray collar.

Prevention

There are important guidelines:

● The owner must never reward barking (e.g. attention, food, play) and must not go to a barking or crying puppy or release it from a cage (unless the puppy is in distress) as this would only serve to reinforce the behaviour.

● Socialise and habituate the dog so that it is accustomed to sounds, situations and people that might initiate barking.
● Basic obedience training and control are important.
● Immediate interruption is required with startle or punishment devices or by training to the 'Quiet' command.

Training to the 'quiet' command

The goal is for the dog to respond to a 'quiet' command when it is barking. This can be accomplished by watching for every time that the dog barks and immediately saying 'quiet!' after the first vocalisation (even if it is just a faint woof), calling the dog, and requesting a sit–stay. Only if the dog sits quietly should a food or toy reward be given. The 'quiet' command and reward process should then be repeated but the dog should be quiet for a few seconds longer each time before the reward is given. Timing is critical in this training as the dog must learn that being quiet (not barking) is the reason for the reward. Shaping is also extremely important and the dog should be required to sit quietly for longer and longer periods before the reward is given.

If the pet ignores the 'quiet' command, the owner should immediately provide a loud aversive stimulus (shake can, foghorn), that is startling enough to stop the barking but not strong enough that it causes it to be reluctant to approach the owner when called.

This technique will not completely eliminate barking. This is important as most owners want to decrease excessive barking and have some verbal control over their pet's vocalisations without preventing it from alerting them when it hears something unusual.

A quick grasp of the muzzle accompanied by a verbal correction may be successful for some owners in interrupting barking and teaching the 'quiet' command if the pet is young and submissive. Releasing the grasp as soon as the dog is quiet is the reward (negative reinforcement) but a food or toy (positive reinforcement) can also be given. If the muzzle grasp is not immediately effective or leads to any sign of anxiety or fear it should be discontinued and alternative techniques used. This approach may be dangerous and should not be tried if the dog is aggressive, dominant or the owner does not have very good control.

Owners that utilise halter training can quickly train the dog to the 'quiet' command by pulling upward on the leash and saying 'Quiet!' each time the dog barks (Fig. 5.5). Release of the leash provides negative reinforcement but food or toys (positive reinforcement) may also be provided.

Case Example

Mr Ed was a 2-year-old neutered male Shetland Sheepdog that barked at virtually any person or pet who approached the property. The owners lived in a townhouse development and the neighbours had recently lodged a complaint. The barking would continue until the person or pet was out of sight or until they came inside and Mr Ed had a chance to greet the visitor. The only way that the owners could stop the barking was to get Mr Ed's tug toy and initiate play. Although the barking was primarily a form of territorial alerting, Mr Ed was not exhibiting any aggression and

seemed more interested in meeting the visitor than in chasing him or her away. Barking only ceased when Mr Ed was rewarded (by the owner's greeting or the arrival of the visitor) or when the stimulus was removed (the visitor or animal was out of sight).

The owner began some basic obedience reward training, but although Mr Ed became much more responsive to commands, the owner was unable verbally to interrupt the barking or train Mr Ed to the 'quiet' command. Mr Ed was then halter-trained and whenever the owners were available to supervise, Mr Ed was left with a head halter and 10-foot remote leash attached. At the instant barking began, the owner would command 'quiet!' and pull on the leash, releasing it after Mr Ed became quiet. If Mr Ed remained quiet (training began with 5 seconds of quiet and was eventually extended to 30 seconds) he was rewarded. Within days, Mr Ed would stop barking on command. However, whenever the owners were out the neighbours would still complain about barking. As there was no way successfully to remove or reduce the sights and sounds that stimulated Mr Ed to bark, debarking surgery and bark-activated devices were discussed. Since the owners would be unable to keep Mr Ed if the barking persisted, surgical debarking was considered, but the owners first decided to test the effectiveness of the antibark devices. A collar-mounted product was chosen since the dog would bark throughout the house and Mr Ed would exhibit anxiety-induced barking if confined. An audible bark collar and an ultrasonic bark collar were both unsuccessful as they were inconsistent and not sufficiently aversive, but Mr Ed responded immediately to the use of a citronella spray collar. Whenever Mr Ed wore the collar, barking was suppressed.

Canine Hyperactivity and Unruliness

Although true hyperactivity disorders are very rare in dogs, hyperkinesis or Attention Deficit Disorder with or without hyperactivity (ADD or ADHD) can usually be diagnosed because of the paradoxical response to amphetamines. (See CNS stimulants at the end of Chapter 4 for details). Most overactive dogs are either genetically predisposed to high levels of energy and activity or have been inadvertently rewarded. Young dogs are generally more playful and active than adults, so that some activity problems may improve as a puppy ages.

Unruliness tends to be a catch-all phrase for dogs that the owners cannot get under control. In addition to the overactive dog, many of the behaviours discussed elsewhere in this text (jumping up, nipping and biting, destructiveness, digging, and some forms of barking) are examples of unruly behaviours that are bothersome for owners. Running away, chasing cars, refusal to come when called and stealing items are also common owner complaints. Obedience training, leash control, head halter training, and other techniques designed to give owners more control over their dogs are required to correct these problems. However, there are great genetic differences between individuals so that training techniques may need to be adjusted to suit the individual.

Diagnosis and Prognosis

Dogs with true hyperactivity disorders exhibit a paradoxical response to treatment with amphetamines. Unlike the CNS stimulation that these drugs produce in 'normal' animals, dogs with hyperactivity disorders become calmer and less active when treated with these drugs. Dogs with hyperkinesis may exhibit overactivity, lack of trainability, aggressive displays and failure to calm down in neutral environments. In suspected cases of hyperkinesis, dogs should be admitted to the veterinary hospital and baseline heart rate, respiratory rate, and activity level should be recorded. The diagnosis can be confirmed by administering 0.2–0.5 mg/kg of dextroamphetamine orally and then observing every 30 minutes for 1 to 2 hours. Dogs with hyperkinesis become calmer and have lowered heart and respiratory rates.

For those cases where a hyperactivity disorder is not the cause, the prognosis will be based on the 'ultimate cause' of the overactivity. Those cases that have been inadvertently rewarded by the owners can usually be improved with behavioural modification techniques, while those with an innately high energy levels and little opportunity to exercise may be much more difficult to resolve.

Management

Treatment of unruliness and hyperactivity must be tailored to the individual pet. The role of genetics, the owner's response to the pet's behaviour, and the amount of previous training (and its responsiveness to training) are all factors in both the diagnosis and the development of an appropriate treatment regimen. The most critical aspect of preventing, controlling or eliminating these types of problems is to identify and address the motivation or underlying cause for the behaviour. Problem situations are likely to occur when the need for exercise, proper social interaction and control are neglected.

Prevention

Dogs, especially puppies and growing dogs, should be provided with appropriate and sufficient amounts of play and exercise to meet the individual's needs (Fig. 5.7). Owners must give no attention and completely ignore their dogs when the pets are exhibiting hyperactive behaviours. Ignoring, walking away and shutting the door or locking up the puppy would be preferable to providing attention. All rewards (play, food, attention) should only be given for calmness and obedience. Since immediately providing a play period or exercise when the pet is acting in an unruly or overactive fashion may reward the behaviour, it is best to apply some distraction that will quieten it for at least 10 seconds prior to engaging it in some form of play or exercise. Head halter training should be considered for dogs that are difficult to manage.

Case Example

Dennis was an 11-month-old 4 kg Toy Poodle, that the owner could never calm down and which would jump from the ground into his owner's arms when he wanted attention. The owner complied by patting Dennis, carrying him around for a few minutes, and sometimes playing ball or giving Dennis a few treats when he was put back down. During the behaviour consulation, Dennis was placed on the office floor but barked excessively, ran back and forth to the door, or jumped on to the owner's lap. He was a very active and energetic young dog. During the course of the consultation the owner was advised to ignore Dennis and a long 10-foot leash was left attached to his body harness. Each time Dennis jumped on the owner's lap or began to bark, an ultrasonic training device, a water rifle or a tug on the leash was used to deter the behaviour. Remote punishment techniques were utilised so that the aversive stimulus was used to interrupt the behaviour (which it did). After several interceptive distrac-

MANAGEMENT OF THE OVERACTIVE DOG	
Method	**Comments**
Exercise	Provide vigorous exercise and play periods to meet the dog's needs for activity and attention. Attempt to provide exercise appropriate to the individual. (Sledge pulling, retrieving)
Rewards	Withhold all rewards except for quiet, calmness and responsiveness to training commands
Extinction	Owner must ensure that attention, rewards, and play are never given on demand. This only serves to reward excitable and pushy behaviour. Ignoring, walking away, or locking up and isolating the dog until it is calm may be successful in some cases. With successful training techniques (*below*), the dog may in time be able to be distracted or calmed with commands
Obedience training	Train calmness and obedience. Slowly extend quiet time during training. Excitable pets may do better in low distraction, quiet environments or even with private lessons during initial training, then moving to group situations. Consider providing an exercise period before training sessions
Punishment/distraction	For dogs that are over active or excitable this approach is seldom successful. It may be possible, in some cases, to identify a device or product that can be used to distract the dog or interrupt the behaviour, so that calmness can be trained. Ultrasonic, audible alarms or a water rifle may be appropriate. If the behaviour is preceded by barking, antibark collars may provide interruption and distraction at the outset
Training devices	No-pull halters, head halters and long leashes are particularly useful in gaining control over exuberant or hard-to-control dogs. Halter devices may actually serve to control and calm some dogs as soon as they are applied (Fig. 5.5)
Drug therapy	Hyperkinetic dogs may respond to amphetamines. Antianxiety drugs and sedatives may occasionally be helpful to gain control during initial training but also interfere with learning. Antidepressants may be useful when high levels of activity are due to anxiety or compulsive disorders

Fig. 5.7 Management of the overactive dog.

tions and 30 minutes of the owner's ignoring Dennis by avoiding eye contact and pulling or stepping on the leash when he tried to jump on the owner's lap, Dennis lay down by the owner's feet and relaxed or slept for the next 30 minutes.

Ignoring and withdrawing all attention and rewards for demanding and excitable behaviour and using interruption techniques were successful in controlling Dennis's unruly behaviour. At home, the owner left a long leash attached, continued to ignore all demanding behaviours, and used interruption devices to deter Dennis. Additional play and exercise periods were provided but only when Dennis was calm and non-demanding. The owner took Dennis to obedience classes where he was too distracted and excitable to respond. The trainer suggested a few private lessons in a quiet environment and Dennis improved considerably, but continued to remain a high-energy, demanding, excitable dog.

Feline Vocalisation

Vocalisation is more common in the Siamese breed but can occur in virtually any cat. In addition to the genetic predisposition of some cats to vocalise, cats may howl and cry for resources, such as social contact, attention or food. Since cats are nocturnal by nature, it is not uncommon to have complaints of nocturnal vocalisation which may either be a form of normal play and communication or attention-demanding behaviour.

Diagnosis and Prognosis

Except in the Siamese, where the behaviour can be highly innate and unrelated to specific stimuli, the prognosis is moderately good for successful correction, provided the owner identifies and treats those factors that are initiating or reinforcing the problem. Knowing the time (nocturnal versus daytime) and situations in which the problem occurs are helpful in making the diagnosis. For diagnosis and treatment, the owner's response to the cat's vocalisation must be determined. Cats placed on weight-loss diets may occasionally vocalise as a demand for food.

Management

The guidelines are as follows:

- Identify the owner's response to the cat's vocalisation and remove any reinforcement (e.g. attention, food, affection, allowing outdoors).

- Identify the stimulus for the cat's vocalisation and limit or minimise access.
- Use remote punishment during vocalisation (water rifle, compressed air device, audible or ultrasonic alarm).
- Provide for all the cat's needs. For nocturnal vocalisation provide play, activity and exercise throughout the evening. Sometimes, obtaining a second playful cat can provide an additional outlet for play. Providing food so that it is available just before bedtime and through the night may also be useful for some cats.
- Cats on weight reduction diets that constantly demand and howl for food should be fed high-bulk diets.
- Drug therapy (benzodiazepines or antihistamines) may be helpful for a few nights to help readjust the cat's day/night sleep schedule.

Prevention

Providing sufficient play and exercise during the daytime and evening will help provide the cat with sufficient attention and may help get it on to a schedule so that it sleeps through the night. Never reward vocalisation by allowing the cat outdoors or providing food, attention or play on demand.

Case Example

Jethro was a 3-year-old neutered male Siamese cat that had always been excessively vocal. Whenever Jethro cried out, the owners tried to determine what Jethro might want so that they could give it to him. Since providing food was the only technique that consistently stopped vocalisation the owners assumed that the cat was constantly hungry.

At the time of consultation, Jethro was 7 kg. He had recently been placed on a diet by the referring veterinarian and the vocalisation problem had further escalated. Rather than buy an expensive prescription food, the owners had merely cut back dramatically on the amount being fed. Because of the diet, Jethro was indeed howling for food. In addition, howling for food was a conditioned behaviour, because the owners had consistently rewarded the behaviour. It is likely that the initial howling was merely the typical overvocalisation of some Siamese cats.

The first step in correction was to satisfy the cat's needs by changing to a high-bulk diet. Jethro was provided with multiple small meals of this diet whenever the owner was home but never on demand. When the owner was out, food was not provided. Whenever Jethro approached the owners and began to vocalise, he was sprayed with a can of compressed air. Whenever Jethro approached the owners and did not vocalise, a catnip treat, affection, interactive play, or a play toy was provided. Although Jethro continued to vocalise, excessively, this was dramatically reduced after only a few days and could be easily interrupted with the compressed air.

Further Reading

Beaver, B. V. (1981) Modifying a cat's behaviour. *Veterinary Medicine Small Animal Clinics*, **76**, 1281–1283.

Beaver, B. V. (1992) *Feline Behaviour: A guide for veterinarians*. W. B. Saunders: Philadelphia, PA.

Campbell, W. E. (1992) *Behaviour Problems in Dogs*. American Veterinary Publications Inc.: Goleta, CA

Coppinger, R. and Feinstein, M. (1991) 'Hark! Hark! The dogs do bark ...' and bark and bark. *Smithsonian*, **21**(10), 119–129.

Hart, B. L. and Hart, L. A. (1984) Selecting the best companion animal: breed and gender specific profiles. In: *The Pet Connection: Its influence on our health and quality of life*. pp. 180–193, Anderson, R. K., Hart, B. L. and Hart, L. A. (eds). University of Minnesota Press: Minneapolis, MN.

Hunthausen, W., and Landsberg, G. (1995) *A Practitioner's Guide to Pet Behaviour Counseling*. AAHA: Denver, CO.

Jones, R. D. (1987) Use of thioridazine in the treatment of aberrant motor behaviour in a dog. *Journal of the American Veterinary Medical Association*, **191**(1), 89–90.

Juarbe-Diaz, S. V. and Houpt, K. A. (1996) Comparison of two antibarking collars for treatment of nuisance barking. *J Am Anim Hosp Assoc* **5**(32), 231–235.

Luescher, A. U. (1993) Hyperkinesis in dogs: six case reports. *Canadian Veterinary Journal*, **34**, 368–370.

Mathews, S. L. (1984) Eliminating barking as an attention-getting device. *Canine Practice*, **11**(1), 6–9.

Overall, K. A. (1992) Recognition, diagnosis, and management of obsessive compulsive disorders. Part 3: A rational approach. *Canine Practice*, **17**(4), 39–43.

Voith, V. L. and Borchelt, P. L. (1987) Advice for clients with overactive dogs. *Veterinary Technician*, September, 25–28.

6

Elimination Behaviour Problems

Canine Inappropriate Elimination

The main purpose of micturition and defecation for the young puppy is to rid the body of wastes. Adult canine elimination behaviour can serve a number of additional functions including communication of information about sexual status, individual identity and territories, and, possibly, social rank. It may also occur in young or adult dogs in a variety of situations as a component of submissive responses, fear, separation anxiety and excitement.

At about 3 weeks of age, most puppies have begun eliminating away from the nesting area on their own. By 5 weeks of age, a general area for elimination is chosen and by 9 weeks the area chosen for elimination becomes more specific. The rationale underlying housetraining strategies involves taking advantage of the dog's innate proclivity to avoid eliminating in its den area and combining this inclination with operant and classical conditioning.

This tendency to keep the home area clean of wastes can be overcome in a number of circumstances. For instance, the dog that is kennelled for long periods has to learn to defecate in the kennel environment. Puppies that are confined to cages or crates for long periods of time will soil their living areas if not given the opportunity to relieve themselves in more appropriate locales. Also, dogs with some medical problems may be unable to control their elimination for entirely physiological reasons. It has been said that some breeds are resistant to housetraining. This section will evaluate elimination problems with a behavioural basis.

Prevention: Housetraining

Most dogs are house pets, so it is very important that they are quickly and dependably housetrained. Housetraining is a simple process but one that must be taught and reinforced in any neophyte owner. Many pets are given up or destroyed because they fail to learn this lesson early and continue to soil their owners' homes.

Owners must understand and work with the dog's natural elimination patterns rather than waiting for the dog to eliminate in inappropriate areas and punishing it. Reward training is far superior to punishment as a means of housetraining. Yet, most owners are quick to punish inappropriate elimination without giving proper credit when a puppy does what is wanted. It is important for dog owners to understand that teaching a dog the correct location for elimination, through repetition and reward, is far more practical than trying to punish it at each of the thousands of locations where it might try to eliminate indoors.

Initially, young puppies (7–8 weeks of age) should be taken outside to eliminate as often as is practical (ideally once an hour when the puppy is awake). Within a short time, the owner will learn to predict the interval at which the puppy actually needs to be taken outdoors. The pet should also be taken outside to the desired area for elimination after eating, drinking, playing and sleeping. A direct route to an easily accessible outdoor location works best. Using the same area allows odours to accumulate and should increase the likelihood that the puppy will return to eliminate there again. If puppies are fed on a regular schedule, rather than *ad libitum*, they also tend to develop very regular elimination habits. The puppy should be praised lavishly or given a small food reward as soon as it eliminates in the appropriate place. If the puppy wants to play or would like to go back indoors, these can also be used to reward the dog as soon as it has completed elimination. Do not wait until the puppy is back indoors to give it a food reward, as this teaches the puppy to anticipate rewards on returning to the home (and not for elimination). By pairing a cue or command with each elimination and then providing the reward, many dogs learn the concept of elimination on command.

Certainly, if the owner views the pet eliminating or beginning to eliminate in an inappropriate location, it should be immediately interrupted with a sharp 'No!'. An appropriately timed verbal correction is helpful, but by itself will not ensure that the pet will refrain from further elimination indoors. Ideally, if the puppy is properly supervised, the owner should soon learn to identify pre-elimination signs (sniffing, squatting, sneaking away) or may be able to anticipate and predict when the puppy needs to eliminate so that punishment is not necessary. In this way the owner can interrupt the puppy before elimination begins and direct it to the appropriate location (where praise and reward can be given for success).

Harsh punishment in the act may teach the dog to:

● Avoid further elimination in that location
● Avoid further elimination in that location when the owner is present
● Avoid all elimination in the presence of the owner

Punishment should **only** be considered if the owner observes the puppy begin to eliminate indoors. A water rifle, shake can or an audible or ultrasonic trainer is preferable to physical techniques or even verbal reprimands, since it is less likely to lead to fear of the owner. When choosing an aversive stimulus for training, the owner must always take the pet's temperament into consideration. In addition, if the owner can remain out of sight while administering punishment the pet may learn to stop eliminating in the area whether the owner is present or not (see Fig. 6.1). Any correction that results in an overly fearful response should never be used, no matter how mild it may seem. Should the pet eliminate in an indoor location with no unpleasant consequence, the dog is likely to return to that location for further elimination. Any area in the home where the puppy has eliminated must be thoroughly cleaned and treated with an odour counteractant to prevent it from returning and soiling again.

Basic housetraining is a combination of reward (for elimination in appropriate areas), preventing elimination in inappropriate locations, identifying pre-elimination signs or anticipating elimination times and directing the pet to the appropriate location, and punishment if the pet is observed eliminating or beginning to eliminate in an inappropriate location. For successful application of these techniques, it is essential that the dog is supervised at all times when the owner is available. Some owners are able to follow and watch their dogs at all times during training, but in most cases this is physically impractical. If the owner cannot stop the pet from wandering away or 'sneaking off', it can be helpful to leave a light, long leash attached to the puppy, either held by the owner or tied to a nearby object. Barricades and strategically closed doors can also be used to keep the puppy in sight. When the dog cannot be supervised, it should be prevented from eliminating in inappropriate locations by keeping it in its crate, room, or run (see *cage training techniques*).

Owners who must leave their dogs for periods longer than those for which they can control elimination will have to consider an outdoor run, or leave the dog in a room or pen with papers on the floor. At first the entire floor (other than the dog's feeding and bedding area) may need to be covered with paper, but the area can gradually be made smaller as the dog begins to use specific locations. Dogs that have been conditioned to eliminate on paper may have a hard time understanding that outdoor elimination is also acceptable.

CANINE HOUSETRAINING IN BRIEF

Teach the puppy where to go by rewarding elimination at the appropriate location. As soon as the puppy eliminates give a social or food reward

Use a direct route to a single convenient area outdoors. The odour and location can then be used to stimulate further elimination at the site

Watch for pre-elimination signals, such as sniffing and circling, and take the puppy to its location immediately when they are observed

Whenever the puppy cannot be closely supervised, it should be confined

The young puppy should initially be taken out to eliminate every hour. When the owner notes that it is not eliminating every hour, the interval between outings can gradually be increased. The goal is to learn to anticipate or predict when the puppy needs to eliminate and to take it to its elimination spot before elimination begins. The pet should also be taken out shortly after eating, drinking, waking and playing, and prior to confinement

Punishment: A sharp, mildly startling verbal reprimand during the act of eliminating in an undesirable area is the only punishment permitted

Any area in the home where the pet eliminates must be thoroughly cleaned and treated with an odour counteractant

Fig. 6.1 The basics of housetraining dogs.

Housesoiling Problems

There are many reasons why a pet might eliminate in the home. The most common reason for housesoiling by young dogs is inadequate training, excitement urination and submissive urination. During adulthood, inappropriate elimination in the home can result from marking and from separation anxiety. Medical problems can occur at any age, but are more likely to be seen in the older pet. Occasionally, you may see a housesoiling problem that occurs spontaneously and may be due to situations where there has been an abrupt change in the owner's schedule, failure by the owner to allow the pet access to the elimination area in a timely fashion, or change in the diet or feeding schedule. It is not uncommon for a dog to develop strong location or surface preferences for eliminating within the home when the problem has been allowed to persist.

Diagnosis and Prognosis

An elimination behaviour problem is diagnosed when a dog eliminates in inappropriate places despite adequate opportunities to use desired elimination areas. A thorough physical examination and laboratory profile should be done to ensure that there is not a physiological reason for the problem (Figs. 6.2 and 6.3). The initial assessment for inappropriate urination should include at least a physical examination, urinalysis and a determination of water consumption and frequency of urination. For inappropriate defecation, the initial assessment should include at least a physical faecal sedimentation test (ova and parasites), an evaluation of stool consistency and frequency, and an assessment of the pet's appetite and eating habits. The pet's age, and the results of the physical examination and laboratory tests may dictate the need for more specialised or intensive testing (e.g. endocrine tests, radiography, ultrasonography, endoscopy, biopsy).

For dogs with elimination problems of a behavioural nature, the prognosis for a full recovery is generally good. For those dogs with physiological reasons for their problems, the prognosis varies with the ultimate diagnosis and chances for curing or managing the underlying medical problems (Fig. 6.4).

Discerning the duration of the housesoiling, how often the problem occurs, the number of areas soiled and the mental state of the pet is pertinent to

MEDICAL CAUSES OF INAPPROPRIATE ELIMINATION

Housesoiling (urine)

Conditions causing polyuria (diabetes, renal disease, hyperadrenocorticism, pyometra, hepatic disease)

Conditions causing pollakiuria (cystitis, calculi, prostatitis, tumours)

Conditions causing incontinence (neurological, urethral incontinence)

Conditions affecting locomotion (arthritis, disc disease)

Cognitive dysfunction

Housesoiling (faeces)

Conditions causing increased frequency/urge (colitis)

Conditions causing soft stools/poor control

Conditions causing painful or difficult defecation (anal sacaulitis, obstipation, constipation)

Conditions causing incontinence (neurological)

Conditions affecting locomotion, positioning (arthritis, hip dysplasia)

Cognitive dysfunction

Fig. 6.2 Medical conditions that might cause or contribute to inappropriate elimination habits.

LABORATORY TESTS FOR ELIMINATION PROBLEMS

Urination Problem

Urinalysis

Complete blood count

Creatinine/urea/glucose

Alanine transaminase, calcium, phosphorus

Serum alkaline phosphatase

Urine creatinine:cortisol ratio or dexamethasone suppression if indicated

Water consumption

Water deprivation test if indicated

Defecation Problem

Faecal sedimentation/saline smear

Complete blood count

Trypsin-like immunoreactivity

Serum alanine transaminase

Amylase/lipase

Serum alkaline phosphatase

Bile acids

Urinalysis

Thyroid evaluation (if indicated)

Fig. 6.3 Laboratory tests that might be indicated for dogs with elimination problems.

DIFFERENTIAL DIAGNOSIS FOR HOUSESOILING

Inadequate or inappropriate training

Submissive urination

Excitement urination

Marking

Separation anxiety

Medical problems

Management-related problems

Undesirable location or surface preferences

FIG. 6.4 Differential diagnosis for housesoiling.

determining the prognosis for successful treatment of a dog that is housesoiling. The prognosis is good for a pet with no cognitive problems and no untreatable medical conditions, and if the problem is of short duration, occurring infrequently in a limited number of areas in the home. The prognosis is also improved if the pet has already been accustomed to a crate or confinement room and the owner is available throughout the day to take the pet outdoors frequently to eliminate.

Management

This section will discuss the management for housesoiling for those dogs with behavioural elimination problems only. Behavioural modification is used for dogs that choose to relieve themselves in inappropriate locations. Dogs that do this have most likely developed the pattern because of self-reward or the owner's lack of intervention. Dogs 'self-reward' when they relieve themselves and do not perceive that the area was inappropriate. They then return to that area on future occasions. Thus, the key to effective housetraining is constant supervision. This allows the owner to prevent inappropriate elimination, redirect the pet to more suitable locations, and to mildly correct the pet if it is observed while eliminating in an inappropriate location. The owner can then reinforce more acceptable behaviour with lavish praise when the dog eliminates in the designated area.

Feeding schedules should be regulated to improve owner control over the situation. Dogs that eat when they wish often need to relieve themselves at a variety of times throughout the day. Dogs that eat two or three scheduled meals each day often void in a very predictable manner. Feeding a low-residue diet may also be of benefit because the dog often has less urgency to defecate and produces less stool.

Owners must not allow dogs with elimination problems into areas they might soil unless the dog is supervised or the area is appropriately booby-trapped (e.g. motion-activated alarm). If the dog is not given the opportunity to make a mistake, the training aspect is greatly facilitated. Accordingly, the owners may elect to keep a long line or leash on the dog when it is wandering in this area so they can exert control. Should the pet begin to eliminate in an inappropriate location, the behaviour must be immediately interrupted with some form of aversion therapy (sharp tug on the lead, water gun, noise maker). The dog should then be taken immediately to an appropriate elimination area and praised when it eliminates there. A single elimination area should be selected outdoors so that residual urine and stool odour will stimulate further use of this area. Owners will get more adept at recognising when a pet is about to eliminate indoors as they consistently interrupt that behaviour. The dog will start to be 'anxious' and sneak away from the owner when it needs to eliminate. Thus, when the owners recognise these tell-tale signs, they should immediately take the dog to the preferred location, allow it to eliminate and praise it when it does so.

This technique is very labour-intensive and requires continual owner diligence and supervision. This will not be possible every moment of the day and is not an option for many owners who are not at home during the day. For those situations, the dog must be confined to an area where it will not eliminate, or do no harm if it does. Dogs will usually not eliminate if kept in a crate, pen or small room. Their den instinct deters them from eliminating in their 'nest'. Alternatively, the dog can be put in a papered room or given access to a 'doggy door'. For those dogs that eliminate only in few inappropriate areas, booby-trapping these areas with detectors, balloons set to pop when disturbed, or aversive tastes and smells may be sufficient to cause the pet to avoid entering these areas to eliminate. Food and water bowls placed at the sites of previous housesoiling may also prevent resoiling of the areas.

When an owner is uncertain which dog in the home has soiled the carpet, aspirin can be given to the dog suspected of inappropriate elimination (5 mg per 15–20 kg). The next patch of urine can then be blotted up with a paper towel and tested with ferric chloride for the presence of salicylate in the urine (turns burgundy).

When dogs have had elimination problems for a protracted period, owners will need to do some additional work. An odour neutraliser should be applied to all areas in the house where inappropriate elimination has taken place. This removes one of the cues that dogs use to select areas for future elimination. Owners that have punished their pets extensively for inappropriate elimination may find that they are now afraid to eliminate in front of them, regardless of location. Crate training is the best solution in this instance. The animal should be kept in the crate overnight, and taken outside on a long lead first thing in the morning. When it does eliminate, it should be praised and allowed to play off-lead. This procedure should not be rushed and owners need to be prepared to wait until the dog eliminates outside. However, if the owner cannot wait any longer, the dog should be returned to its crate and the exercise repeated every hour until it does eliminate. If the pet will not or cannot wait through the night to eliminate, it should not be confined to a crate. It must either be confined to a larger area (small pen or room) or the owner must get up during the night to take it outdoors.

The dog that eliminates in its crate poses special problems. In these troublesome cases, the owner must devise a way of monitoring the dog continually. This might involve monitoring the dog with video equipment or using bedwetting alarms. When the owner observes the characteristic signs that the dog is getting ready to eliminate, the dog should be immediately taken outside to relieve itself. Lavish praise should accompany this response. If the pet attempts to eliminate in its cage the owner might also consider using a distracting stimulus (whistle, water sprayer, audible alarm) to halt this behaviour. Withholding food and water to develop a controlled elimination schedule may also be helpful. Crates and cages are not the ideal training aid for all dogs. Since the purpose of the crate is to provide a safe, comfortable area for the dog to 'curl up and relax', it is not appropriate for dogs that are anxious about entering or staying in their cage. While this can be overcome with training techniques, it may be possible to confine these dogs to a small area such as a laundry room or kitchen where the dog is fed, or a bedroom where the dog sleeps.

This is summarised in Fig. 6.5

SUMMARY OF TREATMENT FOR CANINE HOUSESOILING

Treat or manage underlying medical problems

Reinforce elimination in the desired area

Control the pet's feeding schedule

Close supervision or confinement

Prevent resoiling
  Clean up all traces of odour
  Deny access to areas by moving furniture or closing doors
  Avoidance conditioning (booby traps)
  Move food and water bowls to previously soiled area

Punishment
  Interrupt inappropriate elimination with a mild correction
  Intensity and timing are important
  Avoid physical or delayed punishment

Fig. 6.5 Treatment protocol for housesoiling problems.

Submissive Urination

Submissive urination is a behaviour related to social status. Although this problem can be seen in dogs of any age, submissive urination is most commonly seen in puppies and young female dogs. It occurs when the pet is confronted with certain facial expressions, movements or body postures by a person that it perceives to be socially dominant or threatening. The pet urinates as it shows signs of submissive signalling. Submissive displays are typically used by subordinates to turn off dominant social threats.

Diagnosis and Prognosis

This problem occurs when a person approaches, reaches out, stands over or attempts to physically punish the dog. Stimuli that might trigger urination in submissive dogs include reaching for the dog, patting the dog on the head, excited talk, deep or harsh tone of voice, standing over the pet, maintained eye contact, and physical punishment or scolding. The pet voids urine as it shows signs of submissive signalling, such as ears laid back, horizontal retraction of the lips, avoidance of eye contact, and cowering. Some dogs will roll into a recumbent position on their sides or backs while urinating. The pet may be perfectly housebroken otherwise and may not have a history of having urinated inappropriately in the home. A urinalysis may be performed, but laboratory testing is usually not required unless the dog is also displaying signs suggestive of medical problems.

In young dogs with no concurrent medical problems, the prognosis is good, but when the problem persists into adulthood, resolution may be more difficult. Fortunately, most puppies outgrow these behaviours if the owners change their method of greeting in order to reduce dominant gestures or behaviours that tend to get the young dog excited.

Management

Provided physical problems (e.g. inadequate urethral sphincter tone, ectopic ureters) and medical contributing factors (e.g. cystitis) have been ruled out, the first step is to identify all initiating stimuli. Then, the owner must do whatever is necessary to discontinue these actions so that all urination-eliciting stimuli are removed. It is important that the owner and all visitors interact with the pet in a less dominant or threatening manner.

The pet should be allowed to approach the owner. Kneeling down and speaking softly rather than standing over the dog, and patting the chest instead of the head may help reduce submissive responses. Physical punishment and even the mildest verbal reprimands should be resolutely avoided. In fact, owners who attempt to punish the pet for urinating submissively will make things worse, since punishment tends to intensify fearful and submissive behaviour. When greeting a very submissive dog, the owner may initially need to ignore it completely at greeting, even to the extent of avoiding eye contact.

Counterconditioning can be very helpful in controlling submissive urination. Using this approach, the dog is taught to perform a behaviour that is not compatible with urinating, such as sitting for food or retrieving a toy when it greets someone. When the owner enters the home, the dog can often be distracted from urinating by offering a toy or treat and then encouraged to respond to a previously trained command. If it anticipates food or ball playing at each greeting, it is less likely to eliminate. Food alone will not correct submissive behaviour but is a useful tool. The desired response can be reinforced by shaping. The pet is given food initially on greeting, then only when it sits during greeting in a relaxed fashion and finally only when it sits and is petted.

Prevention

Submissive urination reflects a perceived inferior social status on the part of the pet. A very submissive dog can sometimes be identified with puppy aptitude testing (*see Chapter 2*). Although selection tests are not very specific in their assessment, dogs that are over-submissive or dominant can usually be identified. Advise owners to select puppies that fall between these extremes.

Submissive dogs require patience and confidence building. Obedience training that is based on positive reinforcement is an excellent way for owners to build a non-threatening rapport with their dogs. It is best to avoid stern verbal scoldings. If corrections are used, they should be extremely mild and should be tailored to the individual pet's temperament. Physical punishment should always be avoided.

Excitement Urination

This problem may appear similar to submissive urination, but accompanying submissive behaviours are less prominent or absent. The treatment is basically the same as for submissive urination. For excitement urination, those stimuli that initiate the behaviour should be avoided. During greetings, owners and guests should refrain from eye contact, and verbal or physical contact until the pet calms down. Greetings should be very low-key and words spoken in a low, calm tone. Counterconditioning, distraction techniques and drug therapy might be useful. Caution must be taken only to reward appropriate competing behaviours (e.g. sit up and beg, go lie on your mat, retrieving a ball). Inappropriate use or timing of rewards might further excite the dog and serve as a reward for the excitement urination.

The use of alpha-adrenergics (such as phenylpropanolamine) or a tricyclic antidepressant (such as imipramine) might also be considered as an adjunct to behavioural therapy to increase sphincter tone for refractory cases.

Marking

In most cases, this type of problem involves urinating on an upright object by an intact male. It is likely to occur on or near pheromones left by other dogs. The volume of urine voided is usually less than what is typically voided to empty the bladder.

Confirming the diagnosis involves associating specific territorial or anxiety-eliciting stimuli with the act. For example, the owner may have noted that immediately after barking at a stray dog or visitor in the yard, the pet went to the corner of a couch or side of a plant, lifted its leg and voided a small amount of urine. Anything that causes the pet to become anxious or thwarts a highly motivated behaviour may also trigger marking behaviour. For example, the dog that is denied access to the owner by a closed door inside the home or is unable to accompany the owner outdoors might urine mark indoors.

Consideration should be given to castrating the intact male, preventing exposure to stimuli that elicit urine marking and avoiding situations that make the pet anxious. Castration will eliminate male marking behaviour in over 50% of dogs and spaying is recommended for female dogs that mark during oestrus. Confining the pet so that it is unable to watch other dogs through windows in the home may be helpful. Urine residue must be removed from around doors, windows or other areas where stray dogs have been marking. A stake should be driven into an appropriate area of the garden where marking is permitted. The owner should give food rewards to reinforce marking at the stake and the dog should not be permitted to mark anywhere else. New upright objects that are brought into the home should not be placed on the floor until the pet is familiar with them.

Set-ups involving remote punishment may be attempted. An object, such as a suitcase or grocery sack, can be placed in an area where the owner can observe from out of sight. When the dog attempts to lift its leg to mark, the owner can provide remote punishment by setting off an electronic alarm or tossing a tin can containing pebbles near the pet. The aversive stimulus should be strong enough to stop the behaviour without causing fear and should not be associated with the owner's presence. During training, the owner should closely supervise the pet and confine it to a small area when it cannot be watched. If the male pet marks when another in the home is in oestrus, spaying the female may be helpful.

Separation Anxiety

When a dog has a very close relationship with its owner it may become anxious when it suddenly loses access to the owner. Situations such as changes in the owner's work schedule or returning to work after a long stay at home can lead to this type of problem. The dog with a separation anxiety problem may show signs of either increased activity and anxiety (pacing, restlessness, whining) or depression (lying around, reluctance to move or eat) as the owner prepares to leave. These behaviours occur as the pet becomes aware of certain cues that it associates with the owner's departure, such as picking up a briefcase, reaching for keys or putting on a coat. When the owner returns, the dog usually exhibits high levels of arousal and may show exaggerated greeting behaviours. Separation anxiety can also occur when the owner becomes involved in an activity or relationship that takes a significant amount of attention away from the dog at home. This can occur when there is a new baby or spouse in the home. The anxiety can become a driving force for excessive vocalisation, self-mutilation, destructive behaviour, or housesoiling. Anxiety-based problems, including separation anxiety, tend to occur with increased frequency and intensity in the geriatric pet dog population.

Treatment involves desensitisation to predeparture cues and gradually accustoming the dog to absences by the owner. If the owner can provide a dramatic increase in daily exercise, this will usually have a calming effect. Enriching the pet's environment (rubber toys stuffed with treats) or distractions (another pet, radio) may help, although some dogs experience such high anxiety that food and distractions are ignored. During the early stages of treatment, a small confinement area, a pet sitter or boarding may be necessary and general principles of housetraining should be followed. Drug therapy with benzodiazepines (clorazepate, alprazolam) or tricyclic antidepressants (amitriptyline, clomipramine) may be helpful when the anxiety is intense.

Urinary Incontinence

There are numerous medical and behavioural causes of incontinence. At the very least a urinalysis should be performed on all incontinent dogs, but additional tests may also be required depending on the history and physical examination. When the urination is always in response to specific stimuli, as might be seen in the case of submissive or excitement urination, additional testing might not be required.

However, when there are no recognisable stimuli, such as the dog that exhibits incontinence while relaxing on the owner's bed, walking, or during sleep (enuresis) a thorough medical assessment is required. In some cases, response to drug therapy might be an acceptable diagnostic aid when all laboratory tests are normal. For example, incontinent spayed female adult dogs may respond to therapy with diethyl-stilboestrol.

Examples of medical causes of incontinence are structural abnormalities (ectopic ureters), infections (bacterial cystitis), tumours (transitional cell tumours), neurodegenerative disorders, trauma, an atonic bladder (post-obstruction), hormone-responsive incontinence, partial obstruction (urethral calculi) and conditions causing increased urine volume (diabetes insipidus).

Drugs that might be useful in the control of incontinence include alpha-adrenergics (ephedrine, phenylpropanolamine), hormones (stilboestrol, testosterone), and tricyclic antidepressants (e.g. imipramine) and deprenyl (in elderly dogs).

Miscellaneous Cause of Housesoiling Problems

There are a variety of miscellaneous, unrelated factors that can lead to housesoiling. Changing the time when the pet is fed such that the dog has to eliminate when no one will be available to let it out (moving the meal closer to bedtime or confinement) can lead to housesoiling. Inappropriate punishment that results in fear of the owner can make the dog reluctant to approach the owner to signal when it needs to go outdoors to eliminate. A frightening incident that occurred in the area where the pet eliminates (abuse by a neighbour, severe thunderstorm) or intolerance of inclement weather (rain, wind, snow) may make the dog hesitant to go outdoors and may result in it eliminating indoors. Failure to allow the dog to eliminate just prior to the time it is confined can cause a well house-trained pet suddenly to urinate or defecate indoors. For example, if the owner was not paying attention when the dog was let out into the garden to eliminate just prior to bedtime so that the dog spent the allotted time chasing rabbits instead of eliminating, it is likely that the dog will eliminate in the home during the night.

Case Examples

Case 1

Problem Herman, a 4-month-old Dachshund puppy was eliminating in its cage and throughout the house (but never in the presence of the owner).

History The puppy would eliminate outdoors in the yard and the owner would give appropriate rewards. The puppy would not eliminate indoors as long as a family member was closely supervising, but would occasionally sneak away and eliminate in another room. When the owners found the soiled area, they would immediately take the puppy to the spot, put its nose in the stools or urine and verbally reprimand it. The puppy had also recently begun to eat its own stool. At night Herman slept in the bedroom with the owners and on some mornings the owners would find that he had gone downstairs to eliminate at some point during the night. On weekdays, Herman was left in a cage in the laundry room, from about 8:30 a.m. to 4 p.m. and on most days the owner would find urine or stool in the cage. Whenever the owners found urine or stool in the cage, they would yell at the puppy and put it outdoors in the yard where it was ignored for 30 minutes. The owners were convinced that Herman knew that he was misbehaving because he would act guilty and fearful whenever they arrived home and found that he had eliminated in an inappropriate location.

Diagnosis The puppy had been forced to eliminate in its cage because it was being left for 7½ hours (too long for the puppy to control itself). It had learned that it was safe to eliminate in other rooms provided the owner was not in view. The puppy seemed to act guiltily only because it had learned that it would get abused each time the owner found a soiled area. It was explained to the owners that if the puppy is to understand that the punishment is for elimination, it can only make this association if it receives the unpleasant consequences during elimination. Although it was unlikely that the puppy was eating its stools because the owners were forcing its mouth into the soiled areas, this practice was irrational and unsuccessful.

Management Since it was necessary to provide the puppy with an opportunity to eliminate within 4–5 hours, the owners either had to arrange to allow the puppy outdoors a few hours earlier or provide him with an elimination area while they were out. The owners chose to arrange for the dog to have an additional walk at lunch hour. Since the owners wished to continue to confine the puppy to its crate while out, a cage training guide was provided. The cage was relocated to the corner of the bedroom where the puppy normally slept, and the door was kept closed so that the puppy could not wander downstairs at night. The owners continued to reward the puppy for outdoor elimination and provided diligent supervision when indoors. With the additional walk at lunch hour and the relocation of the cage, the problem was immediately corrected and by 7 months of age the owners attempted to cut out the noon walk. Although the puppy no longer eliminated when left in the cage from 8.30 to 4, after further consultation the noon time walks were resumed to ensure that the puppy had ample opportunity to exercise and eliminate outdoors.

Case 2

Problem An 11-month-old Bichon Frisé would eliminate indoors whenever the owner did not supervise the dog. Even if the dog had been outdoors recently it might sneak away to eliminate. When the owners were away from home, the dog was left in the kitchen where it eliminated on paper. While the owners were outdoors with the dog, it would not eliminate in their presence.

Diagnosis During the first 2 months of ownership the owners would supervise the dog and scream or hit it when it began to eliminate indoors. They would then throw the dog outdoors unsupervised. On occasion, the dog had managed to sneak away from the owners and eliminate in other rooms. The dog had learned to eliminate indoors on paper and had never learned where it was supposed to eliminate. Because punishment had been used without rewards, the dog was fearful of eliminating in the owners' presence regardless of whether it was indoors or out.

Management The first step was to teach the dog that it would receive valuable rewards (food treats, ball playing) whenever it eliminated outdoors. This would be extremely difficult and time-consuming since the

dog was fearful of eliminating in the owners' presence. Rather than send the dog outdoors at each scheduled elimination time, the owners were instructed to go outdoors with the dog until it eliminated (regardless of how long it took). On the first occasion, after a long walk and a half hour of play the dog would not eliminate so the owners returned indoors and continued to supervise the dog diligently. An hour later, the dog was taken out again to its favourite elimination site and with the owner several yards away the dog finally eliminated. As the dog eliminated the owner utilised soft cue words ('Go pee') and rewarded the dog with a piece of meat and a game of fetch. When indoors the dog was constantly supervised or left in the kitchen with paper. The only setbacks were when the dog sneaked away from the owners. This problem was resolved by leaving a 10-foot remote leash attached to the dog so that it could be kept in sight and directed quickly outdoors when pre-elimination signs were seen. At each scheduled elimination time the owner took the dog outdoors and used a 'Go pee' command followed by a food reward and game of fetch whenever the dog complied. In time the dog responded quite well to elimination on command and was not reluctant to eliminate in front of the owners. As outdoor supervised elimination became more successful, indoor paper elimination became less and less frequent.

Case 3

Problem Maggie was a 6-month-old Labrador Retriever that squatted and urinated whenever the owners reached to pet her as they entered the home. If their hands were full so that they could not pet her when she was greeted, the urination did not occur.

Management The owners were told to avoid reaching for her at greeting during the first week of training. Maggie was first taught to sit in response to happy, verbal commands and hand signal cues using food lures. She learned to sit on command by the end of the first week. At that time, the owners were instructed to begin counterconditioning exercises. They were told to wait to start the exercises until she had calmed down following their arrival. Then, they would ask her to do several sits for food rewards in the family room. Next, they moved the exercises to the front door. During the last segment of the conditioning exercises, the owners exited through the door, immediately returned and asked her to sit for a food reward. This was repeated six more times. The exercise was performed once or twice daily until the end of the second week. Each time the pet took the food, the owner calmly patted her with the other hand. During the third week, the owners started the exercises closer and closer to their initial arrival. By the end of the third week they could enter, ask her to sit and pat her without eliciting submissive urination. The food that was given for sitting when greeted was gradually withdrawn.

Feline Inappropriate Elimination

Housesoiling is the most common behaviour problem for which cat owners seek assistance. Undoubtedly, it is also a major reason why some cats become abandoned or eventually killed.

Housesoiling in cats can be due to inappropriate urination or defecation or to spraying. Spraying is a marking behaviour during which urine is sprayed on a vertical object. The incidence increases from 25% in single-cat households to 100% in households with more than 10 cats. Intact males or females in heat are the individuals most likely to engage in spraying.

Litterbox Training

Litterbox training is relatively simple as long as the cat is provided with an acceptable cat litter that is cleaned regularly and placed in an appropriate location. Frequently changing brands of litter and using litter with a strong, fragrant odour should probably be avoided. Sandy, clumping types of litter may be easier to keep clean and seem to be preferred by most cats. When the pet is first brought into the home, it should be closely supervised or confined to one room with its litterbox until the habit of using the box is well established. This may take a few days or weeks.

The box should be placed in a relatively quiet area that provides some privacy. If children or other pets might bother the cat, the box can be placed on an elevated platform or in a room where the only access is through a small cat door. Care should be taken in locating the cat litter appropriately. It should not be placed in the same area where the cat's meals are served and not in an area likely to be invaded by the family dog. Other areas that might deter some cats could be adjacent to a furnace, radiator, doorway, washing machine, toilet or shower stall.

Diagnosis

Successful management of the cat with elimination problems requires a correct diagnosis of the situation. This includes properly differentiating between the cat that sprays vertical surfaces and those that urinate or defecate inappropriately on horizontal surfaces (Fig. 6.6).

Inappropriate elimination on horizontal surfaces is generally caused either by factors that make using the litterbox or location unacceptable (Fig. 6.7) or by factors that make inappropriate areas more acceptable through the formation of surface or location preferences.

Numerous medical problems can contribute to inappropriate elimination, such as lower urinary tract disorders, diarrhoea, arthritis, renal failure, diabetes and constipation. A thorough physical examination and appropriate laboratory tests should be performed on all suspect cats. For inappropriate elimination a physical examination, urinalysis and assessing of water intake and urine frequency should be the minimum work-up. Since some feline urinary conditions (e.g. feline interstitial cystitis) may lead to intermittent or transient dysuria, repeat urinalyses and more intensive diagnostics may need to be performed. These conditions should be suspected in cats that appear to urinate more frequently, appear uncomfortable during urination, or have a history of haematuria

| TYPES OF FELINE HOUSESOILING ||
Spraying	Inappropriate Elimination
Marking behaviour	Elimination behaviour
Most common in intact males and females in heat	Males or females
Adults	Any age
Vertical surfaces	Horizontal surfaces
Urine	Urine and stool
Doors, windows, new objects	Eliminate in variety of areas

FIG. 6.6 Comparison between spraying and inappropriate elimination in cats.

POSSIBLE CAUSES OF INAPPROPRIATE ELIMINATION	
Litterbox aversion	Aversive odour (deodorant, ammonia) Box not cleaned frequently enough Pain/Medical (Feline lower urinary tract disease (FLUTD), constipation, diarrhoea) Unacceptable litter Unacceptable box (too small, sides too high, covered) Disciplined or frightened in the box
Location aversion	Too much traffic Traumatic/fearful experience in the area
Location preference	Another area is more appealing to the cat
Surface preference	Another surface is more appealing than the litter substrate
Anxiety	Owner absence, high cat density, moving, new furniture, inappropriate punishment, teasing, household changes, remodelling in the home
Need for privacy	Nervous or fearful pet
Geriatric problems	Senility, arthritis, polyuria/polydypsia, constipation

FIG. 6.7 Causes of inappropriate elimination in cats.

(with or without crystalluria or bacteriuria). Additional diagnostic tests (e.g., radiography, ultrasonography, endoscopy, biopsy) may also be necessary depending on the results of the preliminary examination. For inappropriate defecation, a physical examination, and stool evaluation, along with an evaluation of eating, drinking and elimination habits would be the minimal work-up. In geriatric cats (and if indicated by the history or urine results) a blood profile including T_4 should also be performed.

The diagnosis can get more complicated in the multi-cat household since it may not be immediately evident which cat is soiling the home. Separation may be necessary to find the culprit. Another method is to give fluorescein orally (0.5 ml of a 10% solution) or by injection (0.3 ml of a 10% solution Sc) in order to trace urine stains to the individual with the problem. The soiled areas should be inspected frequently as the staining persists for at least 24 hours.

Prognosis

For cats with elimination problems, the prognosis varies considerably depending on the cause of the behaviour, the duration of the problem, the pet's environment, the stimuli for elimination and whether stimuli can be identified and controlled. For those with physiological reasons for their problems, the prognosis varies with the ultimate diagnosis and chances for curing or managing it.

Factors affecting the prognosis of the housesoiling cat include:

- Cause of the problem
- Duration of the problem
- Frequency of housesoiling incidents
- Number of areas soiled
- Number of different surfaces soiled
- Number of cats in the home
- Ability to control the arousing stimuli

MEDICAL CAUSES OF HOUSESOILING IN CATS	
Housesoiling (urine)	Conditions causing polyuria (diabetes, renal, hyperthyroidism) Conditions causing pollakiuria (feline lower urinary tract disease, calculi, feline interstitial cystitis) Conditions causing incontinence (e.g. neurological) Conditions affecting locomotion (arthritis, disc disease) Conditions affecting CNS/behaviour (hyperthyroidism?/neoplasia)
Housesoiling (faeces)	Conditions causing increased frequency/urge (Inflammatory bowel disease (IBD)) Conditions causing soft stools/poor control Conditions causing painful or difficult defecation (anal saculitis, obstipation, constipation) Conditions causing incontinence (neurological) Conditions affecting locomotion, positioning (arthritis) Conditions affecting CNS/behaviour (hyperthyroidism, neoplasia)

FIG. 6.8 Medical problems that can contribute to inappropriate elimination in cats.

- Temperament of the pet
- Whether the pet was ever trained to use a litterbox
- Owner commitment to modifying behaviour
- Ability of behavioural consultant/veterinarian to diagnose, explain and treat the problem.

Management of the Cat that Sprays

Urine marking on vertical surfaces is generally referred to as spraying. Spraying indoors is most common in unneutered male cats, followed by unneutered female cats. However, 5% of spayed female and 10% of neutered male cats continue to spray. Spraying is a normal feline behaviour which is a means of social communication. Spraying is most often stimulated by the presence or arrival of other cats into the household or on to the property. Some cats simply spray to 'announce their presence', many spray as a response to new odours (e.g. new carpet, new home, marking of another cat), or new objects or structures (e.g. new furniture, newly planted bushes) in their territory, while some cats spray in response to stressful or anxiety-producing stimuli (e.g. changes in the household, new people in the home). Therapy involves identifying the cause, reducing or modifying the stimuli causing the marking, and modifying the pet's response to the stimuli (Fig. 6.9).

TREATMENT OF URINE SPRAYING	
Goal	**Approach**
Control the stimulus	Eliminate stimulus if possible. For example, if outdoor cats are the stimulus for spraying, discourage their visits with water hose, booby-traps, or humane removal
	Move birdfeeders and rubbish bins that attract cats
	Remove stray cat urine from around windows and doors
	Reduce the number of pet cats in the home
	Prevent children from teasing the pet
Remove access to stimuli	Keep the pet away from windows or other vantage points where it can view outdoor cats
	Use window shades and close doors to prevent the pet from seeing stray cats
	Separate indoor cats
	Confine the pet in an area of the home where visitors will not make it anxious
Surgery	Neutering is very effective for curbing urine spraying. Efficacy has been reported at 90% for males and 95% for females
	Olfactory tractotomy and ischiocavernosus myectomy have been used with varying success. These are extreme measures which should be considered as a last resort when all other approaches have failed and euthanasia is being considered
Confinement	When the cat cannot be supervised, it should be kept confined away from areas that have been sprayed
	Relapses may be reduced by ensuring that the cat is allowed back into previously soiled areas gradually and with constant supervision
Punishment	Punishment, using noise devices and water sprays, can help deter a cat from marking when applied during the behaviour. Use of remote punishment is preferred. Booby-traps can also be considered when indoor cats cannot be monitored or kept away from problem areas
Change the function of location	If a cat only marks certain areas in the home, consider moving its sleeping, feeding or play area there as a deterrent
Access to the outdoors	Some cats will spray less indoors if they have some access to the outdoors, while others will do better if kept indoors all of the time
Drug therapy	Buspirone is effective in 55% of cats. Diazepam is slightly more effective but has greater side effects. Antidepressants (such as amitriptyline, clomipramine, and fluoxetine), other benzodiazepines (such as alprazolam), and progestins are also sometimes effective. About 90% of cats relapse after discontinuing diazepam while only 50% resume spraying when buspirone is discontinued. Antianxiety drugs can reduce fear-dependent inhibitions in a low-ranking individual, and therefore increase social aggression in certain situations. Previous studies have shown that progesterones are effective in approx. 30% of cases, while the effectiveness of diazepam ranged from 55% to 75%. Although diazepam was effective in both sexes, progestins were more effective in males

Fig. 6.9 Treatment of urine spraying in cats.

DRUG THERAPY FOR THE CAT THAT SPRAYS		
Drug	**Dosage**	**Comments**
Buspirone	2.5–7.5 mg/cat PO bid	55% effective with a 50% relapse rate. Does not cause the adverse effects of sedation and ataxia commonly seen with the benzodiazepines. Use for 1–2 weeks and if effective continue for 8 weeks before attempting to reduce dose or discontinue. If ineffective, consider higher dose (within range) or discontinue and consider alternative therapy
Diazepam	1–3 mg/kg bid	Up to 75% improve but most relapse when the drug is withdrawn. Tends to cause sedation, ataxia and hyperphagia. Treat for 2–4 weeks then reduce by approx. 25% of initial dose every 2 weeks if no recurrence. May need to maintain at lowest effective dose in up to 90% of cases if stimuli not removed or minimised
Amitriptyline	5–10 mg/cat/day	May take several weeks to determine therapeutic effectiveness. Sedating and anticholinergic
Alprazolam	0.125–0.25 mg bid	A benzodiazepine that reduces anxiety and potentially may aid in treating anxiety-motivated spraying problems
Megoestrol acetate	2.5–10 mg daily for 1 to 2 weeks then reduce by half every 2 weeks to lowest effective dose	Approximately 30% effective. May respond to antiandrogenic effects of progesterones when antianxiety treatment unsuccessful. (*See Chapter 4 for side effects and contraindications.*)
Medroxyprogesterone acetate	5–20 mg/kg Sc/IM 3 times per year	Long acting. Less effective than megoestrol acetate.

FIG. 6.10 Drug treatment for the spraying cat (*see Chapter 4 for additional side effects and contraindications*).

Factors that might influence a cat's tendency to spray include:

- Hormones
- Temperament
- Feline population density (new cat in the neighbourhood or household)
- Indirect signalling from other cats (e.g. scent on visitor's clothes)
- Changes in the environment (new roommate, remodelling home, new furniture, novel objects brought into the home)
- Moving
- New work schedule for owner
- Owner absences from home
- Owner spending less time with the cat
- Inappropriate punishment.

Management of Inappropriate Elimination (Horizontal Surfaces)

In addition to the medical causes discussed previously, inappropriate elimination on horizontal surfaces can be due to aversion to the litter, litterbox or litterbox area, or a preference for other substrates or locations. Marking might be considered when the urine or stool is found near walls, doors, or windows where the pet can see outdoor cats, or on prominent items such as beds, sofas, or the owner's clothing. These cases will require management with the same techniques and drugs that might be utilised for the treatment of spraying on vertical surfaces (Fig. 6.10).

Litterbox aversion should be considered when the cat does not use its litter for both urine and stools, or when the cat returns to the litter area but eliminates outside the box. Substrate preferences may be the cause when the cat prefers to eliminate on a particular type of surface (carpet, potted plants). Unfortunately, diagnosis is seldom straightforward since mixed factors are often involved. In addition, the cause of inappropriate elimination may be resolved by the time the cat is presented for diagnosis, and other maintaining factors (new surface preferences, learned litterbox avoidance) may now be involved. For example, a cat that begins to avoid litterbox use for urination because of a painful bout of feline lower urinary tract disease (FLUTD) may begin to urinate in a carpeted area, and then develop a preference for carpeted surfaces. A cat in a multi-cat household may utilise the litter when it is clean, but may eliminate in inappropriate areas when it has already been soiled by another cat in the household. The hallmarks of successful therapy are identifying and eliminating the cause, re-establishing

TREATMENT OF FELINE INAPPROPRIATE ELIMINATION	
Goal	**Approach**
Remove the cause	Any medical problems must be addressed
	If the problem is due to litterbox aversion, the box may need to be moved, cleaned more often or litter brand changed. Avoid using harsh chemicals and detergents in the litterbox. Remove scented litter which might deter some cats. The preferred substrate for many cats is finely textured clay litter
	Identify potential deterrents in the litterbox area (noisy central heating boiler, laundry equipment, temperature extremes)
Remove access to soiled sites	Move furniture over the soiled areas
	Close doors to frequently soiled rooms
Re-establish normal litter use	Confine the cat to a small area and only allow it out when it can be supervised 100% of the time
	Confinement should continue for a long enough time for a reliable habit to become re-established. This period should be from 1 to 8 weeks depending on the duration of the problem. The pet should gradually be allowed to have more freedom and less supervision
Decrease desirability of inappropriate sites	Change the surface at previously soiled areas by removing carpet, placing a sheet of plastic or aluminium foil in the area or by placing upside-down plastic carpet runner (nubs up) or double-sided tape
	Place food bowls, bedding, toys or a play centre in the area
	Use environmental punishers (upside-down mousetraps, motion alarms). Lemon-scented room deodoriser will deter some cats
	Remove odour using chemical or enzymatic odour eliminators. Be certain to use a sufficient amount of the product to saturate the entire area
Increase desirability of litterbox	Determine favourite litter by providing a few additional boxes with different substrates (clay, soil, sandy clumping, sand/potting soil)
	Determine favourite box by providing a few different boxes (covered, lower sides, open)
	Determine favourite location by locating boxes in a number of locations
	It may also be helpful to increase the number of litterboxes, and clean them more regularly
Behavioural modification	Desensitisation and counterconditioning may help reduce undesirable responses to anxiety-producing stimuli
	Litterbox can be placed in elimination area and gradually moved to a more appropriate location
Punishment	If the owner catches the pet in the act, it can be punished remotely with a water rifle or alarm
	The cat should never be physically punished and any punishment is contraindicated if anxiety or fear is an important component of the problem
Rewards	Food rewards and play may help reinforce the desirability of litterbox usage. Cats can be followed into the litter area and rewarded for successful use
Drug therapy	Cats that eliminate on horizontal surfaces are unlikely to respond to pharmacological therapy unless an underlying anxiety or territorial aetiology (or medical condition) exists. For these cases, refer to Fig. 6.10. Consider amitriptyline for cats that may also have recurrent inflammatory bladder disease.

FIG. 6.11 Treatment of inappropriate elimination in the cat.

regular litterbox use, and preventing the cat from returning to previously soiled areas (Fig. 6.11).

Case Examples

Case 1

History Morticia, a 6-year-old spayed female cat, suddenly began to urinate in inappropriate locations. Although she continued to use her litterbox occasion-ally, she had also eliminated on a pile of clean laundry, on the owner's bedspread, and in the bathroom sink on three or four occasions. She was taken to her veterinarian who performed a urinalysis and found marked haematuria, pyuria, mild triple phosphate crystalluria, and a urine pH of 7. She was placed on a prescription diet to reduce crystal formation and lower the urinary pH and was given some diazepam to help reduce her apparent dis-comfort. Four weeks later the owner reported a marked improvement but there were still occasional 'accidents', usually in the sink or on the floor just outside the litterbox. A repeat urinalysis at the time revealed a moderate number of red blood cells, but no crystals and an acid pH. Three months after the initial onset of the problem, the cat was referred to a behaviour clinic because the inappropriate elimination continued intermittently.

Diagnosis and Management It was the owner's impression that the cat occasionally vocalised during urination and that there was an increased frequency. A subsequent urinalysis revealed the presence of moderate haematuria, proteinuria with no bacteriuria. Both scout and double-contrast radiographs were unremarkable. At this point the owner declined referral for cystoscopy or exploratory surgery. No environmental or stressful changes could be identified. Because the cat continued to use its litter for all defecation and most urination, it was unlikely that there was a litterbox aversion. However, to rule out the possibility behavioural therapy was initiated. In an attempt to increase the appeal of the litter, the owner added a second litterbox and tried a variety of litterboxes and litter types, without improvement. The owner confined the cat to the washroom with its litterbox when it could not be supervised, but the cat continued to use the sink or the floor in front of the litterbox a few times each week. Confinement in a large cage was successful but when the cat was released from the cage after 3 weeks, the problem recurred every few days. Over a period of another 3 months a number of urinalyses were performed (free flow into a non-absorbable litter) and mild to moderate haematuria was seen on most but not all of the urinalyses. Based on the clinical history, lack of response to behavioural therapy and the recurrent haematuria, feline idiopathic (interstitial) cystitis was considered to be a likely diagnosis. The cat was subsequently placed on 5 mg of amitriptyline daily and after 4 weeks there had been a marked decrease in the problem with only two recurrences.

Amitriptyline has been reported to correct some behavioural causes of inappropriate urination and may help to control feline interstitial cystitis. Over the next year the owner reported that there was infrequent inappropriate elimination (approximately once or twice a month), but when amitriptyline was discontinued for about a month, there were multiple weekly recurrences.

Case 2

History Jasmine, a 3-month-old female kitten that had been obtained at 2 months of age, was using the owner's benjamina plant for elimination. The kitten slept in the bedroom at night on the third floor and the litterbox was located on the first floor in the laundry room. The kitten had used its litterbox for the first few weeks but would no longer use it. The owner had tried a number of litter types and litterboxes with no apparent improvement.

Diagnosis Physical examination revealed a healthy and very alert kitten. Urinalysis and faecal evaluation failed to suggest any organic cause for the elimination problem. The kitten had apparently developed a preference for using the soil in the benjamina plant and had perhaps developed an aversion for the area where the litterbox was kept. Since the kitten exhibited fear of loud noises, it was suspected that the sounds of the washer and dryer could have caused it to avoid the laundry room.

Treatment The owner was advised to prevent the kitten from eliminating in the benjamina plant by covering the surface of the soil with chips of marble. The pet was confined to a small bedroom with its litterbox when it could not be closely supervised. This was carried on for 2 weeks to re-establish desirable litter habits. At that time, the litterbox was relocated to a quiet room away from the laundry facilities. The kitten used the litter consistently and there were no further problems.

Case 3

History Mephistopheles, a 3-year-old neutered male cat, was presented to a veterinary behaviour clinic for urine marking of 2 months' duration. Household diagrams were submitted with the history and it was determined that all urine sites were found in front doors or windows on the first floor. The problem had begun in the early spring and the owner was aware of the sight and smell of new cats on the property outdoors.

Diagnosis Although the cat had been urinating primarily on horizontal surfaces, urine marking due to

FIG. 6.12 The process of investigating and treating housesoiling.

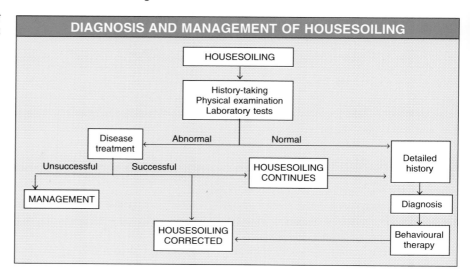

DIAGNOSIS AND MANAGEMENT OF HOUSESOILING

HOUSESOILING

History-taking
Physical examination
Laboratory tests

Abnormal — Normal

Disease treatment

Unsuccessful — Successful

MANAGEMENT

HOUSESOILING CONTINUES

Detailed history

Diagnosis

HOUSESOILING CORRECTED

Behavioural therapy

outdoor stimuli was tentatively suspected as the likely cause of the problem. The medical work-up, including physical examination and urinalysis, were unremarkable. Although the cat resented abdominal palpation, there was no evidence of distended bladder or pain in the area. The history and lack of any physical reason for the problem supported our tentative diagnosis.

Treatment The owner confined the cat into the master bedroom where it slept most nights and had never previously eliminated. The litterbox was relocated to the adjacent washroom and double-sided tape was placed on the window sills to keep the cat from sitting there and watching outdoor cats. The cat used the litterbox for all elimination when confined to the bedroom. When the owner was home, the cat was allowed out of the bedroom and was supervised at all times by the owner. All soiled locations had been treated with a commercial odour eliminator. While supervised, the cat did not attempt to eliminate in the previous spots. After 2 weeks, the owner began to reduce supervision and a new spot was found in front of a sliding door. The owner cleaned the spot and placed vertical blinds on the door to reduce the cat's view of outdoor cats. This successfully stopped further elimination at the location but the cat continued to urinate by the rear doorway. Cat repellents and a motion detector were placed on the back porch to keep outdoor cats away and food bowls were placed at the indoor sites of housesoiling. For 2

months the owners continued to confine the cat when they were not at home and release it when they were. At a 6 month follow-up there had been no further incidents of inappropriate elimination.

Summary

The flowchart in Fig. 6.12 shows how medical and behavioural techniques interact.

Further Reading

Beaver, B. V. (1989) Housesoiling by cats: a retrospective study of 120 cases. *Journal of the American Animal Hospital Association*, **25**(6), 631–637.

Beaver, B. V. (1994) Differential approach to house soiling by dogs and cats. *Veterinary Quarterly*, **16**(Suppl. 1), S47.

Borchelt, P. L. (1991) Cat elimination behaviour problems. *Veterinary Clinics of North America, Small Animal Practice*, **21**, 254–265.

Borchelt, P. and Voith, V. L. (1982) Diagnosis and treatment of elimination behaviour problems in cats. *Veterinary Clinics of North America, Small Animal Practice*, **12**(4), 673–680.

Borchelt, P. L. and Voith, V. L. (1986) Elimination behaviour problems in cats. *Compendium of Continuing Education*, **8**, 197–205.

Buffington, C. A. T and Chew, D. J. (1995) Idiopathic lower urinary tract disease in cats – Is it interstitial cystitis? *Proceedings of the 13th ACVIM Forum*, 517–519.

Cooper, L. L. and Hart, B. L. (1992) Comparison of diazepam with progestin for effectiveness in suppression of urine spraying behaviour in cats. Journal of the American Veterinary Medical Association, **200**, 797–801.

Crowell-Davis, S. (1986) Elimination behaviour problem of cats, I. *Veterinary Forum*, November, 10

Hart, B. L. (1980) Objectionable urine spraying and urine marking in cats: evaluation of progestin treatment in gonadectomized males and females. *Journal of the American Veterinary Medical Association*, **177**, 529–533.

Hart, B. L. (1981) Olfactory tractotomy to control objectionable urine spraying and urine marking in cats. *Journal of the American Veterinary Medical Association*, **179**, 231–234.

Hart, B. L. (1985) Urine spraying and marking in cats. In: *Textbook of Small Animal Surgery*, Slatter, S. H. (ed.) W. B. Saunders: Philadelphia, PA.

Hart, B. L. and Cooper, L. (1984) Factors related to urine spraying and fighting in prepubertally gonadectomized cats. *Journal of the American Veterinary Medical Association*, **184**, 1255–1258.

Hart, B. L., Eckstein, R. A., Powell, K. L. and Dodman, N. H. (1993) Effectiveness of buspirone on urine spraying and inappropriate urination in cats. *Journal of the American Veterinary Medical Association*, **203**(2), 254–258.

Hart, B. L. and Leedy, M. (1982) Identification of source of urine stains in multi-cat households. *Journal of the American Veterinary Medical Association*, **180**, 77.

Hopkins, S. G., Schubert, T. A., and Hart, B. L. (1976) Castration of adult male dogs: effects on roaming, aggression, urine marking and mounting. *Journal of the American Veterinary Medical Association*, **168**, 1108–1110.

Hunthausen, W. L. (1993) Dealing with feline housesoiling: a practitioner's guide. *Veterinary Medicine*, August, 3–7.

Hunthausen, W. (1995) Housesoiling and the geriatric dog. *Veterinary Medicine*, August, Supplement, 4–15.

Korefsky, P. S. (1987) Letter to the editor: 'Identifying source of urine on rugs'. *Journal of the American Veterinary Medical Association*, **191**(8), 917.

Komtebedde, J., and Haupman, J. (1990) Bilateral ischiocavernosus myectomy for chronic urine spraying in castrated cats. *Veterinary Surgery*, **19**(4), 293.

Marder, A. (1989) Feline housesoiling. *Pet Veterinarian*, Sept–Oct, 11–15.

Marder, A. (1991) Psychotropic drugs and behaviour therapy. *Veterinary Clinics of North American*, **21**(2), 329–342.

Mathews, S. L. (1984) A different approach to the litter box problem. *Feline Practice*, **14**(3), 7–11.

Melese-d'Hospital, P. (1996) Eliminating urine odors in the home. In: Voith V. L. and Borchelt, P. L. (eds). *Readings in Companion Animal Behavior*. Veterinary Learning Systems: Trenton, NJ, pp. 191–197.

O'Brien, D. (1988) Neurogenic disorders of micturition. *Veterinary Clinics of North America, Small Animal Practice*, **18**(3), 535.

Overall, K. (1993) Diagnosing and treating undesirable feline elimination behaviour. *Feline Practice*, **21**(2), 11–13.

Ross, S. (1950) Some observations on the lair dwelling behaviour of dogs. *Behaviour*, **2**, 144–162.

Scott, J. P. and Fuller, J. L. (1965) *Genetics and the Social Behaviour of the Dog*. University of Chicago Press: Chicago, IL.

Voith, V. L. (1991) Treating elimination behaviour problems in dogs and cats: the role of punishment. *Modern Veterinary Practice*, December, 951–953.

Voith, V. L. and Borchelt, P. L. (1985), Elimination behaviour and related problems in dogs. *Compendium of Continuing Education*, **7**(7), 538.

Vollmer, P. J. (1977) Inappropriate elimination in an older dog. *Veterinary Medicine Small Animal Clinics*, October, 1577–1578.

Wright, J. C. (1988) Do cats with elimination problems need privacy and escape potential? *Animal Behaviour Consultant Newsletter*, **5**(2), 2–3.

7

Destructive Behaviours

Introduction

Destructive behaviour can occur for a variety of reasons. In many cases it is simply a matter of normal behaviour being directed toward an unacceptable object or area. Preventive counselling, including a thorough discussion of normal kitten and puppy behaviour as well as the appropriate use of confinement and supervision, will help head off many of these types of problem.

Some problems involving destructive behaviour can have more serious and complex underlying aetiologies. Separation anxiety, escape behaviour resulting from an overwhelming phobia, or compulsive sucking and chewing require good diagnostics and well thought-out therapy plans.

Other problems have causes that are basically simple but are somewhat obscure. Chewing and scratching at walls to get at rodents, redirected aggressive chewing at inanimate objects due to territorial arousal, and chewing clothing or carpeting with an interesting odour or taste can all be circumstances that may be difficult to define.

Destructive Chewing by Dogs

Owners frequently complain about damage done to household belongings by pet dogs. In many cases, they contribute to the problem by providing inappropriate chew toys (e.g. old shoes, socks, blankets) and not providing enough appropriate ones. Dogs need to chew; it is a normal behaviour. Puppies are very investigative and more playful than adults. Therefore, the problem is seen less often in adults. Teething in puppies also helps to account for their seemingly endless need to chew. Destructive behaviour by young dogs is generally a training problem, while destructive behaviour by adults can be due to a variety of causes.

Diagnosis and Prognosis

It is normal for puppies to chew. A good portion of their non-sleeping day involves playing, eating and chewing. Destructive chewing is therefore not unusual for puppies and should be expected by owners. Persistent damage reflects a lack of training by the owner rather than a pathological state in the dog. Proper channelling of the need to chew towards acceptable items should be considered a basic component of any dog-rearing programme. The cause of destructive chewing in adult dogs can be more difficult to diagnose and manage successfully. Some underlying causes include lack of stimulation, anxiety, and delayed feeding times. Underlying medical problems also need to be considered. With proper training and adequate supervision, the prognosis for complete cessation of the problem is good to excellent.

Management

For puppies, treatment is relatively straightforward and involves directing the pet towards acceptable chew toys. Do not take desirable behaviours for granted. Dogs can not easily discern which objects are acceptable for them to chew and which are not. This can be particularly challenging if owners play games like 'tug of war' with towels or socks, or give dogs household items like old shoes for chew toys. In all cases, owners should be instructed not to give the dog any household items for its chewing enjoyment.

Chew toys are only appropriate if the dog actually chews them. Durable plastic, nylon and rubber toys are acceptable for some dogs but others may not show interest in them. Coating toys with small amounts of liver paste, cheese spread or peanut butter may increase their desirability. Rawhide chews that can be torn apart are very intriguing to most dogs. Cereal biscuits may promise chewing enjoyment and cleaner teeth but they are too quickly eaten and too high in calories to form the basis for a chewing programme.

MANAGEMENT OF DESTRUCTIVE CHEWING IN DOGS

Step	Comments
Provide acceptable and stimulating chew toys	Owners must provide the dog with every opportunity to chew appropriately. Give the dog a large selection until you can determine preferred chewing objects
	Provide variety in chew toys and offer novel items intermittently
	Playing tug games or fetch with the chew toys may help stimulate interest in the items
	Choose durable toys (rope toys, rubber toys) that can be filled with biscuits or small pieces of meat, or have cheese or peanut butter spread onto or inside them
	Owners must not engage the dog in play with household objects and must not give the dog old household items for chew toys
Rewards	Every time the pet chews on one of its chew toys, it should receive a social or food reward to reinforce the behaviour
Exercise	Lots of vigorous exercise will help the dog burn off excess energy. Consider long walks, retrieving games, or jogging
	Active games such as fetch, retrieving, and catching a ball or flying disc will provide exercise as well as providing mental stimulation
Provide mental stimulation	Some pets may require additional outlets to deter them from destructive chewing. Interactive play toys, additional pets, and obedience training may be helpful
	Hiding stimulating toys and treats throughout the dog's play area can offer an enjoyable and time-consuming activity for the dog
Punishment	To be effective, punishment must be administered during or immediately following the act. A delay of even a few seconds is a contraindication for using punishment
	Remote punishment teaches the pet that chewing leads to punishment whether the owner is present or not
Aversion	Sprays or ointments which taste hot or bitter can be applied to household objects to make them less desirable for the pet to chew
Confinement	Whenever the owner cannot supervise or monitor, the dog should be confined to a crate, exercise pen or dog-proof room so that it does not have the opportunity to fail

Fig. 7.1 Management of destructive chewing in dogs.

Prevention

The best way to prevent destructive chewing is to provide puppies with appropriate chew toys and teach them early which items are theirs to chew, and which are not. Until the owner can trust the pet, it must be under constant supervision or confined to a safe area. Dogs also need ample exercise time for them to dispel some of their boundless energy. Since anxiety can also prompt dogs to be destructive, this or other underlying problems should be promptly addressed (*see Separation Anxiety, below*).

Case Example

Barney was a 9-month-old Labrador Retriever that was presented for his incredible propensity to destroy items around the house. The owners were busy and rarely had time to exercise the pet. During the day, while the owners were at work, Barney was left unconfined in the home. Since he had been adopted,

at 2 months of age, he had eaten holes in the carpet, chewed large holes in two expensive pieces of furniture, destroyed books, chewed spectacles, and had dug up or chewed up every plant in the home.

A dog run was set up in the basement to provide safe confinement when the owners could not supervise the pet. The dog was only allowed out of his run if and when he could be kept within sight. The owners were instructed to provide much more exercise, with the goal of fatiguing the pet. It was suggested that exercise should take place at least three times daily. A professional dog walker was recommended to help out. Several new toys were introduced. They were laced with a small amount of food to make them more attractive than the owner's possessions, and the owners spent time every day playing with the pet and the toys. Barney was taught to play fetch. Whenever the pet initiated chewing on any of its toys, the owners praised it and occasionally gave a small biscuit. Household items in which Barney had shown a special interest were painted with a hot-tasting substance. Small plants were placed out of reach and a small motion alarm was placed at the base of the remaining large plant. Obedience training was also recommended.

Progress was slow. Barney enjoyed his new toys but still managed to destroy several more household items. The owners were justifiably upset but resisted the temptation to punish Barney when he wasn't actually 'caught in the act'. After 4 weeks of therapy, the owners were exhausted but had to admit that Barney now rarely got into trouble. After 2 months, there had only been two incidents when Barney took one of the owner's shoes. However, instead of chewing it, he just played with it in the bedroom and did no real damage. The owner got Barney's attention, gave him a 'sit' command and then rewarded him with a treat. He then offered Barney a chew toy to replace the shoe, which Barney gave up without incident. After 6 months, the owners felt they could truly trust Barney and he was given the run of the house while they were out. No further incidents were reported.

Destructive Chewing by Cats

Cats that chew or suck on objects may cause costly damage to the household or serious injury to themselves (*see also Chapters 8 and 12*). Those that chew houseplants are often indoor cats with little or no access to grass or other vegetable matter. Others, especially kittens, may chew household items as part of their investigation, exploration and play.

Fabric-chewing by some cats may be a form of compulsive behaviour. The damage done by these cats can be quite extensive. There may also be some genetic predisposition to this type of activity. Although sucking or chewing on fabrics can occur in cats of any lineage, Siamese and Burmese cats are especially prone to this type of behaviour. Wool items (clothing, carpets) seem to be preferred.

Diagnosis and Prognosis

The diagnosis is straightforward. Most destructive chewing by cats is attributable to their desire to play and investigate. A familial disorder is suspected in some breeds and for those cats the prognosis is guarded.

Management

The best treatment for destructive feline chewing is to keep the chewed objects away from the cat or make them taste bad, and to provide it with its own chewing alternatives. Cat play areas and activity centres, interactive play toys, such as catnip mice that hang from a cat play centre or are dangled from doors, can keep some cats distracted. Some cats can be encouraged to chew on dog toys or pieces of rawhide, especially if a little cheese spread or fish oil is placed in or on the chew toy. For some cats, it may help to change the diet to a dry, bulky food. This is based on the premise that these cats may actually be seeking additional vegetable matter in their diet. Cats that chew houseplants may be content enough with lettuce, catnip or access to a herb garden. For cats that chew while the owners are out, providing interactive play sessions before departure may help calm and settle the cat while the owner is away from home. For sucking or chewing behaviours that lead to extensive damage, it may be useful to consider providing highly stimulating alternatives such as a microwaved chicken wing.

Environmental punishment using taste aversion or booby-traps may be necessary to deter cats that develop fixations for household items. A plant's leaves can be lightly sprayed with water, and then sprinkled with cayenne pepper. Oil of eucalyptus, menthol and commercial pet repellents can also be used to coat trunks of large plants or saplings to discourage chewing. Motion alarms can be placed near the plants to chase the cat away when it approaches, or hidden under fabric items the pet chews. A hair-dryer, that can be activated by the owner using a remote-control switch, is a useful deterrent. For larger plants or trees, balloons can be tied around the base; when they are played with and pop, they frighten away the cat and act as a deterrent against future incursions. For wool-sucking by oriental and other breeds that is a manifestation of compulsive behaviour, clomipramine or fluoxetine might be considered.

Prevention

The best chance of preventing destructive chewing in cats is to provide them with acceptable chew toys and interactive forms of exercise.

Case Example

Fred, a 1-year-old, neutered male domestic short-haired cat, was presented for chewing holes in the owner's clothing and other fabric objects found around the home. Since both owners worked long hours, Fred spent quite a lot of time alone in the apartment. He had intermittently chewed on a variety of objects since he was adopted at 8 weeks of age, without causing a significant amount of damage. In the 2 months previous to the consultation, the chewing had escalated quite considerably. The primary objects that were chewed were fabric items, although, on rare occasions, he would chew on wooden chair legs, pencils and plastic pens. Yelling at the cat served to distract it temporarily but did not stop the behaviour. Physical examination, faecal examination and routine haematological and biochemical tests failed to reveal a medical reason for the problem. The cause was thought to be behavioural.

The owner was told to keep all fabric items out of Fred's reach except for two or three pieces that had been coated with a commercial antichew spray. Several times a day the items were moved to new positions around the house. Every few days, the type of items was changed. This was done to teach the pet to expect all fabric items, no matter where they are located or what the shape, to have an unacceptable taste. The owner was also encouraged to provide new toys for the pet on a regular basis (including some dog chew toys and some catnip cat toys), and to spend quite a lot more time playing with Fred. A 'kitty condo' was purchased which had crawl spaces, perches and hanging toys to keep him entertained and occupied.

Fred seemed to be doing well until he managed to get into the guest bedroom and discovered the curtains (drapes) there. To stop this behaviour, a light cotton fabric was pinned to the curtains to protect them and a bitter spray was applied to teach the cat to avoid them. After this minor setback, the entire process was recommended and Fred finally relented and became an acceptable housepet. The owners did report that he had the occasional relapse but the damage was not nearly as bad as with previous episodes.

Digging

Digging may be a nuisance, but it is an innate trait for many dogs. Sledge-dog breeds such as Huskies and Malamutes dig holes that provide a cool place for them to lie in and get out of the wind. Terriers and Dachshunds were bred to dig tunnels to flush out prey or to locate rodents. Other dogs may simply dig because their acute senses of smell and hearing inform them that there is something interesting beneath the ground. Since dogs often bury bones, it is not surprising that they should also dig to locate them once again. As a natural escape mechanism, digging is also a good way to avoid confinement.

When dogs become housepets, they often need to leave natural tendencies behind, including digging, if they are to be good home companions. Most dogs have little problem with this compromise, as long as they have sufficient stimulation elsewhere in their lives. However, there are some dogs that are resistant to change and continue to dig despite other adequate outlets. They may dig because of lack of stimulation, to escape or because digging is fun.

Diagnosis and Prognosis

Dogs dig for a number of reasons and, whenever possible, it is important to determine the underlying cause. If not, the dog may respond to punishment in the presence of the owner but resume the behaviour when left unsupervised. Carefully interview the owner as to the circumstances surrounding the digging. For example, does the dog dig to escape from the garden, as a recreational event, or because it has been abandoned without anything more interesting to do?

The prognosis varies considerably with the underlying cause. Understimulated young dogs and intact males with a strong motivation to roam, that have learned that digging provides freedom, can be very frustrating to control. For these cases, keeping the dog indoors in a safe, destruction-proof area or providing a confinement area that does not allow escape digging may be the only viable solution. Discovering the underlying aetiology and having practical solutions available significantly improves the chances for successful resolution.

Management

For dogs that are digging to escape, the motivation for the behaviour should be elucidated and dealt with if possible. If the dog is not getting enough exercise or social attention, this should be provided. If it is escaping to avoid mistreatment, the owner will need to be counselled to correct the situation. If the pet is digging to catch rodents, some thought should be given to capturing and removing them from the yard.

When dogs are digging to create a cool respite, they will usually forsake digging if given a cool, shaded area to lie in, or a wading pool in which they can cool off. Dogs that are digging as a response to fearful stimuli may enjoy the comfort and security of a dog house or other forms of shelter. Another option is to provide a sand/soil digging pit with partially buried toys and bones to encourage digging in one area instead of many. For some dogs, confinement in a secure pen or run may be the best treatment plan

Environmental enrichment is most indicated for those dogs that dig because they have nothing better to do. Whenever the pet is left outdoors unsupervised, it is important to attempt to provide an appealing alternative activity to distract and occupy it. This distraction might include large balls to push around, or wooden boxes and ramps on which to crawl and explore. The success in enriching the environment is variable and may be negligible for some pets. Increased activity, such as vigorous physical exercise (fetch, jogging, speed walking) provided two or more times daily, may often do just as well or better in reducing the amount of time spent digging.

Adding another pet may help, but the owner might also end up with two pets that dig and therefore twice the damage. Digging can be suppressed in the owner's presence by punishment. This is best done by remote means so the dog does not associate the punishment with the presence of the owner. It can be accomplished by monitoring the dog and responding with sprinklers, pulling on an extended leash, a remote collar or booby-traps whenever the dog digs. In most cases, with remote punishment and providing the dog with alternative activities, the digging problems can be corrected. If the dog digs in only one or two specific areas, these can be protected by placing chicken wire over the areas and anchoring it to the ground.

Certain common practices must be discouraged absolutely. These include: delayed punishment; physical punishment; and filling the hole with water or faeces and holding the pet's head in it.

Prevention

Dogs should be closely supervised when outdoors during the first 12–18 months of their lives so that the owner can quickly correct digging behaviour every time it is exhibited. A shake can may be tossed next to the pet each time it starts to scratch the ground in order to discourage the behaviour. Adequate exercise, training and social stimulation are all very important. Digging by young pets that are home alone and allowed to entertain themselves by digging each day can be very difficult to correct.

If there is an acceptable area where the dog may dig in the garden, the owner might consider teaching the puppy to dig in that area soon after it has been brought into the home environment. Toys can be buried in the acceptable area to encourage the pet to dig there. Food or social praise can be used to reinforce the behaviour. To accomplish this, the owner must always be with the pet when it is outdoors so that the correct behaviour can be rewarded and digging in undesirable areas can be punished. Appropriate punishment is very important, because if only positive reinforcement for digging in an appropriate area is used to condition the dog, it may take anywhere from a few months to 2 years before it can be trusted not to dig in unacceptable areas in the garden.

Case Example

Sonic, an entire male Border Collie, was presented for digging under the gate to run in the neighbourhood when the owner was at work during the day. Upon arriving home, the owner would see Sonic, call him, grab him by the collar and punish him for escaping.

The owner was told that punishing the dog when he arrived home at the end of the day, long after the pet had performed the escape behaviour, was counter-productive. In fact, Sonic was starting to avoid the owner when he came home and was more hesitant to come when called. Neutering was recommended to decrease the possibility of sexually motivated escape and roaming behaviour. More exercise by way of jogging and fetch was suggested. The owner purchased several inexpensive soccer balls and encouraged the pet to play with them by throwing and kicking them around the yard. The owner anchored a small sheet of chicken wire along the ground in front of the gate. Whenever he found the dog investigating the ground near the gate, a shake can was tossed near it.

Sonic did extremely well as long as the owner remained attentive to him in the evening. He came to anticipate the play time and was eager for the owner's return home. However, Sonic did have relapses when the owner passed on playtime for a few days in a row, and once when the owner was out of town for 2 days on business. The owner, upon realising the situation, came up with a satisfactory solution for all concerned. He paid several of the neighbourhood children to play with Sonic for at least one full hour on those days when he could or would not spend the time himself.

Separation Anxiety

Dogs bond closely with humans, so it is not surprising that they may have some anxiety when left alone. Some natural canine behaviour associated with being left alone are barking, digging, chewing and housesoiling. These are some of the same manifestations seen with separation anxiety. This is a generalisation, however, because some dogs respond with lowered activity levels. Others may eliminate inappropriately or urine-mark during the owner's absence.

Separation anxiety can result in behaviours that are destructive to the property, dangerous for the pet or annoying for people in its environment, so it must be taken seriously. Owners certainly take it seriously because affected dogs often destroy personal property, especially those items frequently handled by the owner and carrying the owner's scent.

Diagnosis and Prognosis

The onset of problems often coincides with an abrupt change in the owner's schedule that results in the dog being left alone for longer periods or at different times. The destructive activity concentrates on personal possessions of the owner or things they contact, such as hairbrushes, books, clothes and furniture. Owners might believe that their dog is 'getting back at them' for being left alone. They do not always realise that the dog selects those items because they carry the owner's scent. Other foci for destructive behaviour include doors where the owner exits or nearby windows.

Most of the destructive behaviour begins within a few minutes to an hour following the owner's departure when the pet's anxiety and arousal level is highest. In addition to excessive vocalisation, destructive behaviours and inappropriate elimination, dogs may also suffer from hypersalivation, emesis, diarrhoea and self-mutilation. The destructive behaviours most utilised include scratching, digging and chewing.

Separation anxiety must be distinguished from other causes of inappropriate elimination, destructive behaviours, barking and housesoiling. This requires a detailed history from the owner. Typically, the dog that is exhibiting undesirable behaviours due to separation anxiety does not engage in the undesirable behaviours when it has access to the owner. The problem occurs when the pet cannot be with the owner or cannot gain the owner's attention. In most instances, the owner is out of the home, but problems can occur when the owner is at home but ignoring the pet. As the owner prepares to leave, the pet may show signs of either increased activity and anxiety (pacing, restlessness, whining) or depression (lying around, reluctance to move). When the owner returns, the dog ususally becomes extremely active with exaggerated greeting behaviours.

Prognosis is good if the problem is of recent occurrence, if the pet does not have an extremely anxious temperament, and if the owners can be motivated to perform time-consuming exercise as well as change the way in which they interact with the pet.

Initiators of separation anxiety include:

- Change in the owner's routine
- Returning to school or work
- Move to a new home
- Visit to a new environment
- Following a stay in a kennel
- Owner present physically but not paying attention to dog:
    new baby in the home
    new social relationship.

Management

The successful management of separation anxiety includes teaching the dog to tolerate owner absences and correcting the specific problems of chewing, barking, digging, or elimination (Fig. 7.2). (*See also management of barking and destructive chewing.*)

Prevention

When an owner has a very close relationship with the pet and anticipates a major change in schedule or in the amount of time spent with it, some thought should be given to making the changeover as gradual as possible. This will help prevent the anxiety that can

MANAGEMENT OF SEPARATION ANXIETY	
Step	**Comments**
Modify the pet/owner relationship	Teach the pet independence. The pet should not be allowed to get attention on demand. When the pet gets what it wants every time it nudges or whines, it is more likely to be anxious when it is alone and cannot get social attention The owners should know that they can give the pet the attention they desire, but it must always be on their terms, not the pet's
Exercise	Make sure the dog has adequate exercise before each departure so that its energy levels are somewhat depleted during the owner's absence. Exercise also helps dissipate anxiety and tension as well as providing attention. After exercise, it is generally best to allow the dog to calm down for at least a few minutes before the owners depart Providing vigorous exercise two to three times daily can have a very positive effect in many cases
Stimulation	Dogs may be less anxious when they have something to do while left alone. Make sure there are appealing chew toys around or access to the yard with a 'doggy door' For chewing, identify and provide alternative chew items that are equally or more appealing than what the dog has chosen The best toys are those that are highly stimulating and keep the pet occupied. Although many dogs will not chew toys or eat when anxious or stressed, new chew toys (pig's ears, rawhide) or strongly motivating food pieces hidden in the toys, such as meat or cheese, may get the pet's interest. These treats can be hidden inside toys so that they are difficult to remove, in packages that the dog must open, or hidden under bowls around the home In rare situations, having another pet will provide a playmate (or distraction) for the dog
Obedience	The pet should be introduced to the idea that it cannot always be with the owner by frequently being requested to do 'down–stays' and 'sit–stays'. This phase should begin with the pet staying for a very short period before accompanying the owner to various rooms throughout the home. Gradually, the pet should be required to stay for longer periods of time, until it will remain in another room for 30–60 minutes or more. If the dog is confined to a particular room or area during to departure, this is where training (and all good things – food, sleep, toys) should occur
Departure cues and departure techniques	Dogs learn to associate certain cues with the owner's departure. The presence of these departure cues will typically create anxiety about an impending absence of the owner. Until the pet has been desensitised to these cues, they should be avoided whenever possible during actual departures. Putting jacket and boots on in a different room, leaving a briefcase, handbag or keys in the garage, and leaving through a different door while the dog is otherwise occupied or distracted can greatly help reduce departure anxiety Cues that are commonly associated with calmness, food and the owner's presence can be provided during departures to reduce anxiety. During departures, a TV, radio or videotape can be left on, or the dog can be provided with a favourite blanket to lie on. Some owners do not understand the principles of these techniques so that the dog is placed in a cage or a radio turned on only when the owner leaves, so that these cues become associated with anxiety and departure, not calmness The dog should be desensitised to those cues that cannot be avoided during departures. The owner should repeatedly pick up the car keys, open, shut and handle the door, put on a coat or pick up a briefcase so that the pet habituates to these cues and they lose their strength in eliciting anxiety. Placing a dog in its cage, locking it in the kitchen, or opening and shutting the door are events that the dog should be constantly exposed to when the owner is at home, during sit–stay and reward training sessions. After the dog has been desensitised to the departure cues, the owner should practice short mock departures. The pet should be exercised, placed in its resting area, and ignored for 15 minutes prior to departure. The owner should initially leave for a very short period of only a few seconds to a few minutes. The duration should be shorter than the time in which it takes the pet to show signs of anxiety. Periods can be lengthened gradually as dogs respond without associated anxiety. The duration of departure should be lengthened on a variable schedule, so that the pet cannot predict exactly how long the owner will be gone
Preventing destructive behaviour	Confining the dog to a cage or placing a muzzle on it to prevent chewing may rarely be useful as a temporary measure but in most cases is likely to cause increased anxiety
Remote monitoring	To assess the pet's behaviour when the owner is out of sight, remote monitoring can be accomplished using a video recorder, tape recorder or baby monitor
Punishment	Punishment increases anxiety so that it plays no role in the successful management of separation anxiety, except for the occasional item or area that might be booby-trapped or sprayed with an aversive tasting substance. Punishment devices (such as motion detectors) may also be useful to keep the dog out of problem areas when there are not doors that can be closed off. In the rare case that a booby-trap is used, it should be of such mild intensity that it will deter the pet from performing a behaviour without causing any anxiety
Drug therapy	Benzodiazepines, such as alprazolam or clorazepate, are often helpful in reducing anxiety and providing some control as behavioural modification begins Tricyclic antidepressants such as clomipramine and amitriptyline may be useful at reducing departure anxiety that has become chronic, compulsive or stereotypic Other drugs such as barbiturates, propranolol, buspirone, and phenothiazines may also be helpful adjuncts to behavioural therapy techniques. However, on their own, they are rarely successful

FIG. 7.2 Management of separation anxiety.

develop in association with sudden, major changes in the pet's life.

When counselling the owner about a current problem, some time should always be spent discussing similar future situations that might trigger a recurrence and how to best avoid problems.

Case Example

Patsy was a 4-year-old spayed female German Shepherd Dog which started exhibiting destructive behaviour soon after her owner went back to work following an extended illness and stay at home. Patsy was constantly at the owner's side whenever she was home and frequently nudged, pawed or whined to get attention from the owner. When the owner was getting ready to leave, the pet would pace, whine and tremble. While the owner was at work, it would scratch and chew at the front door and would occasionally chew holes in pillows and stuffed furniture. Upon the owner's arrival at the end of the workday, the dog became extremely excited. Dragging Patsy to the areas where she was destructive and spanking her had no effect on curtailing the problem.

Behavioural modification techniques were outlined to the owner but she didn't think they were practical, especially in the short term. Instead, the owner requested drug therapy, as euthanasia was her next consideration. The dog was started on amitriptyline (2.0 mg/kg PO bid) for 4 weeks and then gradually tapered off. The owner was instructed to review the pet's obedience training and to practice stays frequently, leaving the pet for gradually longer periods in a variety of areas throughout the house. During the owner's meals, the dog was given her favourite rubber toy, with a piece of liver and a few dog biscuits placed inside. The dog was taught to lie on its mat in the corner of the kitchen, while the owner turned on a favourite CD. Throughout a meal the dog was taught to stay in place while the owner ate, read a newspaper, had coffee and left the room on a number of occasions. During actual departures the owner was instructed to exercise the dog, return home, and have the dog lie on its mat. The owner then turned on the CD, gave the dog a new rawhide toy and its rubber toy with food and treats packed inside. The owner was to ignore the dog completely, and leave the room once or twice while the dog remained on the mat. While the dog was working on its toys, the owner was to leave and return to the room, and on the second or third

occasion, depart quickly without giving the dog any attention or any indication of departure. This technique provided the dog with an enjoyable distraction, and a departure associated with minimal anxiety. Combined with drug therapy, the dog improved dramatically within the first few weeks.

Feline Scratching

Cats scratch upright objects to pull off exterior layers of nail, to mark upright objects and as a means of stretching. During this behaviour, secretions of glands located on the paws are rubbed on the scratched object. On occasion, the behaviour is directed toward horizontal objects, such as the top or seats of furniture and carpeting. This normal behaviour becomes a problem for the owner when walls, furniture and carpeting are destroyed.

Diagnosis and Prognosis

Diagnosis is straightforward. In most cases, the owner has observed the cat scratching or has found evidence of damage in the home. Some cats that have been harshly punished by the owner when they were scratching may subsequently only scratch when the owner is out of sight.

The duration of the behaviour and the individual cat's inherent drive to scratch directly influence the prognosis. Cats that have been scratching frequently for a long period and individuals with a strong drive to scratch can be very frustrating to correct.

Management

A scratching post must be chosen that is acceptable to the cat. The owner may need to offer several different types until a suitable one is found. Sisal-covered posts and upright fireplace logs are generally well accepted. The post should be placed in a prominent area, perhaps near to where the cat sleeps or plays. During training, the pet should be under constant supervision and covertly punished (watergun) whenever it scratches an unacceptable surface. When the owner cannot watch the cat, it should be confined to a room or portion of the house where the only acceptable surface to scratch is its post. A small treat should be given to the pet whenever it approaches the post and a larger one should be given whenever it actually

DECLAWING STUDIES		
Study	**Reference**	**Findings**
Borchelt and Voith (1987): Aggressive behaviour in cats	*Compendium of Continuing Education*, **1**, 49, 1987	Declawed cats no more likely to bite, bite more times or bite more seriously
Bennett, Houpt and Erb (1988): Effects of declawing on feline behaviour	*Companion Animal Practice*, **2**, 70, 1988	No change in behaviour after declawing. Owners of declawed cats reported higher number of good behaviours than owners of clawed cats
Morgan and Houpt (1989): Feline behaviour problems; the influence of declawing	*Anthrozoos*, **3**, 50, 1989	No difference in behaviour problems (housesoiling, biting) between declawed cats and clawed cats
Landsberg (1991): Cat owners' attitudes toward declawing	*Anthrozoos*, **4**, 192, 1991	Declawing met the objectives of all owners. 70% of cat owners indicated an improved cat–owner relationship. No adverse behavioural consequences noticed by owners
Landsberg (1991): Declawing is controversial but still saves pets	*Veterinary Forum*, October, 67, 1991	50% of cat owners may not have kept their pets if not declawed. As many as 50,000 cats' lives saved per year in Ontario alone

FIG. 7.3 Declawing studies and their findings.

scratches it. More freedom can be allowed once the pet shows a preference for scratching its post and no interest in household items.

If the cat only scratches a few areas, it could have freedom in the home and the appeal of the scratched objects and areas could be reduced by draping a loose covering or attaching double-sided tape to the surfaces, or through the use of aversive scents or humane booby-traps (motion detectors, upside-down mouse-traps). Should the cat continue to choose its own sites and locations, the owner could move the scratching post to the cat's favoured locations, and perhaps even place it directly in front of (or mount it on) the door, wall, furniture, or object that the cat has chosen to scratch. Cleaning the scent left from the footpads may be helpful.

Some owners are unable to train their cats to stop furniture scratching, despite attempts at scratching post training and behavioural modification techniques. These owners may then be faced with the undesirable options of removing the cat from the home, allowing the cat to go outdoors, or constant confinement. Another alternative, which is performed relatively frequently in North America but is condemned and may even be illegal in some countries, is declawing. While the humane and moral implications of declawing are open for discussion, there have now been numerous studies to show that declawing does not cause measurable adverse effects on behaviour or physical health. In countries where it is acceptable, declawing may ultimately increase cat ownership and decrease cat euthanasias. Declawing successfully met the owner's objectives in all cases and many owners of declawed cats felt that they had a better or healthier relationship with their pet (Fig. 7.3).

Prevention

Prevention is accomplished by the same methods used for treatment. Owners should be counselled to avoid allowing cats to scratch old pieces of furniture, as the pet will probably continue to scratch when those pieces are replaced with new pieces.

Case Example

Kermit was a 7-month-old neutered male cat who had been scratching the owner's living room sofa for the past 2 months. The owner was planning to replace the furniture but wanted to stop the scratching behaviour first.

The sofa was covered with plastic while the owner trained Kermit to use a scratching post. A firelog mounted upright on plywood was selected because the cat showed some interest in it and it was dissimilar to the fabric on the sofa. A small amount of catnip was sprinkled on the post to attract the cat. When it approached the post it was given a modest semi-moist cat treat; when it made contact with the post it was given a larger treat. Eventually treats were only reserved for times at which the cat made contact with its paws or actually scratched the post. After 4 weeks, the plastic cover was removed from the sofa when the owner was at home and could watch Kermit. The owner was instructed to toss a key chain near the cat or squirt it with a water gun if it was caught in the act of attempting to scratch the furniture. Within 2 months the owners bought new furniture, supervised closely for the first few weeks, and had no further complaints.

Further Reading

Borchelt, P. L. (1983) Separation-elicited behaviour problems in dogs. In: *New Perspectives on Our Lives with Companion Animals*, Katcher, A. H. and Beck, A. M. (eds.) University of Pennsylvania Press: Philadelphia, PA.

Borchelt, P. L. and Voith, V. L. (1982) Diagnosis and treatment of separation-related behaviour problems in dogs. *Veterinary Clinics of North America, Small Animal Practice*, **12**, 625–636.

Hunthausen, W. L. (1988) Avoiding chewing problems, *Intervet*, **23**(6), 23–24.

Hunthausen, W. L. (1991) The causes, treatment, and prevention of canine destructive chewing. *Veterinary Medicine*, October, 1007–1010.

Landsberg, G. M. (1991) Feline scratching and the effects of declawing. *Veterinary Clinics of North America, Small Animal Practice*, **21**, 265.

Landsberg, G. M. (1994) Declawing revisited. Controversy over consequences. *Veterinary Forum*, September, 94.

McCrave, E. A. (1991) Diagnostic criteria for separation anxiety in the dog. *Veterinary Clinics of North America, Small Animal Practice*, **21**(2), 247–255.

Voith, V. L. (1975) Destructive behaviour in the owner's absence. *Canine Practice*, **2**(3), 11.

Voith, V. L. and Borchelt, P. L. (1996) Separation anxiety in dogs. In: *Readings in Companion Animal Behavior*. Voith, V. L. and Borchelt, P. L. (eds). 124–139. Veterinary Learning Systems: Trenton, NJ.

8

Feeding and Diet-Related Problems

The Physiological Influence of Diet on Behaviour

There has long been a perceived relationship between diet and behaviour but few scientific studies have been conducted to provide any meaningful conclusions. Recently, the term animal psychodietetics has been advanced to describe the relation between nutrition and behavioural changes. It is probably sufficient to realise that nutrients can impact upon the behavioural process in a number of intriguing ways.

It is not unreasonable to assume that some dogs and cats might have behavioural problems related to their diet. After all, many dogs eat high-calorie, high-protein commercial diets, with additives, flavourings, preservatives and other processing enhancements. All of these features have been suspected by different investigators pursuing different aspects of behaviour problems. Until more information is available, it would seem advisable at least to consider a nutritional basis for animals with abnormal behaviour patterns, those that are aggressive, or those that fail to train properly.

In addition, the innate feeding instincts of dogs and cats include hunting and all aspects of prey-stalking, chasing and the kill. Scavenging is also a normal canine behaviour. These activities utilise energy and occupy time in the animal's day. Dogs and cats kept as housepets and fed a highly palatable processed and concentrated food once or twice a day may be receiving a complete nutritious daily ration, but there may be behavioural consequences of this type of feeding regimen.

Most concerns of behaviour specialists focus on the role of protein in behaviour problems. Both the quantity of protein and its quality and extent of processing have recently become suspect. It has been suggested that high-meat diets may possibly result in lowered levels of the neurotransmitter serotonin in the brain, because of the high level of amino acids competing with tryptophan (from which serotonin is formed) for the carrier that transports amino acids across the blood–brain barrier. Low serotonin levels have been associated with aggression in some animals. Reduction in dietary protein content was found to be beneficial in the management of dogs with territorial aggression that is a result of fear. No effect was seen in dogs with dominance aggression or hyperactivity. Recent studies have shown that feeding a reduced protein diet did not significantly change CSF levels of 5HT, norepinephrine, epinephrine, dopamine or their metabolites.

Carbohydrate levels are another area of interest. It is believed that when high-carbohydrate diets are fed, tryptophan reaches the brain in higher amounts and results in the production of serotonin. This may have a calming effect on the animal, making it less aggressive. Supplementing the diet with vitamin B_6 (pyridoxine) might also be beneficial because this aids in the production of serotonin.

Another concern, often posed by dog trainers, is that training problems are more common in dogs fed dry food than those fed a canned ration. If training problems related to dry rations do exist, they are more likely to be related to preservatives than low-moisture content. Since canned food is heat-sterilised before packaging, preservatives are not needed. In dry foods, expected to last for months on store shelves without being refrigerated, many chemicals, especially anti-oxidants and flavour enhancers, must be added to the foods to keep them edible.

Only recently has any scientific research been directed in this area, so little is actually known about the influence of various components of the diet on behaviour. It remains a very intriguing area of applied animal behaviour.

Diagnosis

The hypothesis of high-protein or preservative-rich diets contributing to behaviour problems can be tested by feeding a high-quality but low-protein diet and watching for changes. Prior to placing a pet on a protein-restricted diet, it is essential that there are no abnormalities on physical examination and that routine blood and urine tests are normal. Feeding trial diets must be homemade: canned foods are often very high in protein; dry foods contain large amounts of preservatives; and semi-moist foods are high in sugars. The protein sources that are suitable include boiled chicken, lamb, fish or rabbit combined with boiled white rice or mashed potatoes. This also limits problems that might occur from high-cereal diets (e.g. exorphines), milk proteins (e.g. casomorphine) and preservatives. The meal should be mixed as one part meat to four parts carbohydrate and fed in the same amount as the regular diet. Only fresh water should be provided during the trial. No supplements, treats or snacks should be given. This diet is not nutritionally balanced but that should make little difference for the 7–10 days in which the trial is being conducted.

If there is a response to the diet trial, it will then be necessary to determine whether specific ingredients in the food (allergens, additives, preservatives) or the relative content of ingredients (protein *versus* carbohydrate) are implicated in the changes in behaviour. Therefore, the next step is to challenge the pet for potential offenders. The first test would be to increase the protein component of the diet (50:50) to see if there is a behavioural change. If so, this helps confirm the diagnosis and that it is the protein component that is contributory. At this point a careful reassessment for medical problems such as hepatic encephalopathy might be warranted. If the behaviour problem does not recur with the increase in protein, new protein sources, vegetables, treats and commercial foods can be reintroduced slowly to determine the role of specific ingredients, additives and preservatives to the problem.

Management

For animals that respond to a homemade low-protein preservative-free diet, there are many options available. Regular use of a homemade diet should be discouraged unless a completely balanced ration can be formulated. Low-protein diets are commercially available (such as those prescribed for kidney disease) and are the most convenient option. If owners are selecting their own foods from a pet supply shop, they must look for diets with high-quality protein in moderate amounts and an easily digested carbohydrate source. Start with canned diets, which tend to

have few if any preservatives. Dry foods have the most preservatives. If the condition worsens when the pet is put on to a commercial ration, there are likely to be more problems than just protein content to consider.

For dogs with reactions to preservatives, canned foods are an option and there are also preservative-free diets commercially available. Both of these are usually acceptable but current regulations make it almost impossible to be assured that there are actually no preservatives in preservative-free diets. Manufacturers only need to list on the label those preservatives that they add during ration preparation. However, there is no guarantee that the manufacturer did not purchase the raw ingredients already preserved. If a pet responds well to the homemade diet, and challenge feeding fails to uncover a culprit, consider additives as a likely candidate. When commercial diets cannot be used, homemade diets remain a final option. At this point, it is worth having a diet recipe prepared by a nutritionist to ensure that nutritional requirements will be met. Alternatively, computer software is available so that customised diets can be formulated by practitioners.

Prevention

Since most diet-induced behaviour problems are idiosyncratic, it is often not possible to prevent most cases. There are some general guidelines, however, that might be helpful. Clients do not need to feed their dogs high-protein diets. The average housepet consumes a diet that contains much more protein than is needed for amino acid requirements. The result is a loss of expensive protein in the faeces and urine, or a conversion of the excess energy into fat. Neither of these possibilities makes sense.

It is possible that many pets have reactions to preservatives (e.g. ethoxyquin, Butylated hydroxyanisole (BHA), Butylated hydroxytoluene (BHT), but that most of these reactions are subclinical. This is no different from acknowledging that some people cannot tolerate monosodium glutamate (MSG) in Chinese food, or sulphites at a salad bar. The difference between people and pets is that people dine on these foods occasionally whereas pets consume commercial diets for their entire lives, day after day. If people consumed MSG with every meal, every day, we might find that more people 'cross the threshold' and develop clinical problems. We should strive, then, to provide pets with wholesome diets that do not require extensive preservation. Canned diets contain the least amount of preservatives. Home-delivered, preservative-free, home-prepared and frozen pet foods are all options with which the veterinarian should be familiar.

There is some anecdotal evidence that behaviour problems due to some dietary ingredients may be familial. Some breeds seem to react to preservatives (e.g. Cavalier King Charles Spaniel), some to exorphines (Golden Retrievers), and others to serotonin-influencing factors of different meat proteins. Research remains to be done to confirm these possibilities. Neutering animals with these dietary idiosyncrasies will lessen the contribution of any hereditary factors to the breed gene pool.

Case Example

Willard, a 2-year-old male Doberman Pinscher, was presented with an owner's complaint of 'weird' behaviour. Apparently, Willard would have episodes when he was hyperactive, combined with periods when he slept a lot. When he was hyperactive, he would run in circles in the back garden until he was exhausted. If he was confined indoors, he would press his head against his owners and would not leave them alone. They had tried punishing him with harsh words and locking him in the laundry room, but to no avail. They first noticed the problem at about 8 months of age and felt that it was getting worse.

At the time of his behavioural consultation, Willard was his placid self and demonstrated no evidence of hyperactivity. There were no abnormal findings on clinical examination. The owners felt that he may be worse in the evenings, but they had difficulty pinpointing any pattern to his hyperactivity. Willard was fed *ad libitum*. The differential diagnoses included toxicity (including food reactions, hepatic encephalopathy and copper-induced hepatopathy), forms of epilepsy, and even a variant of normal behaviour. Laboratory testing included a haematological profile, urinalysis and biochemical profile that included bile acids (fasting and 2-hour postprandial), ammonia, serum alkaline phosphatase, glucose, cholesterol, urea, creatinine, and serum alanine aminotransferase.

The results of laboratory testing were not conclusive. There were moderate elevations of serum bile acids with mild hyperammonaemia and hypoglycaemia. Ammonium biurate crystals were only infrequently observed in the urine. Radiographs did not demonstrate a significantly smaller liver than anticipated. In consultation with the owner, it was decided that the case did not warrant liver biopsy and quantitative determination of hepatic copper. The tentative working diagnosis was possible hepatic encephalopathy. A low-protein diet challenge was suggested in which Willard was fed a low-protein homemade diet using chicken and rice with four small meals being fed daily, rather than the *ad libitum* feeding to which Willard was accustomed.

After 5 days on the homemade low-protein diet, the owners felt there was a marked improvement in Willard's behaviour. He still had lots of energy but they did not notice any bizarre behaviours. The owners were advised to feed a high-quality but low-protein commercial ration. After 2 months on this diet, they reported few episodes of hyperactivity. They were happy with the results and chose not to pursue a specific diagnosis with further tests.

Obesity

Obesity is the most common nutritional disorder in North America, outnumbering all deficiency syndromes combined. A sad statistic is that over 25% of dogs in North America are overweight. It is likely that obese pets do not live as long as those of normal weight. They suffer more from heart problems, they fatigue easily, and are at increased risk of developing diabetes mellitus. Obese pets also have a decreased resistance to infection and are more prone to anaesthetic complications should surgery ever be necessary. Links with many other clinical problems have been suggested but have yet to be clearly demonstrated. Today, more than ever, pets are being 'killed with kindness' as their owners allow them to become obese.

Obesity becomes more common as pets get older. Females are more prone to obesity than are males and neutered pets are more likely to become obese than are intact pets. Unfortunately, people that are obese themselves are much more likely to have obese pets, attesting to the significance of environmental factors at promoting obesity. Genetic factors are also contributory. Labrador Retrievers, Cocker Spaniels, Collies, Dachshunds, Beagles, Basset Hounds, Shetland Sheepdogs, and some terriers are more prone to obesity than are other breeds. Some breeds, most notably the German Shepherd Dog, Boxer, Whippet and Greyhound actually have a lower incidence of obesity than other breeds. Although genetics plays a role, clearly the most important factors leading to obesity are providing pets with excessive calories and inadequate physical activity. Obesity is rarely seen in wild animals and only infrequently seen in working dogs. It is the household pet, rarely exercised, confined to the home and fed a high-quality diet that is most prone to obesity.

The petfood industry markets diets with the consumer in mind and provides very palatable, high-calorie diets. The supplement market contributes biscuit treats and fatty acid supplements that are usually calorie-dense. The owner, with a firm emotional bond to the pet, wants to provide a healthy, tasty meal that the pet will devour and ask for more. The veterinarian, in the position of health-concerned middleman, must counsel the owner about what is really in the best interests of the pet.

Diagnosis and Prognosis

Pets are considered obese when they are 20% more than their ideal weight. This can be done by comparing the weight with compiled charts or approximated by visual inspection (fat covering of ribs) and palpation. What is often more critical is to determine the reason for the obesity. In most cases, the owners would rather believe the pet has a medical problem (hypothyroidism is a favourite), rather than consider that they are the most important cause. All obese pets should have a thorough physical examination and laboratory profile (complete blood count, serum alanine transferase (ALT), amylase/lipase, alkaline phosphatase, thyroid profile, urinalysis, cholesterol, creatinine, glucose, insulin) but most cases are due to owner feeding practices.

Owners often find it difficult to believe they are overfeeding their pets. Feeding practices may further complicate matters. The food may be left available to the pet all day, so that feeding can continue all day. Snacks are an important addition to the feeding routine even though most 'treats' contain 60 kilocalories or more apiece. Coat-care supplements of fatty acids are also calorie-dense. Therefore, veterinarians counselling owners of obese pets must be prepared to determine the animal's caloric needs, all

calorie contributors in the pet's diet, and the amount of calorie-burning activities in the pet's lifestyle. Most owners can manage the problem more effectively when they can see, in black and white, where the problem lies. In these cases, the prognosis is good. A poor prognosis is given when owners refuse to admit there is a problem or blame the situation on others.

Management

Obesity can be dealt with intelligently and effectively if pet owners are willing to pay attention to the facts. Owners must be committed to helping their pets lose weight and must realise that the pets will be healthier and happier if they make the effort. All weight reduction programmes should be performed under the supervision of a veterinarian to reduce the risk of complications from obesity or from weight loss.

Regularly scheduled meals and snacks often reduce the client's tendency to overfeed the pet. Making them count calories also makes them more likely to comply with a weight-reduction programme. Several behavioural modification programmes help to reinforce the concepts needed in successful dieting. Clients should be cautioned that when they give in to begging, they only reinforce that behaviour and make weight loss even more difficult. Stimulus control modification is used to regulate the cues that trigger feeding; in other words certain stimuli may have inadvertently become paired with feeding and these need to be carefully managed. Such stimuli might include the owner's arrival home (the dog anticipates a treat), entering the kitchen, opening cupboards, drawers or the refrigerator, or even just sitting in the kitchen. Avoiding these cues, moving food treats to a different cupboard, and changing routines can therefore be an important aspect of behavioural therapy. Another alternative is to insist that the dog performs an appropriate command each time it approaches and begins to beg (e.g. 'down–stay') and to gradually extend the down–stay with each subsequent approach. As a reward the pet can then receive a patting session, a play session, a chew toy, or a walk. This technique does little to decrease approach and begging but does help the owners gain control over the situation. The pet gains no calories from its demands and begging, and the owners learn that there are other rewards that can be just as fulfilling to the pet. Clients must not associate

MANAGING OBESITY IN PETS

Approach	Rationale
Treat the owner	Be aware that owners will feel 'guilty' depriving their pet of food rewards. So, owners must be committed to providing a reasonable amount of calories to their pets, exercising them more, and cutting back on fattening supplements and treats. The management plan will fail if the owner is not completely committed to the process
	For owners who refuse to forego giving treats to the pet, low-calorie foods (cooked vegetables, broth ice cubes) may be suggested to replace commercial treats
Determine ideal weight	Using breed information or empirical evaluation, and allowing for individual variation, reach a consensus with the owner as to what the ideal weight should be. This is critical because the ideal weight will be used to calculate caloric needs
Determine caloric needs	The pet's ideal weight, activity level, age and health status determine its caloric needs. Charts and tables can be found in most nutrition or veterinary texts
Evaluate diet	Select a food that has a moderate amount of protein (20–40% with high biological value) but not excessive amounts of either protein or fat. Muscle can be lost along with fat, so protein restriction is not desirable
	Determine the caloric load of all foods to be fed, including snacks and table scraps
	Reach a consensus with the owner as to how the daily meals are to be apportioned (e.g. a treat after each meal, the amount of food recommended by the veterinarian, and only vegetables from the table). For example, if a dog is to get 750 kcal per day including 2 treats of 75 kcal each, the owner should feed enough of the ration to provide 600 kcal
Restrict calories	The caloric needs determination provides the amount of calories the pet needs on a daily basis. Make the calculation given the food being fed, and contributions from snacks, table scraps and treats. Initially, a feeding regimen must be used that provides about 60% of the normal daily caloric requirements. By creating a calorie deficit of about 250 calories/day, there should be a safe weight loss of about 250g per week (it takes a total calorie reduction of about 3500 kcal for every 500g of weight loss). This will allow pets to lose the required weight over a safe 12-week period. Dogs should have access to their meals for only 30 minutes twice daily and should not be fed between meals
	Cats seem to do better when provided with three or four small meals per day. A very gradual change from the current diet to the low-calorie diet is usually required. Under **NO** circumstances should a cat ever be starved in order to switch it over to a new diet; life-threatening hepatic disease is a likely sequel
Exercise the pet	A severely obese pet will not be able to exercise normally and will quickly become fatigued. The goal should be to accommodate the pet slowly to regular exercise, not stress it to exhaustion. For most pets, a daily walk of 2–5 km is exhilarating and healthy for both dog and owner
	As an alternative, consider teaching the pet to retrieve and using this game for 15–20 minutes twice a day. Instead of treats, reward the pet with an outing instead. Many would prefer the companionship to the treat, anytime
Keep a diary	Supervision and assessment of the progress is easier when the owner keeps a diary of daily food intake, exercise and body weight

FIG. 8.1 The management of obesity.

feeding with 'quality time' for their pet. Thus, the pet should only be given food in its bowl and be fed in only one location. This helps deter the animal from seeking meals and treats elsewhere, and from begging.

Once the weight has been safely lost, it is important not to resort to the old behaviours that resulted in obesity to begin with. It is usually recommended that the calorie content of the diet be left at 90% of requirements rather than 100%, because snacks are bound to creep back into the diet at some point.

Prevention

Obesity is the number one nutritional problem affecting dogs and cats and it is a health concern that is entirely preventable. Pets count on their owners for their health care needs, and calorie restriction rather than caloric excess should be the operative concept. Caloric restriction not only prevents obesity but may lower the risk of musculoskeletal problems and cancer. Unfortunately, weight loss in pets is no easier for most owners than their own diet needs. Proper nutrition requires a basic philosophical change so owners understand the difference between optimal nutrition and overnutrition.

Case Example

Brandy, a 17 kg, 6-year-old English Cocker Spaniel, was seen during a routine annual examination. The owners weren't sure why Brandy was overweight because he only ate one cup of food twice daily, just as recommended by the petfood manufacturer. They thought that perhaps he might have problems with his metabolism because he also wasn't very 'spunky' and that it might have something to do with the fact that he was neutered before 1 year of age.

The physical examination of Brandy was unremarkable other than his obvious weight problem. A worksheet was used to determine 'everything' that Brandy ate on a typical day as well as his usual exercise schedule. Both of the owners worked and Brandy was left alone most of the day. They left food available for him at all times but some of it was still in his bowl when they got home at night. He got three cereal-biscuit snacks in the morning when they left for work, three when they returned and three before bedtime. He also got table scraps occasionally, but not consistently and not in large quantities.

The owners weren't convinced that Brandy was being overfed but agreed to explore the situation with us further. Routine haematological and biochemical tests (including a thyroid profile of free and total levels) were normal or negative. The owner was then given these facts: Brandy should be receiving about 850 kcal daily based on an ideal weight of about 14 kg. The biscuit treats were 90% dry matter (3.60 kcal/g DM) and 25 g each. His nine treats a day amounted to 810 kcal, almost a whole day's caloric requirements! The dry food being fed contained 3.67 kcal/g DM and was 90% dry matter. Further mathematics were unnecessary to convince the owners of Brandy's caloric excess.

The plan was to give Brandy only one treat twice a day, following each of his two meals. Brandy required 850 kcal per day but we decided to create a caloric deficit of 250 calories/day so there could be a safe weight loss of about 250 g per week. Taking into account the owners' wishes, the diet was formulated to account for both pet food and biscuit treats. Therefore, Brandy would be getting 600 kcal per day, 162 kcal from his biscuit treats. The owners did the maths too so they could see that Brandy should

receive only 438 kcal per day from his dogfood, split between two meals. Knowing the caloric density and dry matter of the food (*see above*), this means that Brandy should receive about 132.5 g of food a day, or 67 g with each meal. The owners were informed about specially formulated weight-loss diets but decided they could follow this regimen. They were also going to play fetch with him for 10 minutes each morning before they went to work and take him for a one-mile walk each evening.

On re-examination 12 weeks later, Brandy was a svelte 15 kg and much more energetic. The owners did have some difficulty sticking to the regime and augmented his diet with carrots and popcorn. Brandy really liked the carrots and sometimes preferred them to the cereal treats. They did miss some walks and did not always have time for fetch but, all in all, they were fairly consistent. We decided that Brandy could go on a maintenance diet of 90% of his requirements (about 765 kcal/day) while getting only one biscuit treat daily. This meant that Brandy could get about 207 g of food daily, rather than 132.5g. The owners were happy with the compromise.

Coprophagia

Coprophagia is an ingestive behaviour involving the consumption of faeces. It is not uncommon in the canine population but is rare in the feline population. Dogs may selectively ingest their own faeces, faeces of other dogs, feline faeces, ungulate faeces, other mammalian faeces, or may consume any type of faeces that are available. Whereas adult bitches will consume the faeces of their puppies, all other forms of coprophagia are considered abnormal. The problem tends to be seen more frequently in puppies but most eventually outgrow it. Puppies may indulge in coprophagia as harmless investigative or playful behaviour and owners must be cautious not to inadvertently reinforce the behaviour by giving the puppy additional attention when it consumes faeces. Pets that are underfed or placed on an overly restricted diet may have a voracious appetite which may also include coprophagia. Pets that have been overfed, and those with gastrointestinal conditions such as malabsorption or trypsin deficiencies, may have higher amounts of undigested ingredients remaining in the faeces. These faeces might then be palatable enough to appeal to some dogs. Similarly horse and cat faeces can be particularly appealing to some dogs. It is commonly thought that inadequate exercise and environmental stimulation may make a dog more likely to consume its own faeces.

Diagnosis

The ultimate cause of coprophagia in adult dogs has always been elusive. Some feel that the problem is behavioural while others are convinced there is an organic reason. Recent research has suggested that there may indeed be a medical component to the problem. In a small study of nine coprophagic dogs conducted by two of the authors (GL, LA), all had at least one laboratory abnormality that could explain the problem. The laboratory profile included a complete blood count, complete biochemical profile, amylase, lipase, trypsin-like immunoreactivity, vitamin B_{12}, folate, faecal fat, faecal trypsin, faecal muscle fibre, trace minerals (including zinc, selenium, copper, iron, magnesium, and boron) and faecal sedimentation. Most had borderline to low trypsin-like immunoreactivity (TLI), while others had abnormalities in folate, cobalamin or other nutrients. None of the dogs had internal parasites (determined by faecal sedimentation) or abnormal faecal fat or trypsin levels. In addition, 4 of the 9 dogs showed some benefit when supplemented with a plant-based enzyme supplement.

Management

If the cause of the coprophagia cannot be determined, environmental modifications are the best chance for therapeutic success. Denying access to faeces is the first step. The garden should be cleaned regularly and not in the direct sight of the dog with the problem. On walks, the dog should be kept on a leash or halter and given a stern, verbal correction and a quick pull on the leash when it attempts to sniff or ingest other faeces. The pet must be under constant supervision while outdoors. Tossing a shake can near the pet every time it attempts to consume faeces or painting aversive-tasting (odourless) substances on the underside of faeces may occasionally be effective. However, if the faeces are not consistently coated with the deterrent or the pet is not constantly supervised, the behaviour (which is self-rewarding in the coprophagic dog) will persist. Although generally impractical and excessive, placing nauseants in the stool (LiCl) are the only deterrents that are likely to be permanently effective.

Dietary changes are successful with some but not all coprophagic dogs. Some dogs are less likely to be coprophagic when a more highly digestible diet is fed or when meat tenderisers or proteolytic enzyme supplements are added to the faeces. Most dogs prefer well-formed faeces, so providing a high-fibre diet causes bulkier less formed faeces to be produced. Adding a variety of concoctions to the diet has been advocated but there seems to be no consensus that they work on a regular basis. The exception seems to be the plant-based enzyme supplements but this needs to be evaluated in more dogs before firm conclusions can be made. Products used for reducing stool appeal must be good-tasting or tasteless when initially consumed but suitably aversive when they are degraded in the intestinal tract and appear in the stool.

Coprophagia has always been a difficult condition to treat. However, new studies suggest that veterinarians should always conduct a thorough medical and laboratory investigation before dismissing coprophagia as a behavioural problem.

Case Example

Ginger was a 7-year-old apricot Poodle which had a history of coprophagia spanning many years. The owner had been unable to curb the habit, despite scolding Ginger and adding various noxious agents (such as cayenne pepper) to the faeces in the back yard. At first Ginger was repulsed by the agents, but after a while it seemed that Ginger had actually developed a taste for them. Otherwise, the owner felt that Ginger was a perfect pet.

Physical examination was unremarkable. Laboratory evaluation consisted of routine haematology and biochemistry, faecal sedimentation (rather than flotation), trypsin-like immunoreactivity (TLI), vitamin B_{12}, folate, and faecal trypsin, muscle fibre and fat. There were some striated muscle fibres evident in the faeces and the TLI was low but not in the diagnostic range for exocrine pancreatic insufficiency. It was concluded that there might be a marginal pancreatic enzyme insufficiency as part of the problem.

Treatment consisted of environmental and dietary modification. The owner collected the faeces from the garden on a regular basis and walked Ginger on a leash so she could not consume faeces during walks. The diet was changed to a low-fibre highly digestible ration which was topdressed with a plant-based enzyme supplement (containing bromelain, papain and phytase). Re-evaluation 8 weeks later revealed a dog that was much improved. Although Ginger still occasionally ate faeces, it was not with the same relish that she once possessed. Six months later, the owner reported that Ginger rarely if ever consumed faeces.

Pica

Pica is an abnormal craving or appetite for ingesting non-food substances. While young animals will chew on a wide variety of substances, the items are rarely ingested. Starch-and soil-eating has been documented in humans on severely deficient diets. The cause of pica in pets is unknown. Pica can be a dangerous condition, as well as a nuisance. Some forms of pica such as the wool-eating of cats, 'barbering', or rock-chewing and soil-eating in dogs may be compulsive disorders.

Fabric-eating can be seen as part of the compulsive wool-sucking syndrome exhibited by some cats. The problem seems to appear most frequently in oriental breeds but can be manifested in cats of mixed origin. Many causes have been suggested for this problem, including heredity, early weaning, stress, malfunction of the neural control of appetitive behaviour, separation anxiety and persistence of infant kitten oral behaviour. Woollen items are most commonly chosen but affected cats may well chew on any type of available fabric including cotton, silk and synthetics. The behaviour is most likely to begin during the first year of life and may resolve on its own during early adulthood. (*See also Chapters 7 and 12.*)

Diagnosis and Prognosis

Pica is diagnosed by observing the abnormal behaviour. There are no specific laboratory tests that might provide additional insight, but a full medical work-up is essential, particularly in those cases that are of adult or geriatric onset and where there are no discernible behavioural causes. Medical conditions that lead to nutritional deficiencies or electrolyte imbalances, gastrointestinal disturbances, conditions that lead to polyphagia, and CNS disturbances should all be ruled out. The prognosis is variable, depending on the individual and the material consumed.

Management

By keeping the ingested objects away from the pet, providing appropriate chew toys, or changing the diet to a dry, bulky, nutritionally balanced food, the problem may be corrected. Depending on the pet's level of motivation to chew, taste aversion or booby-traps can be used to keep it away from selected areas or items. Underlying problems that may fuel the behaviour, such as stress or separation anxiety, should be corrected.

Tricyclic antidepressants (amitriptyline, clomipramine) or bicyclic antidepressants (fluoxetine) may be helpful when the pica is compulsive, such as is seen in feline wool-sucking/chewing problems.

Case Example

Rama was a 12-year-old neutered male Siamese cat that had a penchant for climbing underneath one particular sofa, tearing holes in the covering and consuming the stuffing. There were several other pieces of furniture that held no interest for Rama.

The physical examination of Rama was routine. He was a very healthy specimen with no clinical abnormalities. Routine laboratory work-up included faecal assessment, haematology, biochemistry, serum T_4 and viral profiles for feline leukemia virus and feline immunodeficiency virus. No abnormalities were detected on any of the tests.

The first approach involved providing additional oral stimulation and alternative outlets for play and investigation. The owners switched Rama to a dry high-fibre cat food, and provided additional play sessions and cat toys. Although Rama's destructiveness may have decreased, he continued to return to the sofa to chew. Next, the owners attempted booby-trapping the couch with taste aversives and motion detectors, but Rama always managed eventually to get beneath the couch to eat the stuffing. When the owners made a barricade around the base of the couch completely denying access, Rama proceeded to dig between the cushions and tried to chew into the stuffing from the top. Remote punishment with a water rifle was also attempted but Rama continued to return to the area in the owner's absence. Frustrated, the owners finally got rid of the couch. Although they were cautioned that Rama might turn his attention and energy to another piece of furniture, this did not happen. The ultimate cause of the pica was not determined, but the increase in environmental stimulation and removal of the target of Rama's chewing had successfully resolved the issue.

The 'Fussy' or 'Picky' Eater

Both dogs and cats can be finicky when it comes to diet preference. In most cases, the problem stems from previous feeding experiences or heritable responses to feeding situations, although underlying medical problems can contribute. Occasionally, the pet will be reluctant to eat a commercial diet because it has learned that if it waits long enough it will receive more palatable food from the owner.

In truth, the causes of most, true feeding idiosyncrasies are unknown at this time. It is known that odour, taste, texture and temperature can be adjusted to tempt the problem feeder to eat, and that novel foods may increase appetite.

Diagnosis and Prognosis

The diagnosis is usually straightforward but there are some caveats. If the owner complains of a finicky pet, or one that occasionally 'skips' meals, attain an accurate weight of that animal to determine if it is in the normal range. In many cases, these so-called 'finicky' eaters are of normal weight (or even overweight) and do manage to consume all the calories needed on a daily basis. Some dogs may even skip an occasional day with no ill effects. This appears to be a normal mechanism for maintaining optimal weight. It is important to rule out the possibility that the pet is obtaining food elsewhere, either from a neighbour or by hunting. However, this may be a normal mechanism for the individual to maintain its body weight. Make sure to inquire about treats. It is not unusual for biscuit treats to contribute 100 kcal apiece; this can account for a substantial portion of daily requirements.

For pets that are labelled 'fussy' or 'picky' and are underweight, a complete history and thorough medical evaluation needs to be obtained to consider underlying disease processes. Pancreatic, dental, gastrointestinal, kidney and liver disease can all account for 'dietary discrimination'.

Management

All pets with underlying medical problems need to have them addressed. One of the most insidious causes of dietary discrimination is dental disease. Routine dental care is imperative but often under-utilised in practice. It has been estimated that over 85% of dogs and cats have periodontal disease by 4 years of age. It can be inferred from that, that many dogs and cats may have dental pain and discomfort which could interfere with feedings. It is critical that all medical problems be appropriately addressed.

For those healthy animals that continue to turn up their noses at mealtime, there are some alternatives.

THINGS YOU CAN DO FOR THE 'PICKY' EATER

Moisten the food with warm water if you are using dry food. This tends to make hard foods tastier and more chewy

Most dogs prefer the flavours of beef, chicken, pork or lamb rather than vegetable protein such as soy, corn and wheat. Choose a dog food that provides these more desirable ingredients. Cats prefer beef, chicken, fish and pork; select these ingredients for finicky cats

Heating the food in an oven or microwave can enhance the flavour

Add flavour enhancers to the diet, such as liver or poultry broths or bouillon cubes

Consider adding very small amounts of cooked garlic to the food. Use small amounts of cooked garlic cloves, not garlic oil

Add fresh fruit purées as a dressing on the food. Mashed apple or banana are good choices to try first. If necessary, the same effect can be gained by adding small amounts of artificial sweeteners such as aspartame

Add some freshly-cooked food (e.g. hamburger, liver, chicken) to the diet to encourage the 'picky' pet to eat. Slowly wean them off the fresh-cooked food on to the commercial ration

Try a super-premium dog food or gourmet cat food that provides increased levels of protein and fat. Pets need to eat less of these foods to achieve their daily requirements. Owners must be aware that this will not make them less finicky, only assure that even a little bit of food will provide maximal caloric   intake

Add small amounts of commercial catfood to the dog food diet. Cat food has many more flavour enhancers, and is high in fat, high in protein and loaded with B vitamins. Many dogs find it very appealing

Limit treats to the 'picky' pet. Many people that think they have a 'picky' pet really have a dog that fills up on treats rather than his dinner

If the pet is finicky because a new diet is being introduced, add small amounts of the new diet to the previous diet, then gradually increase the proportion of the new diet

Feed small amounts at a time and introduce other foods gradually to foods that are eaten

* Adapted from Ackerman, L. (1996) *What every dog owner, breeder and trainer should know about nutrition*, Alpine Publications

FIG. 8.2 Steps to take with the finicky eater.

The first step is to limit the use of treats and table scraps and see if the owner is pleased with the change. If not, be prepared to calculate the caloric needs of the animal (tables available in nutrition texts) based on its age, weight, and health status and determine the caloric load of the diet being fed. Most commercial diets, especially the gourmet cat foods and the super-premium dog foods, are exceptionally calorie-rich. Because of this, less needs to be fed. Owners often have a preconceived notion of how much their pet should be eating, and it may be completely unrealistic. They tend to try more and more expensive diets (providing more and more calories) and wonder why their pets are getting worse (i.e. eating less). Sometimes, switching to a food that is less calorie-dense will solve the problem because the pet consumes more to achieve its daily caloric needs. Rewards (such as flavoured treats and play) can be given each time the pet voluntarily eats its designated food.

Prevention

Normal, healthy pets rarely try to starve themselves. Most finicky pets actually receive adequate nutrition on a daily basis. Owners should receive veterinary counselling about how much their pet should be eating, based on the food being fed. This requires the veterinarian to be able to determine the caloric needs of the pet, and the caloric density of the food and any treats or table scraps being fed. Everything should be added into the equation.

To help deter pets from becoming 'picky' eaters, they should receive a variety of different food sources so they can develop their 'tastes' while still young. This may significantly impact on food preferences later in life.

Case example

Kwai-Chang was a 3-year old 7 kg Pekingese. His owner was concerned because he almost never completely ate his dinner. She was worried that he might starve to death without her intervention. She was not sure how much he was eating because she fed him dry food by hand. She guessed he was only eating 15–20 pieces of this and only if she handfed him. He wouldn't touch the dry food if it just sat in his bowl. Some days he would only eat his treats and never touch his dry food. She also gave him one fatty acid capsule daily for an undetermined skin ailment.

On physical examination, Kwai-Chang was a healthy and happy Pekingese and not considered underweight. The owner was perplexed as to how he could not be losing weight on such a meagre diet. Together we determined that Kwai-Chang had a daily requirement of about 600 kcal. On average, the owner gave him about six small treats daily, more when he would not eat any of his dinner. Each of the small biscuit treats was about 60 kcal, so six were contributing a total of about 360 kcal to his daily caloric intake. The calories in the fatty acid supplement were considered minimal.

The goal was to lessen the number of treats given daily, substituting a balanced ration. The owner was certain that this could not be done. We decided to commence feeding Kwai-Chang a commercial dry catfood, enough to provide 600 kcal/day. The owner was cautioned not to give any treats to the dog or she would be sabotaging our efforts. She agreed that she would not feed any treats as long as Kwai-Chang ate the food within the first 48 hours. The owner called the next day to say that Kwai-Chang liked the new food but still pestered her for treats. The owner was instructed to ignore the begging (as the behaviour was merely being rewarded by intermittently providing food or attention). Stimuli, situations, and routines that might lead to begging were identified so that begging would be diminished. (*See obesity management for details.*) Since the owners were unwilling to put up with the persistent demands and could not control Kwai-Chang sufficiently to stop the begging, it was decided to use substitute rewards such as toys and play. It was explained that these would also serve to reward the begging but at least Kwai-Chang would learn not to expect food. Each time Kwai-Chang approached they were instructed to have him perform a short 'down–stay' and then go and get a favourite toy and begin a play session. Kwai-Chang's begging quickly diminished, although he still approached for attention and play. The owners were also instructed on methods of stimulus control (*see obesity section above*). Four weeks later Kwai-Chang was still 7 kg and healthy and the owner was convinced he was eating much more than he ever had. She wanted to give him treats again, so three high-fibre low-calorie treats per day (20 kcal each) were added to the daily ration. The owner was instructed, however, to provide the treats only as training rewards and never to give them on demand.

Apetite stimulants

Drugs such as the antiserotenergic antihistamine, cyproheptadine and benzodiazepines such as diazepan, oxazepam or flurazepam may be useful as appetite stimulants on a short term basis.

Further Reading

Ackerman, L. (1993) Adverse reactions to foods. *Journal of Veterinary Allergy and Clinical Immunology*, **1**(1), 18–22.

Ackerman, L. (1993) Effects of an enzyme supplement (Prozyme™) on selected nutrient levels in dogs. *Journal of Veterinary Allergy and Clinical Immunology*, **2**(1), 25–29.

Ackerman, L. (1993) Enzyme therapy in veterinary practice. *Advances in Nutrition*, **1**(3), 9–11.

Annunziata, C., Shell, L., Thatcher, C., Warwick, L., Jones, D. (1996) Effects of a low protein diet on levels of serotonin in canine cerebrospinal fluid. Behavioral abstract in *Am Vet Soc An Beh Newsletter*, **18**(2), 3.

Aschheim, E. (1993) Dietary control of psychosis. *Medical Hypotheses*, **41**, 327–328.

Ballarini, G. (1990) Animal psychodietetics. *Journal of Small Animal Practice*, **31**(10), 523–532.

Blackshaw, J. K. (1991) Management of orally based problems and aggression in cats. *Australian Veterinary Practitioner*, **21**, 122–124.

Brown, R. G. (1989) Dealing with canine obesity. *Canadian Veterinary Journal*, **30**, 973–975.

Buffington, C. A. T. (1994) Management of obesity – the clinical nutritionists experience. *International Journal of Obesity*, **18**(Suppl 1), S29–S35.

Butterwick, R. F., Wills, J. M., Sloth, C. and Markwell, P. J. (1994) A study of obese cats on a calorie-controlled weight-reduction programme. *Veterinary Record*, **134**(15), 372–377.

Diez, M., Leemans, M., Houins, G. and Istasse, L. (1995) Specific-purpose food in companion animals. The new directives of the European Community and practical use in the treatment of obesity. *Annales de Médecine Vétérinaire*, **139**(6), 395–399.

Dodman, N. H., Reisner, I., Shuster, L. *et al.* (1996) Effect of dietary protein content on behaviour in dogs. *J. Am. Vet. Med. Assoc.*, **208**(3), 376–379.

Edney, A. T. B. and Smith, P. M. (1986) Study of obesity in dogs visiting veterinary practices in the United Kingdom. *Veterinary Record*, **118**, 391–396.

Fernstrom, J. D. (1994) Dietary amino acids and brain function. *Journal of the American Dietetic Association*, **94**(1), 71–77.

Gentry, S. J. (1993) Results of the clinical use of a standardized weight-loss program in dogs and cats. *Journal of the American Animal Hospital Association*, **29**(4), 369–375.

Halliwell, R. E. W. (1992) Comparative aspects of food intolerance. *Veterinary Medicine*, September, 893–899.

Houpt, K. A. (1993) Pharmacology and behaviour. In: *Animal Behaviour. The T. G. Hungerford Refresher Course for Veterinarians. July 1993.* pp. 51–59, Postgraduate Committee in Veterinary Science, University of Sydney: Sydney, Australia.

Kallfelz, F. A. and Dzanis, D. A. (1989) Overnutrition: an epidemic problem in pet animal practice? *Veterinary Clinics of North America*, **19**(3), 433–445.

Legrand Defretin, V. (1994) Energy requirements of cats and dogs – what goes wrong. *International Journal of Obesity*, **18**(Suppl 1), S8–S13.

Markwell, P. J., Butterwick, R. F., Wills, J. M. and Raiha, M. (1994) Clinical studies in the management of obesity in dogs and cats. *International Journal of Obesity*, **18**(Suppl 1), S39–S43.

Markwell, P. J. and Edney, A. T. B. (1996) In:

Markwell, P. J. and Edney, A. T. B. (In press) The obese patient. In: Manual of Companion Animal Nutrition and Feeding. N. Kelly and J. M. Wills (eds). pp. 109–116. BSAVA Publications: Cheltenham.

Mugford, R. A. (1987) The influence of nutrition on canine behaviour. *Journal of Small Animal Practice*, **28**(11), 1046–1055.

Neville, P. F. and Bradshaw, J. W. (1994) Fabric eating in cats. *Veterinary Practice Staff*, **6**(5), 26–30.

Norris, M. P. and Beaver, B. V. (1993) Application of behaviour therapy techniques to the treatment of obesity in companion animals. *Journal of the American Veterinary Medical Association*, **202**(5), 728–730.

Quandt, C. (1994) Anorexia and obesity – nonorganic causes and their control. *Praktische Tierarzt*, **75**, 109–110.

Robinson, I. (1992) A taste for survival. In: *Waltham Feline Medicine Symposium*, pp. 55–64, Waltham, Kal Kan Foods: Vernon, CA.

Scarlett, J. M., Donoghue, S., Saidla, J. and Wills, J. (1994) Overweight cats – prevalence and risk factors. *International Journal of Obesity*, **18**(Suppl 1), S22–S28.

Schoenthaler, S. J., Moody, J. M. and Pankow, L. D. (1991) Applied nutrition and behaviour. *Journal of Applied Nutrition*, **43**(1), 31–39.

Wallin, M. S. and Rissanen, A. M. (1994) Food and mood: relationship between food, serotonin and affective disorders. *Acta Psychiatrica Scandinavica*, **89**(suppl. 377), 36–40.

9

Fears and Phobias

There are many reasons why pets experience fears and phobias. Some fear responses are innate (e.g. fear of predators) and are important normal behaviour in safeguarding animals from harm. Problems involving excessive fear responses may be due to an inherited fearful temperament, lack of adequate socialisation, a learned aversion to an unpleasant experience or a combination of these factors (Fig. 9.1). Regardless of the cause, fears and phobias are often reinforced in the animal over time. Whenever a fearful experience leads the animal to perform escape behaviours and it is allowed to escape, the behaviour is reinforced. When a fearful experience prompts an owner to comfort the animal with affection, attention or food, the behaviour is reinforced. In contradistinction, punishing these animals for fearful behaviour only creates more fear and anxiety. The veterinarian must examine the owner's response to the fearful pet to identify and eliminate any potentiating factors. For successful resolution of the problem, owners must be counselled to use appropriate behavioural modification techniques.

Basic Behavioural Modification and the Fearful Pet

Some of the techniques covered in Chapter 3 are particularly relevant to managing fears and phobias, these include flooding, habituation, systematic desensitisation, counterconditioning, shaping and positive

FEAR	
Determinants of Fear	
Genetic	Unconditioned stimuli for fear such as predators, environmental danger, novel situations, and social threats
	Temperament
Environmental	Traumatic experience
	Inadequate socialisation
	Conditioning (reinforcement by the owner or learning behaviours to escape fear-provoking stimuli)
	Sensory isolation during development
Components of Fear	
Physiology	Activation of autonomic and neuroendocrine systems with influence on the cardiovascular system, pupils, piloerection and glucose metabolism
Behaviour	The type of fearful behaviour that is exhibited is determined by genetics (species, breed, individual), experience, type and intensity of stimulus, and presence/absence of conspecifics
	The function of fearful behaviour is to remove the stimulus (threats) or remove the animal from the stimulus (escape behaviour)
Emotion	Although recognised in humans, this has not been scientifically proven to exist in animals

FIG. 9.1 The nature of fear.

MODIFYING FEARFUL BEHAVIOURS	
Step	**Comments**
Identify all fear-provoking stimuli	All stimuli that might evoke fearful responses must be identified to determine the focus for desensitisation and counterconditioning exercises
Identify the threshold for the fear response	The amount, intensity or proximity of the fear-provoking stimulus that is required to elicit signs of fear should be established in order to set a starting point for behavioural modification
Control the pet's environment	Prevent exposure to fear-provoking stimuli or situations that occur outside training sessions
Control the pet's response	The pet must not be allowed to escape or to harm itself or others during behavioural modification. Accomplishing this might include the use of a crate, muzzle or halter. Use of any of these devices is only appropriate if they do not result in increasing the pet's fear
Modify the behaviour	For dogs, it is helpful to use highly motivating rewards such as food, social attention or a favourite toy to reward a 'sit–stay' or 'down–stay' command. Then, combine this command with low-level exposure to the fear-evoking stimulus. Cats can be rewarded with food, patted, played with or groomed during exposure
	When the pet responds well to commands, begin desensitisation with a stimulus intensity just below the threshold that would evoke fear. Rewards are only given when the pet shows no fear response
	Gradually increase the intensity of the stimulus
	Controlled flooding with a stimulus intensity above the threshold for a fearful response can be used for pets with mild problems and good owner control
Avoid reinforcing or punishing fearful behaviour	If the pet is consoled when it is acting fearfully, the fear-related behaviour may be reinforced. If the pet is punished, the state of fearful arousal may increase during subsequent exposures to fear-eliciting stimuli

Fig. 9.2 Behavioural modification techniques used for fearful behaviours.

reinforcement. These can be used individually or together in behavioural modification therapy (Fig. 9.2).

Fear of People

Depending on how a pet was socialised when it was young and the experiences it has with people at any time during its life, it may be fearful of individuals with whom it is not familiar or with those it associates with an aversive experience. In most fearful situations, the animal will attempt to perform behaviours that help it avoid interaction with the fear-evoking stimulus or increase the distance between it and the stimulus. Innate behaviour patterns and conditioning determine whether the animal will freeze, flee or fight. This can prove dangerous if the fear response involves aggression. Any of the following groups may evoke a fear response if the pet has had little exposure to them:

● Babies, children, elderly
● People in uniform
● People whose appearance differs from family members
● Disabled individuals
● Men or women, depending on circumstances

Diagnosis and Prognosis

Fearful behaviour is exhibited with exposure to all types of people or to individuals with specific characteristics. Pets may react quite individually in response to a fearful meeting. Some may respond with aggression while others respond by cowering, remaining motionless, or escaping. Other behaviours that may be seen include trembling, hypersalivation, elimination or dilated pupils.

The prognosis is somewhat variable but is considered good for most cases if the duration is short, the pet was adequately socialised to people, the problem started during adulthood, and the owner can exert control over situations during which the pet

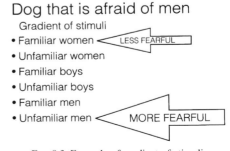

Dog that is afraid of men
Gradient of stimuli
● Familiar women ← LESS FEARFUL
● Unfamiliar women
● Familiar boys
● Unfamiliar boys
● Familiar men
● Unfamiliar men ← MORE FEARFUL

Fig. 9.3 Example of gradient of stimuli.

DOG THAT IS AFRAID OF MEN IN UNIFORMS

1. (a) Female owner wears uniform and approaches
   (b) Second owner or handler gives command, and rewards with treat or toy
   (c) Female owner in uniform gives command, and rewards with treat or toy
2. Repeat with male owner in uniform
3. Repeat with familiar women in uniform
4. Repeat with unfamiliar women or boys in uniform
5. Repeat with unfamilar men with no uniform
6. Repeat with familiar men in uniform
7. Repeat with unfamiliar men in uniform

(Slower progression would be possible by beginning desensitisation to people wearing a portion of the uniform, before the full uniform is applied)

FIG. 9.4 An example of a hierarchy or gradient for desensitisation of a dog that is fearful of men in uniforms.

interacts with people. The prognosis is poor for pets that have shown fear of people as well as other environmental stimuli from an early age without ever being exposed to anything considered aversive in relationship to people or other stimuli.

Management

A variety of techniques can be utilised for the treatment of fear (Figs 9.2, 9.5). Regardless of the method used, successful treatment requires that the owner identify all fear-evoking stimuli so that they can be reintroduced to the pet under controlled, non-fearful situations. Over time, the goal is to teach the pet to associate the stimulus with desirable events. It is important for owners to be aware that reassuring or rewarding the pet when it is fearful will further reinforce the behaviour, while punishment is likely to increase anxiety and further aggravate the fear.

For each fearful stimulus the owner should develop a gradient or hierarchy of stimuli from the least fearful to the greatest. Utilising stimuli that are similar to the fearful stimulus (Figs 9.3, 9.5) and increasing the distance from the fearful stimulus to the pet (Fig. 9.5), are just two methods that can be used to develop this gradient. The pet should be retrained in a friendly non-threatening environment,

MANAGING PETS AFRAID OF PEOPLE	
Step	**Comments**
Identify stimuli and thresholds	It is important to identify specific stimuli that cause the pet to be fearful so that behavioural modification can be completely effective. For example, the pet may not be afraid of all men, just those with beards
	The distance between the pet and strangers, as well as the type of behaviour by strangers that triggers fear, should be identified
Establish a gradient of stimuli	If the distance at which the pet recognises a person is 15 metres (50 feet) and the distance at which it begins to show signs of fear is 8 metres (30 feet), exposure should start between these two extremes
	The pet with a fear of small children might first be introduced to older children. Pets that are fearful of babies can be exposed to blankets with a baby's scent and a tape recording of the baby. Pets afraid of men with beards might be introduced to men with moustaches only, or a family member wearing a false beard. Similarly pets afraid of unfamiliar men in uniform or hats may be first approached by family members or women in uniforms or hats
Desensitisation and counterconditioning	Select a secure location for training. Make sure the pet is controlled and cannot harm itself or others
	Exposure starts with the pet under full control and at a distance from a stranger where it recognises a person but at which it shows no signs of fear. Reward the pet for non-fearful behaviour. Dogs may be asked to sit for a food reward. Cats can be rewarded with food, patted, engaged in play or groomed during exposure
	Very gradually decrease the distance between the pet and the person
	The pet is gradually exposed to people with slightly different characteristics in a variety of situations
Flooding	If the owner has good control of the pet and the fear is mild, the pet can be treated using controlled flooding by being exposed to a level of the stimulus that is just above the fear threshold, while escape is impossible, so that it habituates
	Once the pet shows no sign of fear, rewards should be given and the training sessions can end
	Confinement crates and halters are good accompaniments. Use of any of these devices is only appropriate if they do not result in increasing the pet's fear

FIG. 9.5 Steps in the management of fear of people.

where it can easily be controlled or distracted. The stimuli must be mild enough that the pet can be motivated to perform an alternative non-competing behaviour, such as sitting and taking a food reward or playing with a toy. (*See Figs 9.2, 9.4, 9.5 and Chapter 3 for details.*)

As an example, the pet that is afraid of strangers who enter the home, should first be exposed to people with whom the pet is relatively familiar. It might even be helpful to hold the first session on neutral territory such as the neighbourhood park. At first, the strangers should ignore the pet, and the owners can give treats if no fear is exhibited. Next, the treats can be given by the stranger but only if the pet approaches voluntarily, in a non-fearful manner. It can be counterproductive if the visitor leaves before the pet calms down. Fearful dogs may cower and retreat but some may attack. Therefore the owner should proceed cautiously and slowly with each further session, to ensure safe and successful retraining. A halter and leash works best for dogs, although a leash and basket-type muzzle may be a better means of ensuring safety. For cats, an open carrying cage or a harness and leash should help to ensure control and safety (and prevent escape).

Prevention

Fear of people is relatively easy to prevent by proper and sufficient socialisation. The young animal should be exposed to as many people as possible during its socialisation period, taking care that it is not so overwhelmed as to become fearful. Treats, play, and upbeat social interaction will facilitate socialisation. The veterinarian should be instrumental in reinforcing these notions for all owners.

Case Examples

Case 1

Chimo, a 2-year-old entire female American Eskimo Dog, became panicked whenever someone on in-line skates approached during a walk.

The owner was instructed to review the dog's obedience training, using small titbits of meat for rewards. The meat was only given during training sessions and each time it was given, the owner said 'It's OK' to condition a happy, food-anticipatory response whenever the words were said. As the dog became fearful when it was within 12 metres of skaters, the owner was instructed to walk the pet and take it to between 15 and 22 metres of a skater, say 'It's OK', ask the pet to 'sit–stay' for food, and then walk off in a different direction to look for another skater to repeat the exercise. Gradually, the exercises were performed closer to the skaters. Finally, skaters were asked to toss food to the pet as they skated by it. Within 10 days, Chimo showed no fear of the skaters and even approached them voluntarily, then sat in anticipation of a food reward.

Case 2

Norm, a 3-year-old male neutered domestic short-haired cat, displayed fear aggression towards a teenage member of the household. Whenever he approached, the cat scampered away or would lash out aggressively. Attempts to hold the cat down, pat it and provide food only served to heighten the escape attempts and aggression.

Controlled flooding and habituation techniques using a cage were implemented while exposing the cat to the teenager. The first step in exposure training was to place the cat in a crate in a room with the teenager present. The cat was to be ignored, and the teenager was to go about his daily routines in the presence of the cat. The cat was offered a portion of its daily allotment of food only when the son was close by. Each training session was terminated and the cat released only when its fear subsided. Food and affection were completely withheld by all family members except during training sessions. After a few training sessions the cat showed no fear when the teenager entered the room and would eat food if provided by the owners. At this point the family was instructed that all food and treats should be given only by the teenager. He was to carry favoured (by the cat) treats with him and offer them through the bars of the cage. In time, the cat would voluntarily take food from the teenager through the bars of the cage. Since no other family members were allowed to feed or pat the cat, it soon learned to approach the teenager to solicit food and affection. Amitriptyline at 5 mg once daily was used for the first few weeks of the exposure technique, and was then successfully reduced and terminated over the next month. After a total of 2 months, the cat showed no fear of the teenager and even eagerly approached him for play sessions.

Fear of Animals

Depending on how a pet was socialised and what types of experiences it had when it was young, it may be fearful of members of the same or of other species. This can be dangerous if the fearful pet responds with aggression. Lack of contact or experience with other animals of the same or other species during the socialisation period can result in a pet that is fearful of other animals.

On occasion, a single traumatic event that is associated with another animal can lead to fear of that animal. This seems to be more likely to occur in cats. For example, if one cat in the household hears a sudden, frightening noise while it is resting and looks up to see another pet nearby it may associate the frightening event with that pet and hiss at or avoid it whenever it is nearby. Owners that try to suppress behaviours directed towards other pets (over-exuberance, lunging) by using punishment techniques may cause or further aggravate fearful behaviours.

Diagnosis and Prognosis

Exposure to an individual animal or a certain species consistently elicits signs of fear. Fear may result in aggression by some pets while others respond by cowering, remaining motionless, or attempting to escape. These behaviours may be associated with trembling, hypersalivation, elimination or dilated pupils.

Pets that have exhibited a strong fear response from a very early age (8 weeks or younger) with no suspected exposure to traumatic environmental events, may be very difficult to treat successfully. The prognosis is good for cases in which the pet was adequately socialised to animals, the problem started during adulthood, the problem has existed for a short duration, and the owner can exert control over situations during which the pet interacts with other animals.

Management

Successful treatment requires that the owners first identify all fear-evoking stimuli or situations that elicit a fear response. Next, the owner must take steps to expose the pet to these stimuli or situations under controlled circumstances (Fig. 9.6). It is important that the owners are aware of when rewards are

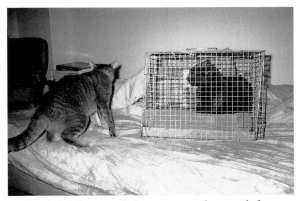

Fig. 9.6 Using controlled exposure to reduce a cat's fear.

appropriate and when they are contraindicated. Rewarding, reassuring or consoling the pet when it is fearful will further reinforce the behaviour. Punishment should **not** be used in fearful situations and can actually make the problem worse. Inhibited nipping by a pet that is mildly nervous when a visitor approaches may escalate to more serious displays of aggression as it learns to expect a beating as the outcome of interactions with unfamiliar people.

In time, pets can turn their animal-associated fears into desirable meetings (Fig. 9.7). This is accomplished by employing desensitisation and counter-conditioning exercises during which the pet receives something highly desirable for being non-anxious in the presence of weak or distant fear-evoking stimuli. The animals that are used as stimuli must be well behaved, well trained and well socialised themselves. There should be sufficient distance between the animals to ensure successful desensitisation. The exercises should begin with the pet being treated at a distance from the stimulus animal that is far enough that the pet exhibits no signs of anxiety. For cats, it is often best to have one or both in crates or on a leash and harness during desensitisation and counter-conditioning sessions. For dogs, the animals should be on a leash or halter, and muzzles may be helpful to ensure safety. The owner should withhold all treats except during training sessions.

Prevention

Fear of animals can be a relatively easy problem to prevent. Proper socialisation is critical for this purpose. The young animal should be exposed to as

MANAGING PETS AFRAID OF OTHER ANIMALS	
Step	**Comments**
Identify stimuli	All stimuli and situations that cause the pet to be fearful must be identified so that behavioural modification can be effective. For example, the pet may not be afraid of all dogs, just large ones, or the pet may be fine in its garden but anxious around dogs in the park. Specific types of behaviour by other animals that triggers fear must also be identified such as barking, quick movements or approaches
Identify the threshold for fear	Identify the distance to other animals at which the pet shows signs of fear or the minimum size of an animal that elicits a fear response
Establish a gradient of stimuli	The gradient should begin below the threshold for fear and should extend in small increments to the strongest presentation of the fear-eliciting stimuli
	Exposure exercises should start between the distance at which the pet recognises another animal and the distance at which it begins to show signs of fear. An alternative approach would be to start with an approaching animal that is smaller than that required to elicit fear and then use larger and larger animals in subsequent trials
	The pet with a fear of large dogs might first be introduced to small dogs. Cats with fear of dogs can be exposed to a tape recording of a barking dog played at a low volume
Desensitisation and counterconditioning	A quiet, non-threatening location with few distractions where the pet feels comfortable should be chosen to begin training, such as the pet's own home or garden. The pet should be under control so that it cannot harm itself or others
	Exposure starts with the pet under full control and at a distance from an animal where the pet recognises it but at which the pet shows no signs of fear. Reward the pet for non-fearful behaviour. Dogs may be asked to sit for a food reward. Cats can be rewarded with food, patted, engaged in play or groomed during exposure
	In subsequent trials, very gradually decrease the distance between the animals
	In later exercises, the pet should gradually be exposed to animals with slightly different characteristics in a variety of situations
Flooding	If the owner has good control of the pet and the fear is mild, the pet can be treated using controlled flooding by exposing it to a level of the stimulus that is just above the fear threshold so that it is very mildly fearful. Escape is prevented until the pet shows no sign of fear
	Once the pet shows no sign of fear, rewards should be given and the training sessions can end
	Confinement crates and head-halters may be helpful accompaniments. Use of any of these devices is only appropriate if they do not result in increasing the pet's fear

Fig. 9.7 Steps in the management of fear of other animals.

many different, well behaved animals as possible during its socialisation period. Adequate supervision and control is important when introducing the pet to other animals in order to insure that the interaction is amicable. The veterinarian should be instrumental in reinforcing these notions in all owners and recommending appropriate social activities such as puppy classes and early obedience training, especially if the animal is the only pet in the home.

Case Example

Tom, a 2-year-old male cat, was recently adopted from a shelter by a family with a 6-year-old female Labrador Retriever. The dog showed no desire to interact with the cat and ignored it for the most part. Whenever the dog entered the room the cat's eyes would dilate, it would hiss, show piloerection and quickly run away.

The owners initially separated the pets at all times except during training sessions. Twice daily, the dog received a long walk to ensure it would be quiet while working with the cat. During the desensitisation and counterconditioning sessions, the dog was attended by a family member and fed at one end of a large room to keep it distracted. At the same time, the cat was brought to the opposite end of the room and fed pieces of chicken and tuna while it was in a crate. During the next stage, the cat was fed in the same area but out of the crate, while it was controlled with a halter and leash. For the course of the remaining sessions, both pets were kept on leashes. Gradually, the pets were moved closer during the sessions. Eventually, the cat was allowed free roam in the house. High resting areas were made available to the cat. In order to continue to associate pleasant experiences with the presence of the dog, the owners were instructed to call the cat and give it a treat whenever the dog entered the room or moved about in the room.

Noise Phobias

Noise phobias are common in animals. Some examples of fear-evoking noise stimuli are thunder, gunshots and fireworks.

Diagnosis and Prognosis

The diagnosis of noise phobia is usually quite straightforward. In most cases, the fear-eliciting sound is loud and quite distinct (e.g. gunshot, thunder). Also, the owner can usually identify exactly when the problem will occur and describe the fearful response of the animal (e.g. hide under couch, run away, attention-seeking).

Many noise phobias can be managed successfully with behavioural modification. The prognosis varies greatly depending on the individual, the duration of the phobia, the ability to control strong stimuli during treatment and the success in finding an effective,

MANAGING NOISE PHOBIAS	
Step	**Comments**
Identify stimuli and thresholds	Make sure that all noises that evoke fear have been identified
	Attempt to isolate the pet from exposure to these sounds during the periods between training sessions
Establish a gradient of stimuli	For flooding and desensitisation techniques, one must be able to control the intensity of the stimuli in order to establish a gradient. For example, an audiotape or videotape of a thunderstorm can be used at varying volumes. A starter pistol in a sound-insulated chamber can provide control of the intensity of a gunshot. Nested cardboard boxes reduce noise
Retrain with rewards	Use a strict retraining programme in controlled circumstances. Teach the pet to respond to verbal commands or sound/visual cues with a 'sit–stay' or 'down–stay' response. Use highly motivating rewards
	By repeatedly associating strong, primary reinforcers such as food with obedience commands and responses, secondary reinforcers are developed. Eventually, these can be used to elicit a state of happy anticipation when the pet is asked to sit in the presence of a likely fear-eliciting stimulus, even when no food is available
Desensitisation and counterconditioning	Select a secure location for training. Make sure the pet is controlled and cannot harm itself or others. Give a training command in a very happy tone of voice and expose the pet to very low levels of fear-evoking sounds. Reward the pet with food for non-fearful behaviour. Very gradually increase the intensity of the stimulus until it approximates actual levels
	If actual fearful situations arise during retraining and trigger a fear response, the pet's behaviour should be ignored. If the pet calms down or can be sufficiently distracted, it should be lavishly praised and rewarded. During the following training session, a lower intensity of stimulus should be used
Flooding	If the owner has good control of the pet and the phobia is mild, the pet can be treated using flooding, by being exposed to a level of the stimulus that is above the fear threshold, while escape is impossible, so that it shows no sign of fear
	Once the pet shows no sign of fear, rewards should be given and the training sessions can end
	Confinement crates or halters may be helpful. Use of any of these devices is only appropriate if they do not result in increasing the pet's fear
Punishment	Under no circumstances should punishment be used
Calm	Keeping the pet calm is an important part of the behavioural modification process. Drug therapy is only one option. Many dogs can be calmed when they are trained with a head-halter. Relaxing music can also be used. Play it when the dog is naturally relaxing and at low levels during training sessions
Drug therapy	Medication may be helpful in managing fearful situations. Drugs prescribed for fears and phobias include antianxiety drugs, antidepressants, propranolol and phenothiazine tranquillisers. In humans, it is recognised that some psychoactive medications may decrease learning or have an amnesic effect. This may occur in animals

FIG. 9.8 Steps in the management of pets with noise phobias.

controllable artificial stimulus to use during exposure exercises. Successful treatment of thunderstorm phobias using only behavioural modification can be very difficult because of the presence of multiple stimuli, difficulty producing an effective artificial storm for desensitisation, and inability to control naturally occurring stimuli during therapy.

Management

An important step in managing noise phobias is to exert control over the pet and the environment (Fig 9.8). Except during training sessions, the pet should not be exposed to the fear-evoking stimuli at all. Sometimes this is beyond the owner's control. For example, during a thunderstorm, it is usually not possible to insulate the pet completely from the noise. In this case, it may be necessary to tranquillise the pet initially, or to train during parts of the year when thunderstorms are not prevalent. Keeping the pet indoors, temporarily relocating the pet when problem situations are expected, or utilising 'sound-proofing' are additional options.

Prevention

The best way to prevent fears and phobias is to expose pets to as many different stimuli as possible while they are still young. As early as 1 week of age, puppies and kittens should be exposed to a wide variety of mild stimuli including different types of noises, lights, handling and movement. Habituation during early, critical periods of development will help prevent many of the fears and phobias that might otherwise occur in adult cats and dogs.

Case Example

The owners were concerned about Bernice, their 3-year-old intact female Bernese Mountain Dog. Bernice became very fearful and distressed around the Fourth of July weekend each year when neighbourhood children were setting off fireworks. She would pant, pace, hypersalivate and whine endlessly.

The owner ensured that all exposure to fireworks was prevented until the dog was properly desensitised. On one occasion, when prevention was not possible, Bernice was tranquillised with aceproma-

zine 2 hours before the fireworks were expected and was kept in the basement with a loud CD playing until the event had passed. A recording of fireworks was made. To test whether the recording would sufficiently resemble the natural stimuli, it was played for the pet starting at a low amplitude, then gradually increased until the pet exhibited the very least sign of anxiety.

At least five times each week the owner would conduct exposure sessions for 15–20 minutes. The tape was played just below the volume that elicited anxiety while the pet was asked to respond to obedience commands for tasty food treats or was engaged in play with the owner. It was also played at a very low volume when the pet ate its regularly scheduled meals. Gradually, the volume was increased until the pet did not become anxious when hearing fireworks. The exercises were held in all rooms of the house and outdoors, with the sound coming from a variety of directions.

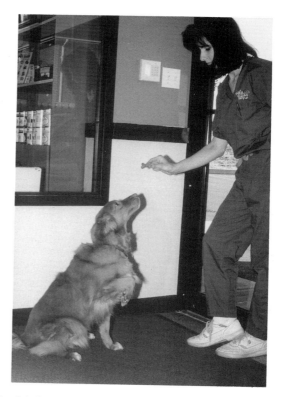

FIG. 9.9 Grace is afraid on her first visit to the veterinary clinic. A technician uses a food lure to request a 'sit-stay' and then 'give a paw'.

MANAGING FEAR OF PLACES	
Step	**Comments**
Identify aspects about the place that elicit fear	Make sure that all stimuli (odours, sounds, visual elements) that evoke fear are identified
	Attempt to avoid fear-eliciting stimuli or places between training sessions
Establish a gradient of stimuli	If the pet is most fearful in a room in a specific building, the gradient would extend from the car park lot or an adjacent property to the room
Retrain with rewards	Teach the pet to respond to verbal commands or sound/visual cues with a 'sit–stay' or 'down–stay' response. Use highly motivating rewards
	Secondary reinforcers can be developed by repeatedly associating strong primary reinforcers such as food with obedience commands and responses, Eventually, these can be used to elicit a state of happy anticipation when the pet is asked to sit near the place that elicits the fear
Desensitisation and counterconditioning	Approach as close as possible to the site that causes the fear response but stop before the pet becomes anxious. In a very happy tone of voice, request and reward an obedience response with a very tasty food reward. Subsequent exercises should take place at closer and closer distances from the problem area
	If a fear-eliciting situation arises during retraining and triggers a fear response, the pet's behaviour should be ignored. If the pet calms down or can be sufficiently distracted, it should be lavishly praised and rewarded. The following training session should occur at a greater distance from the site
Flooding	If the phobia is very mild, the pet can be treated using flooding by taking it to the site that causes anxiety on a leash and preventing it from escaping until it shows no sign of fear
	Once the pet shows no sign of fear, rewards should be given and the training sessions can end
	Confinement crates or halters may be helpful. Use of any of these devices is only appropriate if they do not result in increasing the pet's fear
Punishment	**Under no circumstances should punishment be used**
Drug therapy	Medication may be helpful in managing fearful situations. Drugs prescribed for fears and phobias include antianxiety drugs, antidepressants, propranolol and phenothiazine tranquillisers. In humans, it is recognised that some psychoactive medications may decrease learning or have an amnesic effect. This may occur in animals

FIG. 9.10 Steps in the management of pets who are afraid of locations.

Fear of Places

Pets can become anxious about locations just as they can about people or other animals. Every veterinarian is familiar with the pet that is fearful of the veterinary clinic. Many owners testify that their pet loves to ride in the car but becomes anxious when they approach the clinic or even pass it on the street. Other animals are afraid to be kept in a kennel, or even a crate at home.

Diagnosis and Prognosis

Predictable, recurrent signs of fear or anxiety (shivering, pupil dilation, submissive urination, escape behaviour) when exposed to the same or similar situations is evident when the pet is fearful of certain places.

The prognosis depends on the duration and intensity of the fearful behaviour, as well as how often the pet has to visit the place where it is uncomfortable and endure strong fear-evoking stimuli before behaviour modification is complete. If the pet is fearful of entering the veterinary clinic, repeatedly has to visit for uncomfortable treatments and the owner is unable to work frequently with the pet to reduce fear, the prognosis is guarded to poor.

Management

Exposure techniques involving habituation, desensitisation and counterconditioning are used to treat this problem. The pet should repeatedly be taken near or to the place that causes fear to be given treats or to engage in play (Figs. 9.9 and 9.10). The goal is to provide numerous positive experiences in a controlled, calm manner at the site where fear is experienced and to reduce the occurrence of the fear responses.

Prevention

Frequent exposure to all types of environments should be employed in a controlled, positive way during the early months of the pet's life so that the pet habituates to a variety of environments and situations.

Case Example

Bijou, a young Toy Poodle, shook uncontrollably and crouched against the back of her cage during each visit to the grooming shop.

The owner was instructed to visit the grooming shop two to three times each week for food and play. They started the exercises in the side yard and car park, progressed into the waiting room and finally moved into the grooming shop. At home the owner would frequently turn on an electric razor that was muffled with a towel for short durations while the pet was eating and during play sessions. The owner sent along very tasty treats with the pet when it had grooming appointments. The groomer would frequently give the treats throughout the visit. Within a few weeks, Bijou was allowing the groomer to play with her in the owner's absence, without signs of fear. Within 6 weeks, Bijou could be groomed entirely while showing no evidence of fear.

Further Reading

Baum, M. (1989) Veterinary use of exposure techniques in the treatment of phobic domestic animals. *Behaviour Research and Therapy*, **27**(3), 307–308.

Beaver, B. V. (1983) Fear of loud noises. *Veterinary Medicine, Small Animal Clinics*, March, 333–334.

Hart, B. L. and Voith, V. L. (1976) Fear induced aggressive behaviour. *Canine Practice*, **3**, 14–20.

Hothersall, D. and Tuber, D. S. (1979) Fears in companion dogs: characteristics and treatment. In: *Psychopathology in Animals*, Keehn, J. D. (ed), pp. 239–255. Academic Press: New York.

Russell, P. A. (1979) Fear-evoking stimuli. In: *Fear in Animals and Man*, Sluckin, W. (ed). pp. 86–124. Van Nostrand Reinhold Co.: New York.

Shull-Selcer, E. A. and Stagg, W. (1991) Advances in the understanding and treatment of noise phobias. *Veterinary Clinics of North America, Small Animal Practice*, **21**, 353–368.

Tuber, D. S., Hothersall, D. and Peters, M. F. (1982) Treatment of fears and phobias. *Veterinary Clinics of North America, Small Animal Practice*, **12**, 607–623.

Ursin, H. (1964) Flight and defense behaviour in cats. *Journal of Comparative Physiology and Psychology*, **58**, 180–186.

Voith, V. L. (1979) Treatment of phobias. *Modern Veterinary Practice*, **60**, 721–722.

Voith, V. L. and Borchelt, P. L. (1996) Fears and phobias in companion animals. In: *Readings in Companion Animal Behavior*. Voith, V. L. and Borchelt, P. L. (eds). pp. 140–152. Veterinary Learning Systems: Trenton NJ.

Voith, V. L. and Borchelt, P. L. (1985) Separation anxiety in dogs. *Compendium of Continuing Education for Practicing Veterinarians*, **7**(1), 42–53.

Young, M. S. (1982) Treatment of fear-induced aggression in dogs. *Veterinary Clinics of North America, Small Animal Practice*, **12**, 645–653.

10

Canine Aggression

Aggression is the most common canine behaviour problem for which dogs are referred to specialty counselling centres. It is also the most dangerous problem for owners to deal with because they, family members, visitors or other pets may be at risk. It has been estimated that there are approximately 2 million people bitten by dogs each year in the USA, and 10–16 human fatalities that result. This makes canine aggression a major public health issue as well as a public danger. Pet owners with aggressive dogs are thus urgently in need of help in assessing the extent of danger present in their situations and legitimate advice on how to correct the aggression. However, until these pet owners are receiving appropriate counselling and understand the risks, they should be cautioned to avoid situations that are likely to instigate, precipitate or exacerbate aggressive encounters.

The term aggression is not very specific. In general, it refers to threatening or harmful behaviour directed towards another individual or group. Aggression encompasses a wide variety of behaviours, from subtle body postures and facial expressions to explosive attacks. It is not unusual for dogs to be presented that are exhibiting more than one type of aggression. Although there is some controversy concerning the classification of types of aggressive behaviour, this chapter will examine several different types of aggression, defined according to function. A functional classification approach takes into account the circumstances in which the aggression occurs as well as the organisation of behaviour patterns involved. This allows for inferences concerning the motivation for the behaviour as well as aiding in uncovering the factors leading to the behaviour, thus facilitating the fabrication of a solid prognosis and treatment plan.

The best way to ensure an accurate diagnosis is to combine a physical examination and appropriate diagnostic tests with a complete behavioural history and either direct or video observation of the dog during a typical aggressive display. Since video taping or direct observation are often impractical, most often it is the behavioural history that is used to make the diagnosis. The consultant should determine the dog's facial expressions and body postures, and a description of all situations in which the aggression occurs. In formulating a treatment plan, consideration must be given to the type of aggression, the pet's temperament, and the mental and physical competence of individuals in the pet's environment.

Many types of aggression can be corrected by exposure to the stimulus during desensitisation and counterconditioning sessions. During exposure, the dog must be under complete owner control so that it cannot escape or cause injury. Many owners yell, scream and hit their aggressive dogs, yet they should be instructed that this is not only ineffective but counterproductive. Punishing the aggressive dog increases its fear and anxiety, increases the general level of arousal and increases the risks for family members. Owners also often mistakenly reward their aggressive dogs, albeit unintentionally. They do this by patting and reassuring the dog when they sense that it is aggressive, even offering food rewards in order to try to calm it down and lessen the aggression. The situation can be further complicated when the dog learns that it can get its way by being aggressive. Growling and snapping may very well become an effective way for the dog to avoid an unwanted stimulus or situation (e.g. brushing teeth, trimming claws).

Exposure techniques are used to reduce the pet's response to stimuli that elicit fear or aggression. Counterconditioning exercises teach the pet alternative, acceptable behaviours and condition a calm physiological state. The owner and counsellor must determine all stimuli that cause aggression and formulate an appropriate treatment plan, complete with training sessions.

Factors in determining the prognosis of safe resolution of aggression in dogs are:

- Type of aggression
- Age of onset
- Duration of the problem
- Intensity of the problem
- Degree of danger to people or other pets
- The ability of individual family members to implement the treatment programme safely and effectively
- Whether or not immediate steps can eliminate the risk of injury
- Medical factors (and their treatability).

Although the many forms of canine aggression are described individually below, aggression is often multifactorial or of multiple causes. For example, in cases of possessive or territorial aggression, fear may be a contributing factor. An underlying medical problem may lead to increased irritability, which might further aggravate an existing aggressive problem. Learning is also an important component of many aggressive behaviour problems.

The manifestation of aggressive behaviour may be strongly influenced by the environment, situation or people present. For example, a pet exhibiting territorial aggression at home may be friendly with strangers when at the park; or fear may be exhibited at the veterinary hospital, but not at a hardware store; or a dog may show dominance aggression toward one family member, but not others. The health of the pet can also influence the display of aggressive behaviour. Pain will lower the threshold for aggression and a pet that is normally social may bite when someone reaches to pat its head when it is suffering from a painful otitis condition. Diagnosing and treating aggressive behaviour problems therefore requires an understanding of all of the factors contributing to the problems.

Canine Dominance Aggression

Dogs have evolved from wolves and exhibit social behaviour and organisation similar to that of wolves. This includes a social structure that involves a leader animal at the top of the hierarchy and subordinates with a lower status. The status of members is maintained through an interplay of dominant and submissive behaviours and signals (Fig. 10.1).

CANINE DOMINANT AND SUBMISSIVE BEHAVIOUR

Dominant

Maintained eye contact
Ears erect and forward
Vertical retraction of lips
Head held high
Increased height
Tail above horizontal
Tense, rigid posture
Piloerection
Standing over
Head or paws over neck or body of subordinate
Body slamming
Grabbing the muzzle or neck of the subordinate
Pushing, bowling over
Mounting

Submissive

Avoidance of eye contact
Horizontally retracted lips
Lowered head and tail
Ears flattened
Crouched body position
Lateral recumbency
Submissive urination

FIG. 10.1 Dominant and submissive expressions and signals in dogs.

The condition in which a member of the social group controls situations or the behaviour of others in the group is referred to as dominance. The most dominant animal, the one at the top of the hierarchy, is the one that exercises the most influence or control over other members, social situations and desired resources. For each pair of individuals a dominance–subordinate relationship is established depending on their relative places in the hierarchy. Dominance aggression may be exhibited when an individual dog perceives that it is being challenged or is losing control of a resource or situation to a subordinate (other dog or human). Whether aggression is exhibited is influenced by numerous factors, including the dog's genetic temperament, the relative dominance of the individuals (i.e. near-equal individuals may have more conflicts), the type of threat, and the motivation of the dog to protect or maintain a particular resource. Dogs that have established dominance over a particular person may therefore react aggressively if the person approaches when the pet is resting or eating, or when the person displays dominant social signals (e.g. maintained eye contact, pressure over the top of the head or body, lifting). In these situations, a dominant dog will attempt to signal its dominance by exhibiting

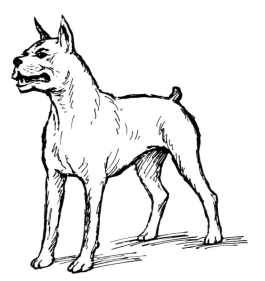

FIG. 10.2 A dominant dog stands with its ears forward and its hackles raised.

various dominant body postures (Fig. 10.2), facial expressions and behavioural signals. If the person does not back off or respond with submissive signals, the dog's aggression may escalate to lungeing, attacking and biting family members. The dominant aggressive behaviour exhibited by the pet is not always consistent. Owners sometimes report that a particular pet will accept patting and direct eye contact on most occasions, but at other times it will resist with aggression. This apparent unpredictability in some cases increases the danger of this form of aggression. The dominant aggressive dog may also be friendly with strangers that it does not consider part of its 'pack'.

Dominance aggression is most common in males and in purebred animals, and signs are usually evident by or before 3 years of age. In recent North American studies, the English Springer Spaniel was the breed referred most frequently to behaviour counsellors for aggression directed towards owners. Cocker Spaniels, Doberman Pinschers and German Shepherd Dogs may also have an increased incidence of dominance aggression relative to other breeds.

Diagnosis

Dominance aggression is diagnosed when historical information or direct observation of pet–owner interaction reveals owner-directed aggression in situations where the dog's perceived position at the top of the hierarchy is challenged.

Problems occur when the owner has attempted to approach, handle or move the dog or when the owner performs a gesture that the pet interprets as a dominant signal that is inappropriate coming from a subordinate human. Attacks may seem to be unprovoked when the owner is unable to recognise subtle dominant signals that usually precede the attack, or when the owner's interaction with the pet occurs too quickly to give the dog a chance to signal. The pet's dominant stare or glare may make the dog appear to have a 'glazed' look before or during the attacks.

The condition itself has two characteristic elements: *aggressive behaviour* and *dominant signalling*. Therefore, the diagnosis is made based not only on family-directed aggression (growling, snapping, biting) but the dog must also demonstrate body postures suggestive of dominance (ears directed forward, elevated tail, staring, mounting the leg, trying to stand above family members). The dominant pet may also frequently 'demand' to be patted or let outdoors and may block the movements of family members within the home. The individual dog may show many of these dominant postures or only a few.

Dogs with a dominant-type personality can become problems for owners who lack the ability or knowledge to assert enough control to become the leader. These pets are likely to be aggressive if disturbed while resting, disciplined, hugged, groomed, patted or stared at. They may be overly possessive of their food, toys and anything else they consider their own. Some dogs are only dominantly aggressive in certain circumstances, while being submissive at other times. Dominant-aggressive attacks are often sudden and seemingly unprovoked. Young children are at high risk living with a dominant-aggressive dog. Some forms of dominance aggression are so severe or dangerous that they have been labelled as 'rage' syndrome (e.g. English Springer Spaniels). Since the problem is often observed in certain breeds with common lineages, there is likely to be a genetic component to the aggression. Although the pathophysiology of this and other forms of dominance aggression is poorly understood, preliminary studies have found that there may be identifiable neurochemical changes in these dogs.

Aggression during one or more of the following situations along with dominant signalling are indicative of, but not necessarily diagnostic of dominance aggression:

- Approached or disturbed while resting
- Protecting resources (food, toys, family members)
- Physical punishment, verbal discipline
- Staring, prolonged eye contact
- Handling by family members (lifting, patting, hugging)
- Restraining, pulling, pushing
- People trying to leave the room
- Family members entering the home
- Placing the pet in a subordinate positions (roll on side, on back).

Prognosis

The consultant must take into account the breed, age of onset, duration of the problem, sex of the dog, familial history (if available), the degree of danger to family members, and the ability of the family to cope with the pet with a dominant personality. Dominance aggression has been identified in certain lines and within certain breeds.

When evidence of dominance aggression appears in the lineage, when infants, the elderly, or infirm are at risk, when dominance aggression is exhibited prior to a year of age, when aggression is unpredictable, when bites are severe, or when the owner is not capable of instituting a safe and effective correction programme, dominance aggression may be difficult or impossible to resolve safely. In a study in the USA, it was determined that dogs over 18 kg were more likely to be euthanased, as were dogs that reacted aggressively to benign dominance challenges by the owner and those reacting unpredictably to stimuli. Family safety has to be the first concern. In some cases, removing the dog from the home is the best solution. Giving the dog to someone else is risky. Although that person may be more authoritative and dominant to the dog, someone may still end up getting hurt. The option of euthanasia should be discussed. Owners must be made aware of all of these factors before undertaking behavioural modification efforts.

Management

The goal of treatment is to stop aggression and prevent injuries by placing the family members in a leadership role in relationship to the pet. This involves major changes in the way the owners view the pet and interact with it. There is not one uniform treatment for dominance aggression and owners must be aware that multiple stages of treatment may be necessary.

Situations and stimuli which elicit aggressive behaviour from the pet must be identified. When the stimuli are identified, they can be eliminated or the pet can be desensitised and counterconditioned. Family members must assume dominance over their pet, but this must be done in a gradual and safe fashion. If too many major changes are attempted too quickly, aggression could potentially increase. Using a trainer or dominant family member is the safest way to begin to gain control of the pet so that behavioural modification can proceed. Behavioural modification, obedience training, surgery, and even drug therapy, may all be required to turn the animal into a suitable pet (Fig. 10.3).

It is important that the dog with dominance aggression has regular re-evaluations. The initial consultation will typically take about 2 hours, and rechecks will need to be planned based on the individual patient. Do not lose touch with these clients; the risk of injury and liability are too great. If after 6–8 weeks of counselling progress is poor or unacceptable, the chances for further rehabilitation may be poor.

Similar Conditions

There has been much research lately on the role of underlying pathology in some dogs with '*apparent*' dominance aggression. Some cases have been likened to episodic dyscontrol (rage), a form of epilepsy. These dogs may respond to antiepileptic drugs such as phenobarbital or primidone. Other dogs may have syndromes similar to attention deficit hyperactivity disorder (ADHD) in people. Dogs with true 'hyperactive syndrome' show a paradoxical calming response to amphetamines. The rationale for the use of amphetamines is that they may mimic the action of noradrenaline or block its re-uptake, thus prolonging its effect. It is believed that the condition might result from a neurotransmitter imbalance that can be alleviated with amphetamine administration. These particular dogs thus have a pathophysiological reason for their aggression and are probably best not grouped into the category of dominance aggression. However, this diagnosis is rarely made because neurotransmitter

APPROACHES TO CANINE DOMINANCE AGGRESSION	
Approach	**Rationale**
Identify and avoid all aggression-evoking stimuli	Review with the owner all situations that might result in aggressive behaviour. Initially, prevent all stimuli that might evoke aggression and avoid further exposure. Be certain that the pet is effectively and safely controlled when exposed to these stimuli
Training	Obedience training is the best way to begin to gain dominance over a dog. This should be done first by a dominant family member or trainer to decrease risk to family members. Head-halter training (Fig. 10.4) and protective devices (e.g. muzzles, see Fig. 5.3) can be used. Slowly condition the dog to assume non-aggressive behaviours while the owner engages in dominant gestures
	Teaching the pet to fetch toys and drop them on command for a food reward can be a way of exerting control over the pet in a non-threatening context
Establish a dominant attitude	The owner must control the dog. This is best accomplished through training. Make the pet defer to the owner before it acquires anything it desires by first responding to an obedience command. The pet should receive **nothing** it values (attention, food, walks, toys, play) unless it first responds to an instruction from the owner
	Owners must avoid rewarding their dog's dominant behaviour by submitting to its demands. For example, when the pet nudges or barks for attention it should be ignored
Control sleeping areas	Pets that are aggressive when resting on the owner's bed or on furniture should not be permitted to have access to these areas
	Leaving a long leash on the pet will permit the owner to get it off furniture with less chance of being bitten
	Motion alarms placed on furniture teach the pet to stay off even when the owner is not present
	If the pet guards a resting area on the floor, the owner might rearrange furniture so it no longer has access to the area, or close the door to the room
	For the pet that has a strong tendency to guard resting areas, it should be prevented from establishing a habit of sleeping in one preferred area. Once the owner notices that the pet is frequenting an area for resting or guarding the area, steps should immediately be taken to prevent access to the area
Control the pet's movement	Once the pet has learned to do a dependable 'stay', the owner should command it to 'stay' for a short period and then release it before it is allowed to enter or exit the home, go up or down the stairs, or follow the person in or out of a room
Rewards	Highly desirable rewards should only be used for obedience, subordinate behaviour, handling, and shaping behaviours
Punishment	Inappropriate behaviour (e.g. barking, nudging for attention) should be punished by completely ignoring the dog for a short period
	A bark-activated citronella spray collar may effectively interrupt the barking, without the need for owner intervention
	Physical punishment is dangerous, unnecessary and should be avoided
Diet	Low-protein diet?
Desensitisation and counterconditioning	**These measures may be dangerous, depending on the temperament of the pet, the gravity of the problem and the assertiveness of the owner. They should only be attempted under the close supervision of an experienced behaviourist**
	In some cases, a dominant dog can be desensitised and counterconditioned to stimuli that elicit aggression, thereby reducing the aggressive response to the stimuli and conditioning an alternative, acceptable response
	If the pet is aggressive when the owner pats its head, exercises should begin with the owner giving a piece of food with one hand and moving the other hand towards the pet's head, stopping at a distance at which no growling would be elicited. During subsequent exercises, the second hand is moved closer to the pet's head until contact is made. Eventually, the dog should associate hand movements and contact on the head with food and the aggression during patting should cease
	Make changes gradually. Progress should be slow enough that no aggression is elicited during training sessions. If aggression results, cease the exercise immediately and resume on the next day at an earlier stage and proceed more slowly
Surgery	Neutering should be considered in **all** dogs with dominance aggression. Dominance aggression has been shown to be sexually dimorphic (approximately 90% of cases are males), with testosterone perhaps acting as a modulator or facilitator of aggression in dogs with a propensity for aggression. While castration alone will rarely eliminate dominance aggression without concurrent behavioural modification techniques, it may increase the changes of successful behavioural therapy and it prevents the possibility of passing on the trait
Drug therapy	Serotonergic drugs (fluoxetine 0.5–1 mg/kg/day or clomipramine 1–3 mg/kg bid) may be useful, particularly if the dog seems to be highly aroused or the aggression seems excessive, out of control or out of context. The aggression may have begun in response to specific stimuli but as the threshold reduces and the stimuli become less specific, therapy with the antidepressants may be a consideration. (These drugs may require several weeks to take effect.)
	Megoestrol acetate: (1–2 mg/kg/day for 2 weeks, then 0.5–1 mg/kg for 2 weeks) or medroxyprogesterone acetate (10 mg/kg IM or Sc)
	Lithium carbonate: 6 mg/kg bid; blood levels must be titrated (*See Chapter 4*.)
	Antianxiety drugs such as benzodiazepines, buspirone and propranolol may also be indicated if there is a fear or anxiety component to the problem, but in most cases are unlikely to help
	Anticonvulsants might be a consideration if aggression is paroxysmal
	Unless drug therapy is combined with behavioural modification techniques, the aggressive behaviour usually returns with the cessation of drug therapy
Safety first!	Do not expose any family member to danger. All exercises should be supervised by a dominant family member or skilled trainer. Drugs, head-halters, muzzles or gloves should be considered. Avoid conflicts and use confinement or 'Time-Outs' as needed

FIG. 10.3 Approaches taken during the management of dominance aggression in dogs.

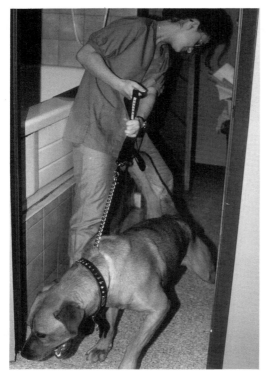 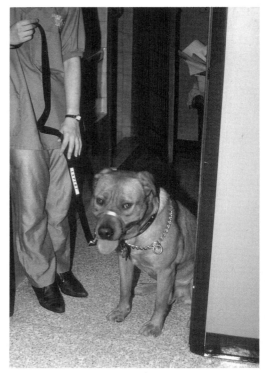

FIG. 10.4 Dog is unruly and uncontrollable as it attempts to attack stimulus (cat not in picture).

After applying head halter dog is controlled in presence of stimulus.

evaluations are rarely if ever done in clinical practice. It is imperative that a full diagnostic evaluation be conducted before considering these diagnoses or administering experimental drug regimens that could, in the event, make the situation worse.

Prevention

Early obedience training, leadership and handling exercises are the best ways to assert dominance over a household pet. Done under the supervision of an experienced trainer, exercises should be safe and effective. Identifying dominance challenges as soon as they emerge and dealing with them promptly and effectively is essential. Dogs that are too dominant to be trained effectively are unlikely to be suitable pets.

Puppy selection tests (*see Chapter 2*) may also be useful in identifying problem puppies before they are welcomed into a home, but dominance aggression does not often emerge until long after testing is performed. These tests can provide an idea of the puppy's present temperament and what the new

owner might initially expect in gaining control and training. There is no evidence that these tests can actually predict adult behaviour.

Case Example

William, a 16-month-old Old English Sheepdog, was referred for aggression toward the husband of the young couple that owned it. The dog frequently growled and snapped at the husband when he grabbed its collar to pull it away from rubbish. Recently, the dog had begun growling at the husband whenever he approached it when it was lying near the wife. When the husband was on the floor watching television, William would occasionally stand over him, stare and growl. The dog's personality was described as 'aloof, independent and irritable'.

The owners were instructed to review obedience training with the dog, require it to sit or lie down before receiving anything it wanted, and request it to 'stay' for a short period whenever it was about to move from one area of the house to another. Feeding was switched from free choice to a regular schedule and the dog had to perform a 'down–stay' for at least 60 seconds before getting the food. In order to ensure that the owners could control and handle the dog in any possible confrontational situations, it was trained with a head halter and leash, and the leash was left attached during training sessions. A pull on the leash was used to correct undesirable responses and it was relaxed or released as soon as the dog complied and showed no threats.

After 2 weeks, the owners were instructed to begin daily exercises to condition the dog to be non-aggressive when the collar was grabbed. Using the head halter to ensure control, they began by lightly touching the collar as they gave a very tasty meat treat and said 'Good boy'. As the weeks went by they very gradually touched the collar more forcefully, grasped it and, finally, pulled it as food was given, thus teaching the dog to look forward to having the collar handled.

To correct the growling when the husband approached his wife, she was told to use a shake can or other loud, aversive noisemaker to correct the growling as the husband approached. The leash and head-halter were used to ensure that if any aggression or threats were exhibited, the dog could be immediately interrupted. The approach exercise was repeated on multiple occasions until the husband could approach without any growling from the dog. Once the dog did not growl when the husband entered, it was told to sit for a very tasty meat reward. This last phase was then repeated at least ten more times before the exercise was finished.

Possessive Aggression

Possessive aggression may be directed at humans or other pets that approach the dog when it is in possession of something that is highly desirable such as a favourite chew toy, food or treat. This condition may occur in conjunction with dominance aggression, but it is not uncommon for a subordinate animal to protect food aggressively or other desirable resources from members it considers dominant if it already has possession of the resource.

Diagnosis and Prognosis

The dog barks, growls or bites when a person or animal approaches it while it is in possession of food,

toys or objects. This problem can occur in puppies but is more common in adults. It occurs equally in both males and females. Defensive aggression shown by a dog that has frequently been beaten for stealing the owner's possessions may appear to be possessive aggression. A detailed history should differentiate the two.

Prognosis is guarded for dogs that show this problem frequently from an early age (first few months of life), for dogs that have exhibited the problems for many years, and in situations where family members are non-assertive. The prognosis is good for a problem of short duration where aggressive incidents have been mild and infrequent, and the owner is assertive.

Management

Behavioural modification techniques are the cornerstone of treatment (Fig. 10.5). A verbal correction that is sharp enough to stop the behaviour without eliciting any sign of fear may be suitable for puppies but is rarely suitable for advanced cases.

It is important to identify all situations in which aggression might occur. The owners are then instructed to avoid these situations or prevent them from occurring until they have more control of the dog and the situations in order to handle them safely.

Prevention

Early obedience training, leadership exercises and handling exercises are the best ways to prevent possessive aggression. Teaching a young puppy to drop objects while playing fetch is a nice way of training object relinquishment. If the owners are clearly dominant in the household, they should be able to take food, toys, or any other items away from the dog. It is best to build this tolerance while the dog is still a puppy rather than trying to convert an already possession-aggressive adult dog.

For dogs that show aggression near their food bowl, the behaviour can be avoided if the puppy is not ignored when it is fed. The owner should also take steps to allay the pet's apprehension that it may lose its meal. This can be done by patting the non-aggressive puppy while it is eating and periodically handling its food (Fig. 10.6). Family and visitors might also handle the food while the puppy is eating, occasionally adding small treats to the bowl. The dog then learns to

MANAGEMENT OF CANINE POSSESSIVE AGGRESSION	
Method	**Example**
Initial considerations for avoiding confrontation	Feed in a separate room
	Do not physically punish the dog for transgressions. This can actually make the situation worse
	If a safe and effective correction cannot be found, it is better to ignore the dog than to risk injury
Deny access to potential problem objects and areas	Keep highly favoured toys, treats and other objects out of reach
	Prevent access to rooms or areas of rooms where problems occur. Control the dog's activity with a leash, baby gate or training crate
Make objects undesirable	Booby-traps
	Application of aversive-tasting substances
Reinforce the owner's leadership position	Obedience training. Use a method that does not require physical force.
	Make the dog respond to a command before getting anything it wants
	Owners sometimes inadvertently reward undesirable behaviour by offering a more acceptable toy while the dog is misbehaving. This only reinforces the bad behaviour
Devices	Use a head halter, long leash or muzzle during problem times.
	Remote punishment devices are sometimes effective
Teach the dog to drop objects on command	Teach the 'drop' command with reward/motivational training
	The family member who is the most confident, assertive and in control of the dog should be the first to begin working with it
	Start by encouraging the dog to hold a toy in its mouth that is not desirable enough to elicit a protective display. Offer a piece of dry food and say 'Drop it!' as the dog drops the toy in order to take the food
	Use different objects, gradually working towards those that are more highly valued, and using food treats that are more desirable
	To ensure owner control and prevent injuries, the dog can be trained with a leash and head halter and a second line or rope can be attached to the object; with these devices, if the dog does not respond immediately to the verbal command, the dog's head can be reoriented away from the object or the object can be pulled away from the pet
	Eventually, the words 'Drop it!' and a hand movement toward the mouth will cause the dog to drop whatever is in its mouth
	The exercises should be performed with a variety of objects in a variety of locations to foster dependability in all situations
Treat underlying problems	Any underlying factors, such as dominance or fear, that are contributing to the aggression problem must be addressed
Drug therapy	Medication is generally not warranted unless the aggression is severe
	Megoestrol acetate (1–2 mg/kg/day for 2 weeks, then 0.5–1 mg/kg for 2 weeks), then gradually reduce
	Antianxiety drugs and antidepressants may be indicated for some cases, depending on the motivation for the problem

FIG. 10.5 Steps in the management of canine possessive aggression.

associate the food-handling with receiving treats, not with the meal being taken away.

Case Example

At 9 months of age, a Cocker Spaniel named Jamie began growling at family members that approached when it was chewing on a rawhide bone.

The owners were instructed to take up all rawhide bones and teach the dog to fetch a ball and to drop it on command using food lures. Once this was accomplished, a variety of objects were used in the fetch game. After about 2 weeks, a new rawhide bone was introduced into the game. After Jamie fetched and retrieved several toys for small meat rewards, the rawhide was tossed a few feet, retrieved, the dog was asked to 'drop it' and it was put away. In subsequent games of fetch, the rawhide was used more and more frequently. The owner was able to establish verbal control of the dog and take objects from it on command. By frequently giving and taking the rawhide away from Jamie, the owner maintained

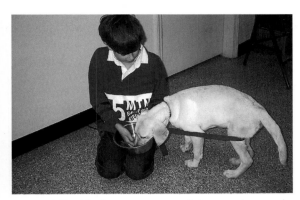

FIG. 10.6 Hand-feeding a puppy can help prevent aggression around the food bowl in the adult dog.

ownership of the rawhide, reducing the likelihood of an aggressive challenge from the dog.

Fear Aggression

Fear aggression is triggered by a fearful stimulus, as perceived by the dog. It is sometimes referred to as defensive aggression. Fear aggression can be displayed when a dog is threatened, punished, or even approached. It usually occurs when the dog is unable to avoid the stimulus that brings about the fear response. Successful removal or retreat of the fearful stimulus further reinforces the response.

Inadequate socialisation and inappropriate punishment are common causes of fear aggression. Fear aggression often is inappropriately rewarded when the owner responds to aggressive behaviour by talking softly to the dog in an attempt to reduce its fear. Aggression associated with a fear response may also be reinforced if it causes the stimulus, such as someone attempting to pat it, to move away.

Genetics can play a role in determining the threshold for a fear response. There is considerable variation in the canine population regarding fear-provoking stimuli. Some dogs require a very strong stimulus to elicit fear, while others become extremely anxious in response to mild stimuli such as a leaf fluttering or any noises that are only the least bit unusual.

A dog with an easily, excitable temperament encountering multiple, strong, fear-inducing stimuli with little chance for escape has a high probability of biting, especially if biting has caused the stimulus to move away during past encounters (Fig 10.7).

Diagnosis and Prognosis

Fear aggression is manifested by fearful facial expressions and body postures (tail down, ears back, crouched body, weight shifted away from the fear-eliciting stimulus) accompanied by aggressive behaviours such as piloerection, growling, barking and biting. Dilated pupils, increased respiratory rate

DETERMINANTS OF THE PROBABILITY OF A BITE FROM A FEARFUL PET	
Factors about the animal	Temperament:
	Genetically influenced behavioural tendencies of the individual
	Although the specifics of genetic influence on fearful behaviour exhibited by dogs and cats have not been worked out, certain individuals seem innately more likely to either flee or fight
	Previous experience and conditioning:
	Aggression used in previous fearful situations has resulted in the removal of the fear-eliciting stimulus
	Owner attention when the pet is acting in a fear-aggressive way may increase its tendency to be aggressive in certain situations
Environmental factors	Number of stimuli
	Intensity of stimuli
	Opportunity for escape. A fearful pet is more likely to be aggressive when it is unable to escape the stimulus that triggers the fear response

FIG. 10.7 Factors determining the probability of being bitten by a fearful pet.

and a rapid heart rate generally accompany an overwhelming fear response.

Factors suggesting a good prognosis include:

- The duration of the problem is short
- The fearful behaviour was acquired as an adult
- All fear-eliciting stimuli are well defined
- Controllable fear-eliciting environmental stimuli
- A relatively high threshold for responding to fear stimuli
- The pet can be protected from strong stimulus exposure during treatment.

The prognosis for safe resolution of fear aggression is generally more favourable than for dominance aggression but adequate care must still be taken. The owners, as well as others, are at risk handling a dog with fear aggression and must be counselled accordingly.

Management

Early recognition and intervention leads to the most effective cures. Fear aggression is best managed with gradual exposure techniques involving desensitisation and counterconditioning exercises (*see fear of people, Chapter 9*). It is crucial that all fear-eliciting stimuli and situations are identified before behavioural modification begins. The goal is to replace the pet's fear response with another response, such as anticipation of food or play. **Safety is very important**. Injuries should be prevented by taking precautions and by proceeding with patience. Owners must be cautioned to avoid consoling the pet or giving treats to calm it down when it acts in a fear-aggressive way or they may inadvertently reinforce the behaviour. **Punishment is contraindicated**.

The appropriate steps to take are:

- Identify fearful stimuli and the intensity or proximity of the stimuli required to elicit signs of fear.
- Obedience training, concentrating on positive reinforcement and owner control. Use a muzzle or head halter and leash during potential problem times so that the dog can be successfully controlled and exposed to the stimuli without escaping, and without causing injury.
- Exposure techniques using desensitisation and counterconditioning.

- Controlled flooding may work if the aggression is mild and both the dog and stimulus are well controlled.
- Drug therapy (benzodiazepines, antidepressants, buspirone, propranolol). (*For more information, see Chapter 9.*)

Prevention

Socialisation and protection of the puppy during early, sensitive months of development is extremely important. The young dog should meet as many different types of people in controlled, positive situations as often as possible during the early months of life. Food treats given by the people the dog meets can help facilitate socialisation. Owners should be encouraged to concentrate on using positive reinforcements rather than punishment for training.

Case Example

Sammy, an 8-month-old Chow Chow, was presented for growling at visitors who reached to pat him. He had been adopted from a neighbour who kept him chained in the backyard and who frequently struck him on the side of the head for barking. Whenever a stranger reached for his head, his ears went down and he growled as he backed away. If he was on a leash or in a chair when reached for, he would snap. When left alone during visits by the owner's friends, he stayed by himself and rested quietly. Although he occasionally cowered when the owner reached for him, he showed no signs of aggression towards her. Traumatic experiences had caused this dog to be fearful of hands extended towards him.

The owner was counselled about gestures and behaviours that visitors should avoid during the initial therapy because they may appear threatening, such as prolonged eye contact, quick movements, loud noise, cornering the dog, and sticking a hand in its face for it to sniff at the initial greeting.

The owner was instructed to use food lures (cooked chicken was used because it was determined to be the most highly valued food) to teach the dog to come and sit on command. Every time Sammy took the food from her hand, she said 'Good boy'. This caused the words to become a secondary reinforcer that could be used to alter the dog's mood when encountering an anxiety-provoking situation. This was the initial step in easing the pet's fear associated with an outstretched hand. The next step was to have a visitor toss the food reward to the dog following each response to the owner's obedience request. Each time the food was given, the owner and visitor would say 'Good boy'. The following step involved having the visitor ask for a command response and give the food as the words 'Good boy' were spoken.

Once Sammy showed no sign of fear or anxiety when a visitor entered the home, it was conditioned to accept patting. The owner began this part of the therapy by patting the dog on the head and saying 'Good boy' at the same it took the food from her hand. After a few weeks an adult friend of the owner took part in working on the handshyness. Each time the dog took food for an obedience response, she would slowly move her other hand an inch or two towards it. As the weeks went by, she was able to slowly move closer and closer until she could pat the dog as it took the food from her hand. The exercises were then repeated with other adults with the attempt being made to include people of varying size and appearance.

Territorial or Protective Aggression

This type of aggression occurs when aggressive behaviour is directed toward a person or another animal that is not considered to be a member of the 'pack'. Aggression may be exhibited towards people or other animals that approach family members or the pet's perceived property. We say 'perceived' property because there is no guarantee that the dog recognises conventional property boundaries. When the dog guards the home or family members too aggressively, a dangerous situation results. Anxiety and fear may also play a role in territorial aggression since threats and aggressive displays are more likely to be exhibited to novel, unfamiliar or fearful stimuli.

Diagnosis and Prognosis

Aggressive behaviours are seen when a person or animal approaches an area (e.g. home, garden, car), person or animal towards which the dog feels protective. This is manifested by typical aggressive postures (ears up, tail held with stiff wagging, assertive stance with weight forward, lungeing and biting) and vocalisations (growling, barking). The

behaviour can be seen in both males and females and usually first appears at less than 3 years of age.

The prognosis is good provided the owner has good control over the dog, and it is not approached in the owner's absence. The prognosis for safe resolution is worse for dogs over which the owner has little control or in situations where it is confined in a home or garden without supervision and allowed frequently to exhibit territorial aggression without any owner intervention to correct the behaviour.

Management

An owner with good control over a dog can usually suppress the behaviour with firm commands and appropriate rewards for compliance (Fig. 10.8). A bark-activated citronella spray collar may be an effective tool if it will suppress the barking that precedes the aggression. Unwary owners may inappropriately reward the bad behaviour by offering food or attention to the dog in order to distract it or to try to calm it. This can be corrected by effective owner education. Punishment may help suppress the behaviour in some dogs, but can have just the opposite effect in others. Although sometimes recommended, castration or spaying is unlikely to affect this behaviour.

This problem is best managed by desensitisation and counterconditioning. Vigilance is very important, because a dangerous situation could arise should the owner become distracted. The owner who does not have sufficient control over the dog should seek additional obedience training guidance and should follow the steps needed to be considered dominant to the dog. A head halter and leash provide an excellent means of ensuring control and progressing throughout

---

MANAGING TERRITORIAL OR PROTECTIVE AGGRESSION

Identify stimuli and prevent or control exposure

Use a muzzle or head halter and leash during potential problem times

Obedience training, concentrating on reward cues and owner control

Devices to control (head halter), distract or interrupt (air horn, ultrasonic device, leash and head halter, bark-activated citronella collar)

Desensitisation and counterconditioning

Fig. 10.8 Steps in the management of canine territorial or protective aggression.

the exposure programme. A pull on the leash can be used to ensure that the dog remains in place without attacking or retreating. Release of the leash provides reward for compliance. Retraining should begin by gradually exposing the dog to stimuli and situations that previously evoked aggression. The stimuli and situations should be controlled and muted so that they are recognised by the dog, but are not strong enough to elicit an aggressive response. Non-aggressive behaviour should be rewarded with food treats. The dog should gradually be exposed to progressively more difficult situations. By withholding food and rewards until strangers arrive, the dog may actually learn to associate the approach of strangers with food and play, rather than fear and anxiety.

Sometimes, training may be accelerated by using an aversive auditory stimulus or distraction device during conditioning sessions. An effective approach for the dog that is aggressive at the front door is to have the owner and dog inside with the pet on a leash with a head halter or muzzle. A person who is unfamiliar to the dog is asked to approach the front door from the garden, knock and enter. As soon as the pet begins to show any sign of aggression, the owner stops the behaviour with the sound of a shake can, airhorn or ultrasonic device. A bark-activated citronella spray collar may also do the trick. At this point, the visitor stops and returns to the starting point. The visitor should continue making approaches until he can enter the house without the dog showing any sign of aggression. When this occurs, the owner should happily request the dog to sit for a very tasty food treat. This stage should be repeated several more times until the dog seems relaxed and looks forward to sitting for food. At this point, the visitor should request the obedience response and toss the food to the pet. While this approach works well for many dogs, aggressive arousal could potentially increase if the owner is not socially dominant over the pet or if the stimulus is too aversive. Any sign of this approach resulting in an increase in aggression should be cause for immediate cessation of the approach.

Pinch collars and shock collars generally make the problem worse by associating pain with visitors and actually raising the dog's state of arousal.

Prevention

Adequate early socialisation and a firm, dominant owner can reduce or eliminate protective aggression in dogs. Owners should be encouraged to take control over their dogs by establishing a strong leadership position for themselves at a very early age. Veterinarians should strongly recommend obedience training, puppy parties, and other ways for dogs to interact with people in an appropriate manner. However, it is true that some breeds and certain individuals are genetically more territorial and more difficult to control. These dogs require even more socialisation and training, not punishment.

Case Example

A 5-year-old neutered male German Shepherd Dog named Rufus was presented for aggressively barking and lungeing at visitors who entered the home. Rufus had not bitten anyone because the owner always had firm control with a leash. After the visitor entered, Rufus was banished to the basement or backyard. When the owner was at work, he was confined in the backyard where he spent the most of the day lungeing and barking at passers by at the fence line.

The owner was told to keep Rufus indoors to eliminate the daily displays of territorial aggression. The owner was told to review obedience training with the dog, using tasty food rewards. A distraction/counterconditioning exercise was set up to discourage undesirable aggressive displays and replace them with acceptable social behaviour. The exercises involved having a visitor approach the front door, knock and enter. The owner had Rufus under control in the entry way, using a leash and head halter. Each time the visitor approached and the pet responded with any aggressive behaviour, it was interrupted with a loud blast from a compressed airhorn, at which time the visitor would go back to the starting point in the front yard. Each time the exercise was repeated, the dog waited longer before starting the aggression and the intensity of the aggression decreased. Once the visitor was able to enter the home and stand for 60 seconds without any sign of aggression from the pet, Rufus was asked in a happy tone to sit for a tasty food reward. This stage of the exercise was repeated until the dog appeared relaxed and automatically sat and looked to the owner for the food as the visitor entered. The next stage involved having the visitor give the command to sit and the food reward after entering. Following this, the exercise was repeated with a wide variety of people of differing appearance.

Predatory Aggression

Predation is a normal instinct in dogs. It is in their nature to chase and hunt prey. However, when this instinct is applied to family and other domestic animals, it causes problems that need to be corrected.

Predatory behaviour involves stalking, chasing, catching, biting, killing and eating. Domestic dogs may go through the whole sequence or may stop at any stage. Predatory behaviours may be stimulated by the movement of joggers, cyclists, playing children, or moving automobiles. Auditory stimuli, such as the cries and screams of babies or young children, may also elicit a predatory response. Predation is not preceded by threats because it represents a normal instinct to hunt and kill, during which the performance of warning or threat behaviour would be counterproductive. This aspect, along with the fact that killing and feeding are parts of this behaviour, can make it an extremely dangerous problem.

Diagnosis and Prognosis

Predatory aggression may be exhibited by dogs of either sex and any age. A quickly moving stimulus is the usual target. The response of the dog is to chase, bite and, potentially, kill its perceived prey. Pre-attack vocalisation is rare. Dogs that show an extremely unwavering focus directed toward the movements or vocalisations of a baby should be suspect and watched very closely. In some dogs, counterconditioning, punishment and aversion therapy are effective, but not in others.

The prognosis is quite variable. The manifestation of a high arousal level, a strong focus on the prey object and difficulty in distracting the dog during the behaviour all suggest a poor prognosis. Since this is an instinctive behaviour, it is difficult to override in many cases. Correcting dogs that chase and kill game animals is typically more difficult than correcting dogs that chase cars. Regardless of the chances for eventual correction, if a dog attempts to prey upon people or pets the prognosis for safe correction should be considered guarded to poor.

Management

Punishment, desensitisation and counterconditioning techniques are considerations for therapy of dogs

---

MANAGEMENT OF PREDATORY AGGRESSION

Identify all stimuli that elicit the behaviour

Deny exposure to any stimuli that elicit behaviour, except during training

Keep confined or under complete owner control

Obedience training, concentrating on reward cues and owner control

Desensitise using exposure techniques and counterconditioning

Consider remote punishment

FIG. 10.9 Steps in the management of canine predatory aggression.

---

that chase moving targets, including joggers, cyclists and playing children (Fig. 10.9). An owner with very good control may be able to prevent or interrupt the behaviour with training commands, distraction or punishment devices. To be effective, the punishment must be considered aversive and the dog must associate the punishments with its predatory actions. Do not underestimate the extent of punishment necessary to curb this instinctive behaviour. Dogs will repeatedly attack porcupines and skunks, regardless of the consequences, because this trait is so strongly instinctive and difficult to override. In some cases, the predatory instinct is so strong that it cannot be suppressed, regardless of the training technique. Although remote shock collars may be more successful than other corrections, their use can cause other problems and should be avoided if at all possible.

For some dogs exhibiting predatory aggression, the only sure way to prevent the behaviour is to keep the animal strictly confined. Walks should only be taken with a lead and halter. Continuous outdoor supervision under full control is obligatory. The owners must understand that if the dog gets loose, it may cause injuries for which they have full liability.

Prevention

Predatory aggression is difficult to prevent because it is an instinctive behaviour. The fact is that some dogs are born with more predatory drive than others. Obedience training is a must, and may be sufficient for the dog with mild to moderate predatory instincts. These dogs should always be on a lead when outside. Young dogs should not be encouraged to chase squirrels and other small animals.

Case Example

Emma, a 3-year-old female mixed breed dog, was presented for attacking a young female cat which had recently been adopted by the family. The cat was about one-third the size of Emma, who had a history of frequently chasing and occasionally killing small wild mammals in the backyard. The first attempt to introduce the two pets to each others resulted in Emma immediately rushing to the cat without warning, grabbing it in her mouth and shaking it. The owners immediately intervened to save the cat. The owner attempted to reintroduce the two on the following day by carrying the cat into the room with the dog. As soon as Emma saw the cat, she immediately lunged and attempted to grasp the frightened cat out of the owner's arms.

Because of the dog's history of predatory behaviour, the quickness of intense attack behaviour and lack of warning, the owners were urged to place the cat in another home. Although they were hesitant to do so, after another attack (and a large bill from the veterinary emergency clinic), they agreed.

Pain-induced Aggression

All veterinarians are aware of pain-induced aggression, even in the most sociable and docile animals. Any handling that elicits pain or discomfort can lead to this irritable aggression. This can happen when an individual attempts to manipulate a painful area, even if that manipulation is just patting, grooming or applying medication. The presence of pain may lower the threshold for the manifestation of other types of aggression, such as fear or dominance aggression.

Diagnosis and Prognosis

The diagnosis is not usually difficult. When the dog with a painful area is touched or anticipates being hurt, it reacts aggressively. The dog might growl or bite people who seem intent on causing it pain. If the dog perceives that biting accomplished its goals (i.e. stopped the pain or interaction), it might use aggression when similar situations arise in the future, whether or not the pain is still present. Thus, the situation must be corrected so that routine care such as nail trimming, home dental care, medicating and grooming can be accomplished without triggering aggressive episodes.

MANAGING PAIN-INDUCED AGGRESSION

Eliminate or reduce the source of pain

Adjust the treatment approach so it is more tolerable

Be patient and gentle when handling the dog and consider muzzling for protection

Promote owner control with training

Desensitisation and counterconditioning to accustom the dog gradually to handling the sore area

Avoid any type of painful punishment

Fig. 10.10 Steps in the management of canine pain-induced aggression.

Management

Ideally, if the dog is in pain, it would be best not to manipulate the area and cause further pain. However, this is not always possible, especially when medications may need to be applied, or physical therapy utilised. Thus, the approach must be to treat the pain, avoid eliciting further pain, and employ desensitisation and counterconditioning exercises to increase the dog's tolerance to being handled (Fig. 10.10).

Prevention

The best way to prevent pain-induced aggression is to anticipate it and handle the dog in such a way that pain does not occur or is minimised. Handling exercises that are performed when the pet is a puppy may help increase the individual's threshold for pain-elicited aggression. These can be done at dinner time. While the dog is being hand-fed, the owner can handle all parts of its body. As days go by, the intensity and variety of handling should increase. Grooming and nail trimming should occur during these exercises. Although it is not possible to anticipate the effects of all painful stimuli, the dog that is trained to be handled, have its claws trimmed, its teeth brushed and its anal sacs expressed (without complaint) will also be more likely to tolerate handling when it is in more severe pain.

Case Example

Babe was a 5-year-old Labrador Retriever with recurring painful ear problems. Over the past year, she had progressively become more and more irritable when treated at home by the owner. Two days ago she had bitten the owner who had lifted Babe's ear to instil medication.

Recommendations were made to address the problem on two fronts. Babe was sent to a dermatologist for further evaluation of the recurrent ear problem and the owner was instructed in behavioural modification techniques for allowing access to the ears.

The owner was counselled about paying closer attention to the ears so that cleaning and treatment was begun before the problem reached a painful stage. She was told to say 'Hold still' in a happy tone and give a meat reward several times each day. Between treatments, she was instructed to touch the ears frequently in a very gentle manner, and say 'Hold still' in a very happy tone as she gave the food reward. Eventually, 'Hold still' became a secondary reinforcer that could be used to reduce the pet's apprehension during ear treatments. The handling exercises gradually changed from simple, gentle handling to handling that closely approximated actual ear treatments until the owner was able to treat the ears with no problem.

Play Aggression

Play aggression is a normal behaviour in young dogs that needs to be controlled because of potential danger to family members and other pets. Dogs typically 'play hard' with each other but quickly learn by the process when they are actually causing pain. The same rules must be taught to the housepet.

Puppies that do not get adequate amounts of exercise are the most likely to become a problem. Uncontrolled playful aggression may possibly lead to dominant and learned forms of aggression as the dog matures, as well as being dangerous for young children and adults with fragile skin.

Diagnosis and Prognosis

Play aggression is typically seen in puppies and young dogs and is accompanied by playful, yet threatening postures. Prolonged, deep-tone growling associated with staring and stiff body postures may indicate that the behaviour is more serious than simple play aggression. This behaviour can mimic dominance, possessive, protective, and predatory forms of aggression.

MANAGING PLAY AGGRESSION

Avoid 'tug of war' and teasing

Provide plenty of vigorous exercise

Provide early obedience training

Promote owner leadership and control

Use toys and games, such as fetch, to channel the puppy's energy in a positive direction

Correct playbiting by using a startling verbal reprimand followed by redirecting the pup's attention to other types of play

Head halters will give all family members, even young children, control over the dog

FIG. 10.11 Steps in the management of canine play aggression.

The prognosis for correction is good for puppies living with assertive adults. Prognosis for safe resolution is guarded for puppies living with families that have young, active children and poor adult supervision.

Management

Play aggression can be effectively managed with exercise, obedience training and behavioural modification (Fig. 10.11). The more exercise the puppy receives, the less energy it will have to expend on playbiting behaviour. Long walks and games of fetch should be provided several times daily. Setting up regular play sessions with another social, active young dog may be helpful. Puppies can learn obedience commands as early as 7–8 weeks of age, so training should begin shortly after the puppy is brought into the home. The puppy should be enrolled in a formal puppy class at 8–10 weeks of age. When the owner has trained the puppy to respond to commands reliably, it can be controlled in a variety of situations.

Hitting the puppy on the nose, or other forms of physical punishment that the owner may use to attempt to gain control, should be discouraged. These techniques are generally not successful and may lead to other problems such as handshyness and fear aggression.

Prevention

Play aggression can be effectively prevented by providing adequate exercise, appropriate socialisation and early obedience training. Exercise is very important and vigorous exercise should be encouraged several times during the day. The more opportunity the puppy has to burn off excess energy, the less likely it will be that the owner will have problems with play aggression. (*See Chapter 2 for more information on working with new puppies and kittens and on socialisation and habituation.*)

Case Example

Simon was a 4-month-old Standard Poodle presented for biting his owners. Both of the owners spent long hours at work. Simon's only opportunity to exercise was when he was let out into the backyard. The husband would often tease the puppy with a towel and Simon would respond by lungeing at the towel and occasionally at the owner's hand. In the evening, the puppy would come up to the owners, bark, lunge and nip at any available body part. Attempts at verbal and physical discipline only seemed to aggravate the situation.

Puppy training and socialisation classes were suggested. Daily long walks were advised and the owners were taught how to teach Simon to play fetch. The husband was told to stop engaging the puppy in all biting games. Any attempts at nipping and biting were to be treated by ignoring the puppy or walking away until he calmed down. A variety of toys were kept on hand at all times to distract the puppy into acceptable behaviour. The owners were not happy with what they considered a slow rate of progress, but with some encouragement they persevered in their efforts. Although they resented having to change their approach to satisfy Simon, after 3 weeks they were happy with the results.

Maternal Aggression

All mothers have protective instincts towards their offspring. Maternal aggression refers to aggressive behaviour directed towards people or other animals that approach the bitch with her puppies. Bitches that experience pseudocyesis (false pregnancy) may also display maternal aggression despite the lack of puppies.

Diagnosis and Prognosis

The diagnosis is not difficult. The animal is a newly whelped bitch or one with pseudocyesis. She barks, growls or attempts to bite humans or other animals

---

MANAGEMENT OF MATERNAL AGGRESSION
Provide a quiet, low-stress environment
Avoid eliciting the aggression by minimising approach and handling of puppies
Improve owner control by reviewing obedience using reward training
Desensitisation and counterconditioning
Use a leash and head halter, or muzzle as needed
Drug therapy for pseudocyesis – mibolerone, megoestrol acetate

Fig. 10.12 Steps in the management of canine maternal aggression.

that approach the puppies, puppy surrogates (for those that were pseudopregnant) or nest area.

The prognosis is good and there is usually spontaneous remission as the puppies age. Behavioural modification can be used if the puppies need to be handled while the mother is still very protective.

Management

Some bitches are more protective than others and gentle handling by trusted family members is the best way to allay apprehension. It is best to minimise handling of the puppies during the first few days when the bitch tends to be most protective. The well trained bitch is most likely to allow her puppies to be handled, especially by trusted family members. Alternatively, muzzling the bitch for short periods before the puppies are approached and handled may be the most expedient way of minimising danger when she is most likely to be aggressive. Desensitisation and counterconditioning are the cornerstones of behavioural modification for maternal aggression (Fig. 10.12).

Prevention

The best way to prevent maternal aggression in dogs not kept for breeding is to have bitches ovariohysterectomised (spayed) before their first heat. This prevents actual maternal aggression as well as that resulting from pseudocyesis. In breeding animals, extensive socialisation, handling and obedience training starting at an early age are the best ways to minimise the risks of maternal aggression.

Case Example

The owner of Helga, a 2-year-old intact female Rottweiler, reported that her dog had been acting aggressively when visitors were present since giving birth to six healthy puppies 3 weeks ago. Helga showed mild signs of agitation when the doorbell rang, then growled and barked when she saw the visitor. Prior to this she had been friendly to visitors and never exhibited any sign of aggression. This was the pet's first litter.

The owners were told to keep the dog's environment as quiet as possible and limit the number of visitors. Desensitisation and counterconditioning exercises were recommended to change the response to the doorbell. First, the doorbell was muffled until it was barely audible. Then, the owners would ring the bell and give Helga a small chunk of canned dog food. The exercise was repeated until the dog showed signs of happily anticipating food whenever the bell was rung. Gradually, the loudness of the bell was increased. The next step was to have friends quietly visit in an area of the home that was farthest from the dog. During the visit, a family member would accompany the dog and give a small portion of canned food every time it was alerted by visitors' voices at the other end of the house but did not act aggressively.

Redirected Aggression

Redirected aggression occurs when aggressive behaviour is directed to a person or object that is not the stimulus for the aggressive arousal. The most common example is the person who gets bitten trying to break up a dog fight. In this case, the aggression becomes redirected from the original target to a person that did not initiate the aggression. The target is therefore an 'innocent bystander' that gets caught up in an aggressive act.

Diagnosis and Prognosis

The diagnosis of redirected aggression is usually not difficult. The history suggests victim interference when the dog was threatened or fighting. The dog growls or bites the person who was not the original target. Males or females may exhibit this type of problem and it is more common in adult pets.

MANAGING REDIRECTED AGGRESSION

Identify stimuli that trigger aggression

Avoid or prevent exposure to stimuli

Place a leash and head halter or muzzle on the dog when stimulus exposure is likely

Distract the pet's attention from the stimulus with an auditory stimulus (horn, whistle)

Carefully remove the dog from the stimulus and confine until calm

Treat underlying problems such as territorial aggression that result in states of high aggressive arousal

Desensitise and countercondition response to stimuli

Obedience training for more owner control

FIG. 10.13 The management of canine redirected aggression.

The prognosis is good for cases in which there have been few incidents, bites have been inhibited and the underlying motivation for aggressive arousal can be controlled. Prognosis is generally poor to guarded for dogs that manifest an exceptionally high level of aggressive arousal in social or territorial situations. These are usually dogs that become so focused on the stimuli that it is next to impossible to distract them or get their attention.

Management

It is important to educate owners in detail about the nature of the problem so that they can avoid interfering with the pet when there is a realistic chance of getting bitten (Fig. 10.13). Treatment requires a clear understanding of the problem, and identification of all stimuli that might arouse the dog and lead to aggression. It is important to treat underlying causes of aggressive arousal such as territorial aggression, interspecies aggression and predatory aggression. Desensitisation and counterconditioning the pet's response to stimuli that elicit aggression is the behavioural modification approach of choice. Owner control of the pet is important as is anticipation and avoidance of stimuli that arouse it.

Prevention

The best ways to prevent redirected aggression is to socialise the pet adequately when it is young, establish control through early obedience training and treat any type of aggression as soon as it appears.

Owners should be cautioned not to intervene in aggressive situations. Good handling and training skills should allow the owner to control the dog safely before an aggressive episode occurs. In early cases, situations that lead to high arousal states can be prevented from getting worse but using desensitisation and counterconditioning behavioural modification techniques (*see Chapter 3*).

Case Example

A young couple owned a neutered, male German Shepherd Dog cross that weighed 35 kg. The dog spent each day in a fenced backyard while the owners were at work. Their home was on a corner lot and the dog spent most of the day barking at various noises and movements in the neighbourhood. He charged the fence line and lunged aggressively at most of the passers by just outside the fence.

One day, the husband was talking to a friend who was standing on the other side of the fence when the dog charged out of the house, ran to the fence and aggressively lunged towards the neighbour. The owner reached for the dog and grabbed it by the scruff of the neck. The dog turned and bit the owner's wrist, causing two deep lacerations. Prior to this incident, the pet had no history of exhibiting aggression toward either of the owners.

The cause of the bite was redirected aggression. The stimulus for the high state of aggression was the visitor. When the attack was thwarted, the pet's aggressive energy was directed to the owner's arm. The underlying problem was territorial aggression. Since territorial aggression is somewhat of a self-reinforcing behaviour, it was desirable to stop the frequent displays of aggression that occurred throughout the day. The owners were instructed not to allow the dog in the backyard unsupervised and to confine it to the basement when they were not at home. The owners were encouraged to enroll in obedience training to give them more control of the pet. Desensitisation and counterconditioning exercises were recommended to decrease the pet's high arousal state when it saw someone (*see territorial aggression*). A head halter was used to reduce the likelihood of an injury occurring during training exercises and to ensure control of the dog during periods of high arousal. A decrease in territorial aggression was noted within 2 weeks and within 6 months the territorial aggressive displays could be controlled or minimised in the owner's presence.

Intraspecies Aggression

Dogs can be aggressive towards other dogs for many of the same reasons that they are aggressive towards people (dominance, territorial, possessive, redirected). Inadequate interaction with other dogs during sensitive periods of development and socialisation can be an underlying cause of intraspecies aggression.

In most cases, dogs are aware of their status in the hierarchy and can settle their differences without injury. However, with some forms of aggression, injuries may occur and behavioural modification is necessary. Dogs that have not received adequate social contact with other members of the species during early sensitive periods of development may never get along with other dogs.

Diagnosis and Prognosis

Intermale Aggression

Male–male aggression often results from hormonally driven competition, but dominance or fear may also play a role. This is usually first evident in males 1–3 years of age and they may respond by barking, growling and attempting to bite other male dogs they encounter. Sometimes dominance and/or fear postures are exhibited. The prognosis is fair and treatment may involve surgery, behavioural modification and drug therapy. The prognosis is guarded for males that will not be neutered and for males that show the problem after they are neutered.

Interfemale Aggression

Female–female aggression may also have a hormonal involvement. The aggression is usually directed to another female dog in the same home. Typically it is first seen in intact bitches between 1 and 3 years of age. Females show the same posturing and vocal responses as described for male–male aggression. In most cases, the problem results from an unstable social hierarchy. The condition is sometimes hormonally driven and may worsen during oestrus and pseudocyesis.

The prognosis is guarded to fair and treatment may involve behavioural modification, drugs and sometimes surgery. In general, female–female aggression among pets in the same household is more difficult to resolve than is male–male aggression.

Social Status Aggression

Another form of intraspecies aggression is seen when two dogs inhabit the same house and have nearly equal social status. This competition is usually resolved without injury as the dogs sort out the social hierarchy through social posturing and minor skirmishes, but not in all cases. Competitive aggression is usually most intense when feeding, resting areas, highly desirable chew items, or owner attention is involved. Competitive rivalry can be successfully resolved if a stable dominance hierarchy can be established amongst all the dogs in the household. A very strong leadership role for the owners in respect to all dogs is extremely important.

Social status among housedogs can change when:

- A new dog is introduced to the household
- A family dog returns from surgery, boarding or vacation
- An existing pack leader becomes ill, aged or dies
- A younger dog matures and challenges the pack leader for dominance.

Management

Advanced cases of intraspecies aggression can be very difficult and frustrating problems to control. The

MANAGEMENT OF INTRASPECIES AGGRESSION	
Method	**Rationale**
Neuter	Neutering males reduces or eliminates intermale fighting in about 60% of cases
	Spaying may eliminate hormonally driven interfemale aggression
Re-establish stable dominance hierarchy with the owner well established at the top	Dogs usually coexist peacefully within their own hierarchy. Owner must assert full dominance to control social status in the home. The more absolute control the owner has, the better the prognosis
	The owners must determine which dog should be dominant and reinforce its dominance by ensuring it is the first to receive food, play, and attention. In conflicts the subordinate should be reprimanded or pulled away
Avoid all potentially aggressive situations	Minimise the possibility of conflicts and competition
	Feed the dogs in different parts of the house
	Do not allow the dogs to greet visitors excitedly together
	Do not allow the dogs to run the fence line aggressively together
	Deny free access to highly desirable objects (rawhide, bones)
Safety	Use whatever devices are necessary to ensure that no family members or pets are injured, such as a muzzle or head halter
Leash/distraction devices	Use leash control or distraction devices to prevent dogs from contacting one another and instigating competitive contests and aggression
Confinement	Sometimes it may be necessary to confine dogs in crates or separate rooms if there is a risk of aggression. This should be done so that they are unable to see each other. If they are allowed to growl aggressively and posture toward each other over or through a barrier, the level of aggressive arousal may increase
Punishment	Light punishment (auditory or leash corrections) may be effective at suppressing aggression by correcting the subordinate when it does not properly defer to the more dominant dog
	Painful punishment of either pet is likely to escalate the aggression
Desensitisation and counter-conditioning	The dogs should be on leashes and under absolute control. Each handler and dog moves to a distance that is just beyond that at which either pet shows any sign of aggression. The pets are asked to respond to obedience commands for food rewards. The distance between the dogs is gradually decreased
Drug therapy	Progestins may be useful when treating dogs for intermale aggression. Megoestrol acetate (1–2 mg/kg for 2 wks then 0.5–1 mg/kg for 2 wks) or medroxyprogesterone acetate (10 mg/kg IM or Sc not to exceed three administrations per year) may be effective
	Buspirone and fluoxetine might also be considered

Fig. 10.14 Steps in the management of canine intraspecies aggression.

owners need to be sufficiently educated about canine social behaviour and to be committed to training (Fig. 10.14).

Prevention

Intraspecies aggression can, in part, be prevented by neutering dogs while they are not yet fully mature. This is most effective for intermale aggression but may also be helpful for interfemale aggression that is associated with oestrous cycles. Some behaviourists believe that aggression may actually increase following ovariohysterectomy in a small subset of female dogs, but this is debatable and information needs to be collected from a larger number of animals to appraise this notion accurately.

The owner should practice obedience skills so that all dogs are under dependable verbal control. Care should be taken to ensure that all family pets are well socialised to other dogs during the first few months of life. Frequent social interaction with adults and peers can help facilitate normal social communication. Dogs that have been well socialised and allowed to engage in a lot of play as puppies are much less likely to do serious damage to another dog in a fight because they learn bite inhibition during play. They are very aware of the pain caused by a hard bite and are less likely to use excessive force in a hierarchical struggle. Taking a puppy away from its littermates and preventing interaction with other canids prior to 6 weeks of age may impede its ability for normal social interaction with other dogs throughout life. Owners should understand the concept of social hierarchies and be sure to be the dominant pack members.

Case Example

Annie was a 5-year-old spayed Dalmatian cross who had been adopted from the dogpound by her owner 6 months previously. The owner complained that although the dog acted fine with people it became very aggressive every time it saw another male or female dog. Aggressive lunges by the pet were so forceful that the owner was occasionally pulled off her feet.

To provide the owner with some control, Annie was fitted with a head halter and was taught to sit on command. Since the dog seemed to be able to recognise another dog at 45 metres and became aggressive when it was within 22 metres, the owner was told to take it for walks and look for other dogs that were at a distance of 22–45 metres away. Every time it saw another dog at this distance and showed no signs of aggression, it was asked to sit for a very tasty food reward. The owner gradually performed the exercises closer and closer to other dogs until Annie was counterconditioned to be non-aggressive whenever she saw another dog. The owner was instructed to proceed sufficiently slowly in decreasing the distance between dogs during training, so that no aggressive responses would be elicited. If Annie did show any sign of aggression, the owner was instructed to give an immediate verbal correction, quickly turn around and walk her pet away from the other dog.

Other Forms of Aggression

Pathophysiological Aggression

Pathophysiological aggressive disorders are those that have an underlying medical cause. These conditions may arise at any age, may have a sudden onset, and may not fit neatly into the other aggressive behaviour categories already described. Many of these are described in Chapter 3 in the discussion of the medical examination. Some of these are shown in Fig. 10.15. In most cases, a combination of behavioural factors and medical problems are necessary for the aggression to be fully clinical.

The treatment for pathophysiological aggression is to address and correct the underlying problem. This type of aggression is occasionally drug-responsive but often poorly managed by behavioural modification techniques alone.

SOME PATHOPHYSIOLOGICAL CAUSES OF CANINE AGGRESSION	
Underlying Cause	**Example**
Infectious agent	Rabies
Endocrinopathy	Hypothyroidism
Neurological disease	Epilepsy
Painful conditions	Dental disease, otitis, arthritis, wounds
Other medical problems	Sensory loss, fatigue

Fig. 10.15 Some examples of canine pathophysiological causes of aggression.

Idiopathic Aggression

A diagnosis of idiopathic aggression is reserved for those dogs that have been thoroughly assessed by a competent behaviour consultant and no identifiable stimulus for the aggression can be found. Some cases of idiopathic aggression may represent unusual types of pathophysiological aggression for which the cause has not yet been determined. In addition to 'idiopathic aggression', the terms 'rage syndrome', 'idiopathic viciousness', and 'mental lapse aggression' have also been used to describe aggression that has no other discernible diagnosis. However, these terms often become a catch-all for aggression that has not been (or cannot be) accurately diagnosed or categorised. Any cases of aggression for which a solid diagnosis cannot be made or for which the stimuli for aggressive attacks cannot be ascertained should be considered very dangerous. For most of these, euthanasia is the appropriate choice.

A specific category of idiopathic aggression, 'mental lapse syndrome', was described by Dr Bonnie Beaver in 1980. A small number of cases have been reported in young adult dogs of popular breeds. Affected dogs seem to undergo a dramatic personality change between 18 months and 2 years of age, changing from amiable to aggressive.

The aggressive incidents are sudden, dramatic and seemingly unprovoked. Affected animals exhibit an abnormal electroencephalogram with a low-voltage fast activity pattern. The EEG pattern has been described to more closely resemble a wild animal than a domestic dog. It is a very dangerous type of aggression with no known treatment.

Learned Aggression

Learned aggression can result from teaching dogs to be aggressive. However, it can just as easily result when other causes of aggression are unintentionally reinforced by the owner. For example, the owner who talks softly to the fearful dog that is growling is conditioning the growling behaviour. A dog that growls and stops the owner from grooming it not only learns to control grooming sessions but may generalise the behaviour to control other interactions with the owner. In fact, any time a dog's threats or aggression result in removal or withdrawal of the stimulus, the behaviour is further reinforced.

In addition, dogs that are threatened or punished for aggressive displays can learn to associate pain or fear with the stimulus and become even more aggressive each time the situation recurs.

The problem is managed by first educating the owner about how to stop conditioning the behaviour. Depending on the type of aggression, other considerations might include handling exercises, and desensitisation and counterconditioning to correct the specific type of aggression that is being conditioned (e.g. fear, dominance, territorial, protective).

Further Reading

Beaver, B. V. (1980) Mental lapse aggression syndrome. *Journal of the American Animal Hospital Association*, **16**(6), 937–939.

Beaver, B. V. (1983) Clinical classification of canine aggression. *Applied Animal Ethology*, **10**, 35–43.

Beaver, B. V. (1993) Profiles of dogs presented for aggression. *Journal of the American Animal Hospital Association*, **29**(6), 564–569.

Beaver, B. V. (1994) Differential approach to aggression by dogs and cats. *Veterinary Quarterly*, **16**(Suppl. 1), S48.

Borchelt, P. L. (1983) Aggressive behaviour of dogs kept as companion animals: classification and influence of sex, reproductive status and breed. *Applied Animal Ethology*, **10**, 45–61.

Borchelt, P. L. and Voith, V. L. (1996) Aggressive behavior in dogs and cats. In: *Readings in Companion Animal Behavior*. Voith, V. L. and Borchelt, P. L. (eds) pp. 217–229. Veterinary Learning Systems: Trenton, NJ

Borchelt, P. L. and Voith, V. L. (1996) Dominance aggression in dogs. In: *Readings in Companion Animal Behavior*. Voith, V. L. and Borchelt, P. L. (eds) pp. 230–239. Veterinary Learning Systems: Trenton, NJ

Crowell-Davis, S. L. (1991) Identifying and correcting human-directed dominance aggression of dogs. *Veterinary Medicine*, **86**(10), 990–998.

Dodman, N. H., Miczek, K. A., Knowles, K. *et al.* (1992) Phenobarbital-responsive episodic dyscontrol (rage) in dogs. *Journal of the American Veterinary Medical Association*, **201**(10), 1580–1583.

Feddersenpetersen, D. (1994) Reduction of aggressive behaviour in dogs. *Praktische Tierarzt*, **75**, 104–108.

Hopkins, S. G., Schubert, T. A. and Hart, B. L. (1976) Castration of adult male dogs: effects on roaming, aggression, urine marking and mounting. *Journal of the American Veterinary Medical Association*, **168**, 1108–1110.

Joby, R., Jemmett, J. E. and Miller, A. S. H. (1984) The control of undesirable behaviour in male dogs using megestrol acetate. *Journal of Small Animal Practice*, **25**(9), 567–572.

Landsberg, G. M. (1990) A veterinarian's guide to the correction of dominance aggression. *Canadian Veterinary Journal*, **31**(2), 121–124.

Landsberg, G. M. (1990) Diagnosing dominance aggression. *Canadian Veterinary Journal*, **31**(1), 45–46.

Marder, A. (1989) Aggressive types. Managing canine aggression depends upon diagnosing the type involved. *Pet Veterinarian*, November/December, 8.

Marder, A. (1990) Aggression Rx. Make a specific diagnosis and use specific management methods. *Pet Veterinarian*, May/June, 43–46.

McKeown, D. and Leuscher, A. Canine competitive aggression – a clinical case of 'sibling rivalry'. *Canadian Veterinary Journal*, **29**(April), 395.

Overall, K. L. (1993) Canine aggression. Part 1. *Canine Practice*, **18**(2), 40.

Overall, K. L. (1993) Canine aggression. Part 2. *Canine Practice*, **18**(3), 29–32.

Overall, K. L. (1993) Treating canine aggression. *Canine Practice*, **18**(6), 24–28.

Overall, K. L. (1994) Prevention of aggressive disorders. *Canine Practice*, **19**(1), 19–22.

Overall, K. L. (1995) Sex and aggression. *Canine Practice*, **20**(2), 16–18.

Polsky, R. H. (1996) Recognizing dominance aggression in dogs. *Veterinary Medicine*, **91**(3), 196.

Reisner, I. R. The biting dog: diagnosis, prognosis, and resolution of canine aggression: a case study. Presentation to the AVMA Annual Conference, July 1995.

Reisner, I. R., Erb, H. N. and Houpt, K. A. (1994) Risk factors for behaviour-related euthanasia among dominant-aggressive dogs: 110 cases (1989–1992). *Journal of the American Veterinary Medical Association*, **205**(6), 855–863.

Reisner, I. R., Mann, J. J. and Stanley, M. *et al.* (1996) Comparison of cerebrospinal fluid monoamine metabolity levels in dominant-aggressive and nonaggressive dogs. *Brain Research*, **714**, 1–2.

Voith, V. (1982) Treatment of dominance aggression of dogs toward people. *Modern Veterinary Practice*, **63**, 149–152.

Voith, V. L. and Borchelt, P. L. (1982) Diagnosis and treatment of dominance aggression in dogs. *Veterinary Clinics of North America, Small Animal Practice*, **12**(4), 655–663.

Vollmer, P. J. (1978) Modifying aggressive behaviour in the older dog. *Veterinary Medicine Small Animal Clinic*, **73**, 282.

Vollmer, P. J. (1978) Socially influenced aggression; the alpha syndrome. *Veterinary Medicine Small Animal Clinic*, **73**, 141.

Young, M. S. (1982) Treatment of fear-induced aggression in dogs. *Veterinary Clinics of North America, Small Animal Practice*, **12**(4), 645–653.

11

Feline Aggression

Aggression is the second most common feline behaviour problem referred to veterinary behaviour consultants. Only housesoiling is more prevalent. Aggressive cats are risky to have at home because they pose a significant danger to family and visitors. Problems can vary from the cat that hisses and avoids interacting with the family to one that aggressively attacks people. Owners with aggressive cats are thus urgently in need of solid advice on how to correct this type of problem. Initially, they should be cautioned to avoid situations that are likely to instigate, precipitate or exacerbate aggressive encounters until they receive appropriate counselling and fully understand the risks involved.

In general, aggression refers to threatening or harmful behaviour directed towards another individual or group. Aggression embraces a wide variety of behaviours from somewhat subtle body postures and facial expressions to violent attacks. This chapter will examine several different types of aggression, defined according to function, and how each can most successfully be prevented or managed. Although diagnostic considerations for each type of aggression may be clear-cut and straightforward, clinical cases of aggression may be multifactorial. As with every behaviour case, it is essential that the veterinarian first assesses the cat's physical health to determine if there are any medical problems that might have caused or contributed to the aggression (and to determine the effect that these problems might have on treating the problem). Painful conditions (e.g. arthritis, anal sacculitis, dental disease), conditions affecting the central nervous system (e.g. brain tumours, meningitis) and endocrine imbalances (e.g. hyperthyroidism) could all have a direct effect on behaviour. Alternatively, they might act in concert with environmental, genetic and other health factors, to push the cat beyond the threshold at which aggression would be exhibited. Therefore, treatment of the medical condition alone may not be sufficient to resolve the problem. Conversely, for those medical conditions that cannot be treated or resolved, behavioural modification and environmental manipulation may still be successful.

Combining a complete behavioural history with either direct or video observation of the cat during a typical aggressive display is the best way to ensure an accurate diagnosis. This is ideal but not practical in most situations. Therefore a detailed history is most important, including a description of the cat's facial expressions and body postures, and a description of all situations in which the aggression occurs. In formulating a treatment plan, consideration must be given to the type of aggression, the cat's temperament, and the mental and physical competence of individuals in its environment.

Factors in determining the prognosis of safe resolution of aggression in cats include:

- Type of aggressive behaviour
- Age at onset of the aggression
- The length of time the problem has existed
- The degree of intensity of the problem
- Degree of danger to people or other pets
- Successful diagnosis and treatment of concurrent medical problems
- Ability of each family member to implement the treatment programme safely and effectively
- Whether immediate steps can eliminate the risk of injury.

Desensitisation and counterconditioning exercises are frequently used in treating many types of aggression by exposure to the stimulus. During exposure, the owner must provide complete control of the cat so that it cannot escape or cause injury. Many owners yell, scream and hit their aggressive cats; they should be instructed that this is not only ineffective but counterproductive. Punishing the aggressive cat increases its fear and anxiety and increases the risk of injury for family members. Owners also often mistakenly reward their aggressive cats, albeit unintentionally. They do this by patting and reassuring the cat when they sense that it is aggressive, even offering food rewards in order to try to calm it down and lessen the aggression. The situation can be further complicated when the cat learns that it can get its way by being aggressive. Growling, scratching and biting may very well be effective ways for the cat to avoid an unwanted stimulus or situation (e.g. brushing teeth, trimming claws).

Exposure techniques are intended to reduce fear and anxiety, as well as to teach the cat that aggressive displays are not successful at eliminating the stimulus. It is important that the owner and counsellor work together to determine all stimuli that cause aggression and formulate an appropriate treatment plan, complete with training sessions.

Play Aggression

Play aggression is a normal behaviour in kittens and young cats. It is the most common type of aggressive behaviour that cats exhibit towards their owners. Although the name implies a rather benign behaviour, play aggression can result in a variety of injuries, and needs to be controlled to reduce the potential danger posed to family members and other pets.

Situations that warrant treatment of play aggression include:

- The play is directed toward the face of a young child
- Biting or scratching is deep and non-inhibited
- The behaviour is directed towards a family member with fragile skin
- The target is someone with an immune-deficient disorder
- The behaviour is upsetting for a passive or fearful pet in the home
- Nocturnal play keeps family members from sleeping.

Kitten play contains elements of play and of intra-species aggression. There may also be predatory components, including stalking, chasing, attacking, and biting. The behaviours exhibited include: exploration and investigation; stalking, chasing, attacking, pouncing and leaping sideways; fighting, wrestling, swatting and biting. Vocalisations are rare and bites are usually inhibited. Kittens typically 'play hard' with each other but quickly learn when they are actually causing pain; the bitten kitten will either stop playing or react with defensive responses. Bites tend to become inhibited and swatting is done with claws retracted. The amount of actual inhibition varies between individual kittens, with some biting quite hard. When a kitten grows up without appropriate social interaction that discourages hard biting, it may bite without inhibition into adulthood and be quite dangerous. Owners often contribute to the problem by playing with kittens in a way that encourages attacks towards hands and feet. Unless encouraged, the behaviour tends to wane as the cat grows into adulthood.

Diagnosis and Prognosis

Play aggression is typically seen in kittens and young cats (Fig. 11.1) and is accompanied by threatening postures given in a playful context. The cat typically targets moving objects, such as hand movements, foot movements and the owner moving through the home. Occasionally, the unwanted attention is directed exclusively toward one family member. In most cases, these problems are seen in single-cat households where the pet does not have the opportunity to engage in normal play with conspecifics. The play usually involves inhibited biting and, occasionally, scratching. It is often associated with stalking, pouncing and hopping sideways.

The prognosis for correction is good but if left unchecked or handled improperly, play aggression can develop into more severe forms of aggression that are less amenable to correction.

FACTORS FAVOURING FELINE PLAY AGGRESSION	
Age of cat	Kitten or young cat
Play experience as a kitten	Encouraged to chase and attack hands and feet
Number of cats in the household	Sole cat
Type of play with owners	Teasing, rough play
Amount of time spent alone	Spends little time with humans or other pets

Fig. 11.1 Factors favouring feline play aggression.

Management

Play aggression can be effectively managed by behavioural modification while cats are still young (Fig. 11.2). The most important consideration is to provide and encourage plenty of exercise that involves acceptable chase and attack behaviour. Toys that bounce, flutter or move in such a way that entices the cat into play should be provided. Teasing and any interaction with the cat that encourages attacks directed towards the owner should be avoided.

Owners should be discouraged from using any type of physical punishment to correct the behaviour because other problems, such as fear or defensive aggression, are likely to develop. If an aversive stimulus is required to stop a play bout, the hissing noise made by releasing compressed air from a canister used to clean photographic lenses will generally work without being too disagreeable. For bolder cats, audible alarm devices (e.g. foghorns or battery-operated alarms) may be necessary. Owners should be taught to anticipate play attacks so they can prevent them by engaging the cat with toys or control them with aversive responses. This is one of the few behaviours that can be corrected by adding another pet to the home. Adopting a young cat of the same size and temperament may very well take care of the problem in a quick fashion with little energy required on the owner's part.

Play aggression is usually a problem between the cat and a family member, but it can be a source of problems between two cats in the home. This is likely to be the case if the other cat is old, weak or very passive. In those situations, the owner must keep the pets separated whenever they cannot be very closely supervised. Behavioural modification sessions should be set up during which the kitten is squirted with a water gun each time it begins to direct any assertive or aggressive play behaviour toward the other cat. During the same sessions, the kitten should receive a tasty food reward every time the other pet moves and the kitten exhibits no attempt to go after it.

Prevention

Play aggression is effectively prevented by routine socialisation, appropriate exercise and avoidance of inappropriate play with the kitten. (*See Chapter 2 for more information on working with new puppies and kittens and on socialisation and habituation.*)

Case Example

Although the owners loved Cameron, a feisty little 4-month-old kitten, they were about ready to get rid of him because of the intensity of his play. Their arms and ankles were full of scratches and teeth marks and they could hardly relax without him playfully attacking them. Swatting the kitten, tossing it to the floor or thumping it on the nose only served to increase the intensity of the attacks.

Treatment included a substantial increase in owner's play with the kitten, involving tossing and dragging toys for him to chase. Play attacks were discouraged by directing a blast of compressed air at him from a compressed air canister used to clean the owner's camera lenses. The owners were also told to stop using physical punishment.

Fear Aggression

Fear aggression results when a cat is exposed to a fearful stimulus, especially when there is no opportunity to escape. The more threatening the stimulus (to the cat), the more heightened is the fear response. Fear aggression can be displayed when a cat is threatened (Fig. 11.3), punished or even approached (especially if it is confined in some way). Fear aggression is sometimes referred to as defensive aggression.

Inappropriate punishment is one of the most common causes of fear aggression. Another cause is inadequate socialisation. It is also not unusual that fear aggression can be inappropriately rewarded if the

---

MANAGING FELINE PLAY AGGRESSION

Avoid engaging the cat in aggressive play

Redirect play to appropriate objects (e.g. moving toys)

Appropriately punish undesirable behaviour (e.g. compressed air, water pistol, foghorn)

Avoid all physical punishment (swatting, thumping on the nose)

Drug therapy:

  The sedative effect of antihistamines may be helpful on occasion, but not as a regular protocol, for cats performing nocturnal play behaviour

  Anxiolytics are sometimes prescribed but rarely indicated

Consider getting a second cat of similar age and temperament

Fig. 11.2 The management of feline play aggression.

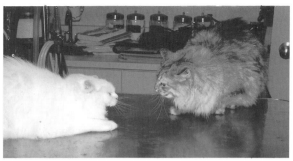

F<small>IG</small>. 11.3 The cat on the right approaches with an offensive threat, while the cat on the left holds its ground and displays defensive aggression.

owner responds to the fear aggression by talking softly to the pet in an attempt to calm it down. The aggression may also be reinforced if the stimulus for the fear response moves away when the cat acts aggressively.

Another important factor in determining the threshold for a fear response is the genetic make-up of the cat. There is considerable variation in the feline population. Some cats require a very strong stimulus to elicit fear, while others become extremely anxious in response to mild stimuli such as something falling or any noises that are only the least bit unusual.

Diagnosis and Prognosis

Fear aggression is typified by a variety of facial expressions and body postures. The cat usually displays a combination of defensive behaviour (ears back, body hunched) and aggressive behaviour (piloerection, growling, swatting, biting and scratching). Pupillary dilation is also usually present. Defensive signals include:

● Hissing, spitting, growling
● Teeth bared
● Ears laid back, flattened against the head
● Crouched body position, body lowered, legs tucked under body, rolling to the side, tail tucked.

The prognosis for fear aggression depends on a number of factors. If the problem occurs first in adulthood, is of short duration and mild, and the cat can be protected from fear-evoking stimuli during treatment, the prognosis is favourable. The owner is still at risk handling a cat with fear aggression and must be counselled accordingly. The cat may attack the owner because of something about the owner that elicits a fear response or it may attack due to redirected aggression when it is fearful of some other stimulus.

Factors suggesting a good prognosis include:

● Problem of short duration
● Adult onset
● All fear-eliciting stimuli are well defined
● Exposure to fear-eliciting stimuli can be controlled
● The cat can be protected from strong stimulus exposure

MANAGING FELINE FEAR AGGRESSION	
Steps	**Comments**
Identify fearful stimuli	Identify all fear-eliciting stimuli and the threshold (intensity or distance) at which that fear is manifested. During treatment, it is important that the cat be insulated from anything that would cause anxiety or fear
Desensitisation and counterconditioning	If the threshold for fear is a man within 3 metres of the cat, the man should be visible but further away than that when desensitisation exercises begin. The owner provides a reward when the cat is not fearful. Very gradually, the man moves closer. It may be helpful to use a halter or pet carrier for control (only if this does not lead to more anxiety). This process must not be rushed
Flooding	Use only when the fear response is mild
	The cat is placed in a cage in a room with the person that triggers a fear response until all signs of fear or aggression have stopped. Exposure continues until the cat habituates
	Food can be used to accelerate exposure training, but must only be given when there are no longer any signs of fear or aggression
	The fear may get worse if the person leaves before signs of fear or aggression have ceased
Drug therapy	Drug therapy is sometimes necessary. Prescription agents such as benzodiazepines, buspirone and tricyclic antidepressants may be helpful in reducing fear and anxiety to a level that is low enough to allow behavioural modification to begin

F<small>IG</small>. 11.4 Steps in the management of feline fear aggression (*see also Chapter 9*).

- The threshold for fear responses is relatively high
- The owner is capable of controlling the cat for training applications.

Management

Fear aggression is best managed with gradual exposure techniques (Fig. 11.4) involving habituation, desensitisation and counterconditioning. Flooding may be effective when the fear is mild or when the cat and the stimulus can be well controlled. Early recognition and intervention leads to the most effective cures.

Prevention

Owners should be advised to adopt a kitten by 7 weeks of age from a family situation that has provided an adequate amount of gentle handling and interaction. In most cases, fear aggression can be effectively prevented by encouraging owners to socialise their cats adequately. Selecting a friendly sociable kitten can also be extremely helpful, as kittens that exhibit fear and aggressiveness may be difficult to socialise. Veterinarians should educate owners about the concepts of socialisation and behavioural development, and how they can prevent such problems.

Case Examples

Case 1

Brenda was a 5-year-old spayed female domestic long-haired cat who was adopted by her owner at 8 weeks of age from a friend at church. The woman lived by herself and had few visitors, most of whom were women or children. The cat was playful and confident at home alone with its owner, but became nervous and usually hid when a visitor entered the home, especially when the visitor was a man. The owner had recently begun a relationship with a man named Ralph whom she met at work. She was disconcerted about the fact that Brenda had not taken to her new friend. In an attempt to facilitate the relationship, she encouraged Ralph to attempt to pick up the cat during each visit and give it a food treat. Each time he did this, Brenda would become very agitated, hiss, growl, flail its legs and occasionally bite to get released. Instead of getting better, Brenda's behaviour worsened. The cat became more nervous around Ralph and frequently hissed at him when he visited.

The owner was told that, while her intentions were good, she had tried to encourage a relationship between the cat and the new boyfriend too quickly. To make Brenda less anxious, Ralph was told to enter quietly, maintain a distance from the cat, avoid eye contact, and not move toward it when he was in the apartment. Whenever the cat ventured out from hiding, Ralph was instructed to casually toss a very tasty piece of food toward it without looking directly at or reaching for the cat. Initially, Brenda ignored the treats, so food was taken up about 8–12 hours prior to his visits in order to increase her appetite. After one week, the cat was eating the food tossed to it, and Ralph was instructed to toss the food so that it would land closer and closer to him. Two to three weeks later, the cat was willing to take food from his hand. Next, the food was offered on the sofa next to Ralph and then closer to him. Through subsequent trials, Ralph gradually moved the non-feeding hand closer and closer to Brenda until he was able to stroke the cat gently when he was feeding her. This last step took about 5 months.

Case 2

Elaine and Jerry lived in a large home with their cat Cosmo. When the children were grown up and had moved out of the home, Elaine and Jerry decided to take in a boarder. Although the boarder, whose name was George, lived in the finished basement, he shared the kitchen facilities with Elaine and Jerry. If George entered the kitchen when Cosmo was present, the cat would back fearfully into a corner and begin to hiss. If George approached, Cosmo would lunge and swat with a paw. Attempts by George to talk reassuringly to Cosmo or to offer food did nothing but increase Cosmo's fear and threats.

Cosmo had an open wire cage which was used for travelling and where he was placed when company came over. Elaine and Jerry were instructed to place Cosmo in the cage near the kitchen table and to have George come over after dinner to spend a few hours in the kitchen with Elaine, Jerry and Cosmo. Cosmo was to be ignored and when there was no apparent fear or anxiety, the cage was to be moved closer to the table. After 1 hour, Cosmo was still anxious and fearful whenever George arose or moved in the cat's direction. After 2 hours Cosmo showed no further anxiety, but the owners decided to call it a night, and requested an antianxiety drug for further retraining sessions. Because alprazolam (0.125 mg/cat PO) had been used successfully on previous occasions (e.g. veterinary visits), it was redispensed.

The next evening George was invited up for dinner and drinks. Cosmo was not fed all day and was given the alprazolam 1 hour before George arrived. The cage was placed about 1 metre from the table and after about 30 minutes Cosmo showed no further anxiety. The cage was moved progressively closer to George throughout the evening so that after 2 hours the cage was situated at George's feet. At this point George was able to toss a few cat treats into the cage which Cosmo ate willingly. By the end of the evening, Cosmo was taking the treats from George through the bars of the cage. On subsequent evenings, the exposure techniques were repeated without the alprazolam, and during the fourth session, Cosmo was released from the cage. Cosmo ate his dinner and showed no fear even if George left and re-entered the room. George was instructed to offer cat treats to Cosmo but not to approach him, and after a few more evening sessions, Cosmo would approach George and take food treats from his hand.

Predatory Aggression

Predation is a highly motivated, instinctive behaviour for cats. It is in their nature to chase and hunt prey. However, when this behaviour is directed toward family or other animals, it causes problems that need to be corrected. In many cases where cats are kept for rodent control, predation is a desirable behaviour. Predation is not preceded by threats because it represents a normal instinct to hunt and kill, not warn. This makes it an extremely dangerous behaviour problem when it is misdirected.

Diagnosis and Prognosis

This type of aggression can be found in cats of either sex and any age. A quickly moving stimulus is the usual target. The response of the cat is to chase, bite and, potentially, kill its perceived prey. Thus the extreme danger is when the prey target happens to be a child or another pet. True predation directed toward humans is extremely rare, but play aggression which contains elements of predation is very common.

The prognosis for complete resolution of this type of problem is generally quite poor, especially when directed toward small mammals or birds. It is an instinctive behaviour that is very difficult to override. Pets that are most at risk are birds, rabbits, hamsters, gerbils and the like. Owners may also want to prevent access of wildlife to the yard so that they do not succumb to their cat. Outdoor motion detectors and other booby-traps may be successful at repelling potential prey that might wander into the garden.

Management

In most cases the predatory instinct is so strong that it cannot be suppressed, regardless of the training technique. Therefore, the best approach is to prevent the cat's access to its intended prey. Although putting a bell on the collar may be sufficient for many cats, most require confinement indoors to guarantee that the predation will cease. Declawing seldom reduces a cat's ability to hunt or kill prey. Constant outdoor supervision may be the only practical course of action for cats that continue to go outdoors.

Prevention

The development of predatory aggression is difficult to prevent because it is primarily an instinctive behaviour. A portion of hunting behaviour is learned from the queen, so that keeping a queen indoors with no access to hunting until after the kittens are weaned (and adopted) may prevent the learned components of the hunt and kill from developing. Selecting a kitten from parents that do not hunt may also be helpful. The fact is that some cats are born with more predatory drive than others. These cats should either be kept inside if predatory behaviour is a problem, or only allowed out when on a halter and leash.

Case Example

Amos was a 3-year-old neutered male Siamese cat. Whenever he could get into the children's room, he spent a large part of the day sitting next to the hamster cage, batting at the hamsters and trying to get into the cage. Although the children were repeatedly advised to keep the door to their room shut, this was extremely impractical as they played and did their homework in their room, and were constantly coming and going with their friends.

The hamsters were temporarily moved to a different cage in the basement. This was done without the cat watching. An electronic mat was placed on the table next to the cage where the hamsters were kept in the children's room. When Amos jumped up on the table, he received a harmless but uncomfortable stimulus (shock). The cat avoided the table top even after the hamsters were placed back in the original cage.

Petting-Induced Aggression

Some cats have the disheartening habit of accepting their owner's attention only to respond by biting when they have had enough. Apparently, these cats do enjoy the attention and even seek it out. However, they seem to have a certain threshold for the amount of physical attention they can tolerate. When they have no more tolerance for stroking, they bite and run off. Another possibility is that these cats are being assertive and letting the owners know in no uncertain terms when they have had enough. (*See status aggression, below*).

Diagnosis and Prognosis

The observant owner can often tell when a bite is about to occur. The cat will usually become tense, lean away, flatten its ears against the head and stiffly twitch its tail. It may even hiss and retract its lips before biting.

The prognosis for correcting this problem behaviour is fair to guarded, depending on the duration of the behaviour, the pet's threshold for physical interaction and the patience of the owner. Young children are at a greater risk, as they do not 'read' the signs.

Management

The cornerstone of treatment is to identify the threshold of tolerance for the cat and gradually to condition the cat to accept more stroking, while avoiding the risks of attack. To do this, the owner must determine how long the cat can be stroked before it attacks. Food treats should be restricted to training sessions (Fig. 11.5). In addition, the owner must not initiate the training, and should not physically restrain the cat during petting. Training starts only when the cat approaches the owner for affection.

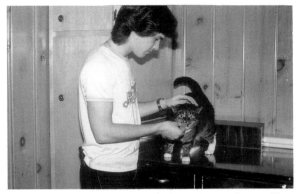

FIG. 11.5 Hand-feeding is one method of managing stroking-induced aggression.

Petting should then take place for a short period of time and stop before the threshold is reached. The cat can then be given a food treat if it does not show any evidence of nervousness or aggression. The cat must not be held or confined in any way; it is more desirable for it to jump down on its own rather than become aggressive. The sessions can gradually be lengthened as the cat learns to tolerate longer and longer stroking sessions in anticipation of a food reward. Conditioning can be facilitated by feeding on a schedule and holding the sessions just prior to meal time.

Physical punishment should be avoided. Hitting the cat on the nose, swatting it or forcefully tossing it to the floor invariably make matters worse.

Prevention

Early socialisation, grooming and handling of the young kitten may help to prevent this problem.

Case Example

Harry was a 2-year-old domestic short-haired cat who would rub against the owner's leg, jump into her lap and purr as she stroked him. After about 5–10 seconds of petting, he would suddenly bite her and run off.

The owner was instructed to avoid absentmindedly petting the cat and only to stroke him when he solicited attention. She was cautioned to watch for pre-bite behaviours and to stop well before a bite might occur. Whenever he jumped in a chair beside her or in her lap for attention, she was instructed only to stroke him for 4 seconds and then give a very tasty food treat. Harry was then to be ignored or placed on the floor until he voluntarily approached again. The petting sessions gradually increased in duration as Harry learned to allow himself to be groomed in anticipation of getting a food reward.

Status (Assertion) Aggression

Some cats may display aggression towards their owners or other cats when displaying assertiveness. This type of aggression is infrequently described in the veterinary literature but is a consideration in those cats that bite or attack their owners or other cats in order to control a situation (Anderson, 1996; Overall, 1994a,b,c). Biting during stroking, when the cat is lifted or approached, or when the owner attempts to remove the cat from a worktop or piece of furniture may all be expressions of the cat's assertiveness. Cats that solicit attention or play through biting may also be displaying assertiveness.

Diagnosis and Prognosis

The diagnosis may be difficult as this condition is poorly described in the literature and the cats may be displaying other forms of aggression (fear, territorial, redirected, predatory, play) in combination with status aggression. Cats that display assertive or status aggression may bite or threaten when the owner attempts to approach or handle them. This biting is an attempt to control the situation. Assertive displays, soliciting attention and play through attacks or biting, and attempts to control the environment by blocking access to doorways and refusing to be moved from perches or sleeping areas may be displays of social status. Although some cats exhibiting this behaviour may be overly demanding, vocalising or constantly soliciting affection from the owners (on their own terms), others may appear aloof and independent, preferring to be left alone when the owner attempts to initiate affection or attention. The prognosis is guarded and variable as these cats may be dangerous and the problem may have both innate and learned components.

Management

The goal of management is that the owners gain control over the cat (Fig. 11.6). Much like the dominant aggressive dog, the owners can best gain control by identifying and avoiding those situations that might lead to aggression and training the cat that all rewards (all play, all food, all affection, all attention) must be earned.

MANAGING FELINE STATUS AGGRESSION	
Step	**Comments**
Identify stimuli leading to aggression	Avoid stimuli such as approach, stroking and handling that might lead to aggression
Training	Although difficult for some owners cats can be taught simple commands such as 'come' or 'sit' by enticing, directing or encouraging the cat to perform these behaviours, whenever the cat is 'in the mood' for food, affection, or play
Withhold rewards unless earned	The cat should be taught to defer to the owners for any treats, affection, or play
	Play, affection and treats must never be given on demand but can be given if the cat accepts a small amount of handling, holding, or lifting or responds to a trained command
Desensitisation and counterconditioning to handling and approach	After withholding rewards begin to offer all food, affection and play only if the cat begins to accept very small amounts of the approach or handling that would cause aggression. Then, progress in small increments only. (See petting-induced aggression for details.)
Interrupt or deter undesirable behaviour with devices	Physical punishment must be avoided but any undesirable behaviour can be interrupted or deterred with inanimate devices such as alarms, water guns or a can of compressed air
Control devices – 'confront and win'	A harness and long leash can be left attached to the cat to ensure control without the need for physical contact
Safety and success	A cage or leash and harness can be used to allow the owner successfully to handle cats when they must be approached or handled. Biting and escaping must be prevented as this would only serve to reinforce the status aggression

Fig. 11.6 Steps in the management of feline status aggression.

Prevention

From the outset, the owner should never accede to the cat's demands but should insist that all play, feeding or handling be on the owner's terms. Hand-feeding may be helpful since the cat can be taught to perform a command or accept some handling before any food or treat is given. Teaching a few basic commands can also help the owner gain control. Petting and handling should be practised regularly for short periods and play or food rewards can be given after each session. Any demanding, pushy or aggressive behaviour should not be tolerated and should be dealt with immediately (*see above*).

Case Example

Napoleon was a 16-month-old male neutered domestic short-haired cat who would lunge and bite at the owners whenever they attempted to remove him from any chair, table or worktop where he had 'parked' himself. Napoleon would growl and bite when the owners attempted to lift or stroke him, but would solicit and enjoy a few minutes of petting whenever he was in the mood. Napoleon's aggression had become so severe that the owners were afraid to approach him even when he was lying on their bed, sofa, or kitchen worktop.

Napoleon was fitted with a body harness and a 3-metre lead was attached whenever the owners were at home (except for night-time). The leash was then used to remove Napoleon from his resting areas without confrontation or injury. The owners were instructed not to feed, play with, or stroke Napoleon except during training sessions. At scheduled feeding or play times the owners were to hold out the food or toy, call Napoleon to come, pet him for a few moments and then provide the reward. Each day Napoleon was taught to be held, stroked or lifted a little longer than the previous day before the rewards were given. Whenever Napoleon approached the owners for play, food or affection he was to be ignored. However, a few minutes later the owners were to hold out a food treat or a play toy, use the come command and have Napoleon approach for a short handling session before the reward was given. The owners also were taught to identify any signs of impending aggression so that they could avoid the situation or use a small can of compressed air to deter the behaviour. After a week Napoleon had learned to come when called and would tolerate a minute or more of handling before receiving his play or food. When he had to be moved from a piece of furniture he could either be enticed to leave with a command and food reward or, at the very least, removed with a leash and harness. In short order Napoleon learned to tolerate approach and several minutes of handling without aggression, and would voluntarily get off of the furniture without showing aggressive displays.

Redirected Aggression

Redirected aggression occurs when the object of the animal's aggression is not the stimulus that triggered the state of aggressive arousal. This problem usually results when a person or animal intervenes in aggressive activity taking place between two other animals. The most common examples include a person getting bitten trying to break up a cat fight, or intervening when a cat is threatening or afraid. In these cases, the aggression becomes redirected from the original target to a person or pet as an 'innocent bystander'. It is also not uncommon for a cat that is highly aroused by external stimuli (e.g. other cats on the property) to become aggressive to an owner (or other pet) merely by approaching the cat during this aroused state.

Diagnosis and Prognosis

The diagnosis involves recognising a stimulus that aroused the cat and resulted in a nearby person being bitten. In general, the history suggests victim interference when the cat was threatened, afraid or fighting. But the diagnosis of redirected aggression in cats can be problematic in occasional cases. This is because some cats may stay in a state of aggressive arousal for hours after the stimulus has disappeared. This makes elucidation of the specific stimulus for arousal difficult, thus leading to a very disconcerting situation for the owner. Not knowing that the cat was exposed to some earlier stimulus that triggered the redirected aggression can make it seem to the owner that the cat has suddenly 'gone mad'. Stimuli that can cause redirected aggression include:

- Sight, sound or odour of another cat
- Sight, sound or odour of other animals
- Unusual noises

- Unfamiliar people
- Unfamiliar environments.

Males or females may exhibit this type of problem and it is more common in adult cats. The cat scratches or bites the person who was not the original target. Owners can often describe the posturing that occurs during a state of aggressive arousal. Typically the cat exhibits growling, yowling, nervous pacing, piloerection, tail lashing, dilated pupils and a fixed gaze. These situations are quite dangerous and typically result in multiple, deep, bite wounds.

Diagnosis made by identifying the arousing stimuli, associating the arousing stimuli with attacks, and by ruling out pathophysiological problems.

The prognosis is good for a single event but is poor if the cat is frequently and easily stimulated to a state of aggressive arousal. When the stimuli are difficult to identify or control, or the aggression is intense or prolonged the prognosis is much more guarded. Family members who are unable to recognise when the cat is aroused are in particular danger. Factors influencing the prognosis of redirected aggression include:

- Frequency
- Severity of the aggression
- Ability to identify arousing stimuli
- Ability to reduce exposure to stimuli
- Ability of all family members to recognise and avoid the aroused cat.

Management

Redirected aggression is best managed (Fig. 11.7) by avoiding interference if there is a realistic chance of getting bitten or scratched. Treatment requires a clear understanding of the problem, and identification of all stimuli that might arouse the cat and lead to aggression. If at all possible the underlying cause of aggressive arousal should be corrected. Habituation, desensitisation and counterconditioning are the behavioural modification treatments of choice. When it can be done safely, the cat should be confined to a darkened quiet room when it is very aroused until it calms down. Sometimes the cat can be successfully interrupted using a device such as an audible or ultrasonic alarm, compressed air, or spray of water (rather than physical or verbal punishment). This teaches the cat that there are unpleasant consequences for the behaviour, but causes no fear or anxiety toward

MANAGING FELINE REDIRECTED AGGRESSION
Identify stimuli for aggressive arousal
Avoid or prevent exposure to stimuli
Interrupt the behaviour using a distraction device (whistle, airhorn, water gun)
Carefully remove the cat from the stimuli
A blanket, towel or gloves may provide some safety when moving the pet
A leash and body halter can be left on the pet for control and to safely guide it into a quiet room when it becomes aggressively aroused
Confine in darkened quiet room until calm
Desensitise and countercondition the pet's response to aggression-provoking stimuli
Antianxiety drugs (benzodiazepines, buspirone) or tricyclic antidepressants (amitriptyline) may be considered to decrease high states of arousal

Fig. 11.7 The management of feline redirected aggression.

the owner. Interruption should be done carefully because additional stimuli may actually increase the level of arousal in some cats.

If the aggression is continual or if family members cannot recognise and avoid the aroused cat, removing the pet from the household may be the best solution.

Prevention

Prevention of redirected aggression involves early recognition of stimuli and situations that trigger aggression, followed by desensitisation and counterconditioning to change the pet's behaviour. Prevention of attacks involves knowing how to recognise and avoid the cat in a high state of arousal, as well as taking steps to prevent exposure of the cat to these stimuli.

Case Example

The owner was sitting in the living room one evening watching television when he heard a cat howl outside the apartment. B. G., his 2-year-old spayed domestic short-haired cat, sprung to her feet, appeared very agitated and hissed. As the owner quickly got up, the pet turned toward him, yowled and viciously attacked his leg. Before the owner was able to shake the cat loose by striking it several times, B. G. had delivered a number of deep bite wounds. The cat ran off into the guest bedroom and hid under a chair where it hissed and growled every time the owner entered the room.

An animal control officer was called to pick up the stray intact male that was howling outdoors. As is often the case with redirected aggression, fear aggression developed due to the owner's response to the attack and it was very important that this be addressed. The cat was kept confined to the guest bedroom immediately after the incident and was placed on diazepam (1 mg P0 bid) for 10 days and gradually weaned off during the following 10 days. For the first few days, the owner was instructed to leave a large bowl of food and water and two litterboxes for the cat in the room, to keep things quiet around the apartment and to stay out of the room other than to check occasionally on the pet. After 3 days, the owner was instructed to enter the room numerous times during the day and casually toss pieces of chicken or tuna to the cat. When the cat became calm and stopped showing signs of apprehension, the door was left open for the pet to leave at its own will. For the following week, the owner continued to limit his interaction with the cat, only tossing food when it approached. Within 3 weeks, the cat was back to acting normally.

Although desensitising and counterconditioning the pet to the stimulus of a yowling cat would have been ideal, it was not practical. The owner was educated about redirected aggression and made aware of signs of arousal so that he would know when to avoid the cat. It was suggested that the pet not be allowed out on to the balcony to observe outdoor cats and that if the owner should ever hear a cat call outdoors and notice that the pet focuses, but does not become aroused, he should praise it or reward it with food.

Territorial Aggression

Unlike dogs, cats rarely fight to protect family members except for females protecting their young. However, they do guard their own turf, and this is most often a problem when a new cat is added to the family or when a neighbourhood cat visits the garden. In the wild, scent-marking with urine, faeces and, possibly, with sebaceous skin secretions, serves to acknowledge the presence of individuals and provides a way for recognition of occupation of an area and

thus facilitate avoidance. This helps reduce aggressive interactions. In the confined area of the home, avoidance is less likely and aggression becomes more probable. Territorial aggression might also erupt when one cat in the household returns home from the veterinary hospital or groomer and smells or acts differently than it did before.

Diagnosis and Prognosis

Territorial aggression is most often seen when a new cat is added to the household. The resident cat typically swats, chases and attacks the newcomer and this can quickly evolve into relentless pursuit. Territorial aggression can also be directed against visitors. The cat may be bold and approach or lunge at the person. Although there may indeed be fear components to the behaviour, territorial aggression generally differs from fear aggression where the cat tries to avoid an encounter and is only aggressive when it cannot avoid the person or other cat.

Territorial aggression directed at humans generally has a good prognosis. Territorial aggression directed toward other cats usually has a significantly poorer prognosis. The likelihood of a favourable outcome depends on the duration of the problem, the social experience of the cat, its temperament and its threshold for arousal in response to territorial stimuli.

Management

Territorial aggression is best managed by desensitisation and counterconditioning. Drugs are often necessary not only to control the behaviour of the aggressor cat, but also to decrease the defensive posturing and vocalising of the cat that is being threatened. Defensive signalling and frantic escape behaviours tend to elicit aggressive attacks and chasing from the bolder cat in these situations.

Unwary owners may inappropriately reward undesirable behaviour by offering the aggressive cat food or attention to try to calm it down. This can be corrected by effective owner education. Light punishment (using an inanimate device such as an alarm or water gun) may help suppress the behaviour in some cats, but can have just the opposite effect in others. Castration or spaying is unlikely to affect this behaviour. Antianxiety mediations and antidepressants (amitriptyline, fluoxetine) may occasionally be helpful as an adjunct to therapy.

Treating territorial aggression towards a recently adopted cat should begin with isolating the cats in confinement areas where they are unable to see each other. The owner should then alternately release one cat at a time to roam in the house. Once any initial anxiety dissipates, desensitisation and counterconditioning can begin.

Under controlled situations, the cats should gradually be exposed to each other. This should be done with the cats in carriers or controlled with a harness and leash at opposite ends of the largest room or longest hallway in the home. During the sessions, the cats are fed highly palatable food or engaged in play. During following sessions, the cats are slowly brought closer together. By withholding food and rewards except for training sessions, each cat may learn to associate the presence of the other cat with food and play, rather than fear and anxiety. Once the cats are showing no tension during the sessions at close proximity to each other, the owner can attempt to allow them to have freedom in the same room. A high-power, compression water gun may be used to correct unacceptable behaviour by the aggressor cat. Conditioning can take months and requires considerable patience and time on the part of the owner. In some instances, the most expedient and safe way to end the conflict is to remove one of the cats from the household.

Aggressive threats and brief 'spats' between cats are to be expected as cats attempt to gain or maintain control over resources. However cats should not be allowed to 'fight it out' as these fights rarely settle conflicts and may make the situation worse. Holding the pets to introduce them is commonly attempted by owners and should also be discouraged.

Prevention

Adequate early socialisation can reduce the manifestation of territorial aggression in most cats. However, certain individuals are genetically more territorial and more difficult to control. In all cases, it is best to have an initial separation period when introducing a new cat to a household. A useful way of doing this is to establish the cats in separate rooms and then, periodically, switch the rooms. This allows the cats to become familiar with the scent of each other before they are actually introduced. Next, one cat can be given freedom of the entire home, while the second is kept to its own room. The situation is then reversed. The cats should then be slowly introduced during meal time, being fed at opposite ends of the same room. They should be more intent on eating at that time, than on fighting. If there are any signs of aggression, the cats should be separated at a slightly greater distance during meals, or the cats can be confined to separate metal cages or controlled with harness and leash. When there are no signs of aggression, the cats can be given more freedom to be together in the home. If aggression is seen when the cats are placed together at meal time, it might be necessary first to place the cats in separate metal cages during meal time and switch cages at each subsequent meal. When the cats reach the stage where they are both allowed to run free in the home, at least two litterboxes and two feeding stations should be made available in relatively open areas. This will allow one cat to see the other approaching without getting surprised.

Case Example

When the owners' elderly male cat died, they decided to adopt a 4-month-old female to keep the remaining 5-year-old female cat, Carley, company. As the owner carried the kitten into the home, Carley immediately focused on the kitten, walked deliberately towards it, yowled and jumped to attack it in the owner's arms. The owner turned and was badly bitten on her leg by Carley. The kitten was confined to a bedroom and during the following 2 weeks Carley sat outside the bedroom door, hissing and rattling the door. Two attempts to introduce the cats resulted in Carley immediately hissing or growling and attacking the kitten. The kitten was becoming increasingly more anxious and exhibited some hissing and withdrawal when the owners entered the room in which she was confined.

Carley was given buspirone (5 mg every 12 hours) and the cats were separated in such a way that Carley was unable get near the door to the kitten's confinement room. During the second week, each cat was allowed to roam in the house while the other one was confined. By the end of that week, both cats had started to settle down and acted much less anxiously. During the third week, the owners started desensitisation and counterconditioning exercises. Body harnesses and leashes were placed on the cats and they were taken to opposite ends of a long hallway and fed pieces of chicken for 15 or more minutes, at least five times each week. Every few days, the distance between the cats was decreased by small increments. After 4 weeks, the cats could be fed a few feet apart, on leash, without any sign of aggression or anxiety. The feeding exercises were carried out in various areas of the house over the following 2 weeks. Following this, the pets were fed and allowed to move about on their own while under close supervision for short periods after feeding for another 2–3 weeks. During that period, they were allowed freedom in the home and Carley was gradually taken off the buspirone.

Pain-induced Aggression

Even the most sociable and docile animal may exhibit this form of aggression. Any handling that elicits pain or discomfort can lead to this irritable aggression. This can happen when an individual attempts to manipulate a painful area, even if that manipulation is just stroking, grooming or applying medication.

Diagnosis and Prognosis

The diagnosis is usually straightforward. The cat has a painful area and reacts aggressively when it is hurt or anticipates being hurt. It might hiss, snarl and growl or bite people who seem intent on causing it pain. It is important to remedy the situation because, if the cat perceives that biting accomplished its goals (i.e. stopped the pain) it might use aggression when similar situations arise in the future, whether or not the pain is still present. Thus, the situation must be corrected so that routine care such as claw trimming, home dental care, medicating and grooming can be accomplished without triggering aggressive episodes.

Management

If possible, it is best not to manipulate the cat when it is in pain. However, this is not always practical, especially when medications may need to be applied, or physical therapy utilised. Thus, the approach must be to control the pet to reduce danger to the handler; avoid eliciting pain, treat the pain, and employ desensitisation or counterconditioning exercises to increase the cat's tolerance of being handled (Fig 11.8).

MANAGING FELINE PAIN-INDUCED AGGRESSION
Eliminate or reduce the source of pain (medical therapy/drugs)
Modify treatment to be less aversive
Handle the patient gently and consider muzzling for protection
Promote owner control with reward cues and training
Desensitisation and counterconditioning to gradually accustom the cat to handling
Painful punishment is contraindicated

Fig. 11.8 The management of feline pain-induced aggression.

Prevention

Handling exercises performed with a kitten may help raise its threshold for pain-elicited aggression. These can be done at feeding time. While the pet is being hand-fed, the owner can gently handle all parts of the pet's body. As days go by, the intensity and variety of handling should increase. Grooming and claw trimming should occur during these exercises. Although it is not possible to anticipate the effects of all painful stimuli, the cat that is trained to be handled, have its claws trimmed, and its teeth brushed (without complaint) will also be more likely to tolerate handling when it is in more dire pain. The best way to prevent pain-induced aggression from a cat that has been hurt is to anticipate the problem and handle the pet in such a way that pain does not occur or is minimised.

Case Example

Zeke was an 18-month-old neutered male domestic short-haired cat who received a painful bite wound over his right shoulder. As part of the treatment, the owner was instructed to cleanse the area gently three times daily.

To make Zeke less anxious about having the shoulder treated, the owner gave him a small piece of tuna 15–20 times each day as she touched the opposite shoulder and said 'Good boy'. When she treated the wounded shoulder, she gave him a large piece of tuna and repeated 'Good boy' as she applied the compress.

Maternal Aggression

Protective instincts to offspring are present in virtually all mothers. Maternal aggression refers to aggressive behaviour directed towards people or other animals that approach the queen with her kittens. This type of aggressive activity is believed to be a function of the hormonal state of the female during lactation as well as the presence of the young.

Diagnosis and Prognosis

The diagnosis involves observation of a queen that hisses, growls, and attempts to bite humans or other animals that approach the kittens or nest area.

For well socialised queens, the prognosis is good since there is usually spontaneous remission as the kittens age. The prognosis for quick resolution of the problem is guarded.

Management

Although regular handling of newborn kittens is regarded as beneficial for their development, it might be necessary to avoid handling them for the first few days, as this is when the queen tends to be most protective. Gentle handling by trusted family members accompanied by tasty food offerings is the best way to allay apprehension. The well socialised queen is most likely to allow her kittens to be handled, especially by trusted family members. Subduing the queen by gently wrapping her in a towel or applying a cat muzzle when she absolutely has to be handled or enticing the queen to leave her kittens with food or toys may be the most expedient way of minimising the dangers during the short period when she is most likely to be aggressive (Fig 11.9).

MANAGEMENT OF FELINE MATERNAL AGGRESSION

A quiet, low-stress environment should be provided

Avoid approaching and handling of the kittens if the queen appears agitated

Muzzle or gentle restraining device (blanket/towel) when the queen needs to be handled

Distract or entice the mother to leave the litter before the kittens are handled

Desensitisation and counterconditioning

Fig. 11.9 Managing feline maternal aggression.

Behavioural modification can be attempted if the kittens need to be handled while the queen is still very protective, although the maternal behaviour usually runs its course in perhaps the same or less time than would be required to complete a desensitisation and counterconditioning program.

Prevention

Early socialisation and handling of young, female kittens should reduce the likelihood of maternal aggression. For breeding animals, the owner should provide extensive socialisation and handling from kittenhood into adulthood. Gentle handling of the queen and hand-feeding of food throughout pregnancy and after parturition may also be helpful.

Case Example

After giving birth to a healthy litter of six kittens, Sheba, the 2-year-old queen, became very protective and hissed or growled at anyone who approached, except one teenage girl in the family. Prior to this time, the cat appeared very social and exhibited no signs of aggression.

The family was told to provide a quiet environment and to keep visitors to the home at a minimum. The teenager fed canned food to the pet four to six times daily. Each time she entered the room with food, she rang a bell very softly. Within a few days the cat would leave the litter and approach the owner when she heard the bell. After 2 weeks, other family members would accompany her into the room, ring the bell and provide the canned food.

When the kittens were 4 weeks old, the family attempted to have a friend visit the litter. The mother hissed, so visitors were discouraged from entering the room with the litter for another 2 weeks, after which time the maternal aggression had abated.

It was a bit unfortunate in this case that socialisation of the kittens with strangers had to be delayed until 6 weeks of age. Handling by visitors starting earlier is generally more effective in promoting socialisation to humans.

Intermale Aggression

Aggression between male cats is one of the most common forms of feline aggression. This evolves out

MANAGEMENT OF FELINE INTERMALE AGGRESSION	
Method	**Rationale**
Castration	The most successful approach
	Neutering reduces or eliminates intermale fighting in approximately 90% of cases. Neither the fighting experience nor the age at time of surgery seem to affect the success rate
Avoid all potentially aggressive situations	Minimise the possibility of conflicts and competition. Feed cats in different parts of the house
Confinement	Sometimes it may be necessary to confine cats in crates or separate rooms if there is a risk of aggression
Behavioural modification	Success rate is low when used by itself
	Desensitisation or counterconditioning
	Light punishment (watergun) may be effective at suppressing aggression by either cat
Drug therapy	Progestins may be useful when treating cats for intermale aggression
	Anxiolytics (benzodiazepines, buspirone) or antidepressants (TCAs, fluoxetine) may be helpful
	Effects tend to be temporary and the behaviour usually resumes after the drug is discontinued

FIG. 11.10 Steps in the management of feline intermale aggression.

of a normal behaviour of challenge that takes place as cats mature sexually and behaviourally. It is particularly common during the mating season.

Diagnosis and Prognosis

Male–male aggression often results from hormonally driven competition, but territorial interests or fear may also play a role. This problem usually develops after sexual maturity in males 1–3 years of age. They may respond by hissing, growling, scratching, and biting. Elaborate and ritualised threat displays may precede the events. The prognosis is fair.

Management

Treatment may involve behavioural modification, surgery and drug therapy (Fig. 11.10).

Prevention

Intermale aggression may be prevented by neutering in some cats. Care should be taken to ensure that all family pets were well socialised during infancy. Also, cats that have been well socialised may be more likely to get along and less likely to do serious damage to another cat in a fight.

Case Example

Barney was a 13-month-old male Persian cat that the owner, a part-time cat breeder, had been raising for breeding stock. Six months earlier the owner had purchased Fred, a 1-year-old Himalayan male, also for breeding purposes. There were also two adult female Persians and one Himalayan female in her home. When the owner was out, the Himalayans were housed in one room and the Persians in another. Whenever the owner was home, the cats had always played and eaten together. Approximately one month earlier, the owners had noticed that one of the male cats had begun to spray on a few of the walls in the kitchen and family room. The owners started to separate the males so that most of the time only one of the males was allowed to roam freely at a time and this had been successful at reducing the spraying. However, with play time, feeding times, cleaning times, and many family members and visitors in the home, it was impractical to keep Barney and Fred away from each other at all times. Now, the cats had begun to fight whenever they saw each other, and even hissed and growled 'through' the closed door at each other. Barney had just returned from the referring veterinarian for treatment of a deep abscess on the side of the face.

The owners were extremely reluctant to neuter either cat, so exposure and counterconditioning techniques were discussed. The cats were kept apart except during feeding times when they were placed in separate metal carrying crates where they could see each other. Although some aggressive displays were exhibited, the cats soon ate in their separate cages without incident, even if the cages were side by side. The owners then attempted to allow one cat out at a time during feeding and there was only the occasional threat (when Fred was the one out of the crate). However, when both cats were allowed out (a harness and leash was attached to each cat to maintain control and ensure safety), threats and attacks resumed whenever the cats got within a few feet of each other. Toys, catnip and food could be used to occupy the cats without aggression for very short periods, but as soon as the cats investigated or approached each other the aggression recurred. The owners decided that the most practical solution for their household was to have one of the cats neutered. It was likely that Fred was the instigator of the aggression and the one most likely to spray. Also, it was in the owners' best economic interest to attempt to neuter Fred first and to use Barney for breeding. If this was not successful, they would have Fred adopted out into another home. Within 1 week of the neutering, spraying stopped and aggressive displays between the two cats were almost entirely eliminated.

Other Forms of Aggression

Pathophysiological Aggression

Pathophysiological aggressive disorders are those that have an underlying medical cause. These conditions may arise at any age, may have a sudden onset, and may not fit neatly into the other aggressive behaviour categories already described. Many of these are described in Chapter 3 in the discussion of the medical examination; some are listed in Fig. 11.11. In some cases, the medical problems alone may not cause the problem, but a combination of behavioural factors and medical problems may be necessary for the aggression to be patent. Underlying medical problems need to be addressed for successful treatment of pathophysiological aggression. This type of aggression is occasionally drug-responsive but is often poorly managed by behavioural modification techniques.

FELINE PATHOPHYSIOLOGICAL AGGRESSIVE DISORDERS	
Underlying Cause	**Example**
Infectious agent	Rabies
Endocrinopathy	Hyperthyroidism
Neurological disease	Epilepsy
Painful conditions	Dental disease, otitis, arthritis, abscesses
Other medical problems	Sensory loss, fatigue

Fig. 11.11 Some examples of pathophysiological causes of aggression problems in cats.

Idiopathic Aggression

Idiopathic aggression is a catch-all category for aggressive behaviour that appears unpredictably and for which the underlying cause is not known. The diagnosis is reserved for those cats that have been thoroughly assessed by a competent behaviour consultant without revealing an identifiable stimulus or motivation for the aggression. Redirected aggression or fear aggression that has resulted from circumstances that the owner did not observe are likely to end up in this category.

Learned Aggression

There may be a learned component with many types of feline aggression. Learned aggression can result from intentionally and repeatedly provoking cats to be aggressive. In other cases, the owner may have unintentionally conditioned the aggression. When the owner attempts to soothe a cat exhibiting fear aggression, the aggressive behaviour is reinforced. In addition, pets that are threatened or punished for aggressive displays can learn to associate pain or fear with certain stimuli and become even more aggressive each time the situations recur. Behavioural modification is the treatment of choice.

References

Anderson, R. K. (1996) Feline aggression. In: (eds): *Cat Behavior and Training: Veterinary Advice for Owners.* Ackerman, L., Landsberg, G. and Hunthausen, W. (eds). TFH Publications: Neptune City, NJ.

Overall, K. (1994a) Feline aggression (part 1). *Feline Practice*, **22**(4), 25–26.

Overall, K. (1994b) Feline aggression (part 2). *Feline Practice*, **22**(5), 28–31.

Overall, K. (1994c) Feline aggression (part 3). *Feline Practice*, **22**(6), 16–17.

Further Reading

Ackerman, L., Landsberg, G. and Hunthausen, W. (1996) *Cat Behavior and Training: Veterinary Advice for Owners*. TFH Publications: Neptune City, NJ.

Askew, H. R. (1993) The treatment of aggression problems in cats. *Kleintierpraxis*, **38**(1), 35.

Beaver, B. V. (1989) Feline behavioural problems other than housesoiling. *Journal of the American Animal Hospital Association*, **25**, 465–469.

Beaver, B. V. (1994) Differential approach to aggression by dogs and cats. *Veterinary Quarterly*, **16**(Suppl. 1), S48.

Blackshaw, J. K. (1991) Management of orally based problems and aggression in cats. *Australian Veterinary Practitioner*, **21**, 122–124.

Blum, S. R. (1979) Aggressive behavior. *Feline Practice*, **9**(2), 9.

Borchelt, P. and Voith, V. L. (1982) Diagnosis and treatment of aggression problems in cats. *Veterinary Clinics of North America, Small Animal Practice,* **12**(4), 673–680.

Borchelt, P. and Voith, V. L. (1996) Aggressive behavior in cats. In: *Readings in Companion Animal Behavior*. Voith, V. L., Borchelt, P. L. (eds). pp. 208–216. Veterinary Learning Systems: Trenton, NJ.

Borchelt, P. and Voith, V. L. (1996) Aggressive behavior in dogs and cats. In: *Readings in Companion Animal Behavior*. Voith, V. L., Borchelt, P. L. (eds). pp. 217–229. Veterinary Learning Systems: Trenton, NJ.

Chapman, B. L. and Voith, V. L. (1990) Cat aggression redirected to people: 14 cases (1981–1987). *Journal of the American Veterinary Medical Association*, **196**(6), 947–950.

Hart, B. (1977) Aggression in cats, *Feline Practice*, **7**(2), 22.

Hart, B. L. and Barrett, R. E. (1983) Effects of castration on fighting, roaming and urine spraying in adult male cats. *Journal of the American Veterinary Medical Association*, **163**(3), 290–292.

Heidenberger, E. (1993) Aggressive behaviour of household cats. *Tierärztliche Umschau*, **48**(7), 436.

Marder, A. R. (1993) Diagnosing and treating aggression problems in cats. *Veterinary Medicine*, August, 8–13.

Matthews-Cameron, S. (1987) Diazepam treatment of fear-related aggression in a cat. *Companion Animal Practice*, **14**, 4–6.

Reisner, I. R, Houpt, K. A., Erb, H. N. and Quimby, F. W. (1994) Friendliness to humans and defensive aggression in cats – The influence of handling and paternity. *Physiology and Behaviour*, **55**(6), 1119–1124.

Schwartz, S. (1994) Carbamazepine in the control of aggressive behaviour in cats. *Journal of the American Animal Hospital Association*, **30**(5), 515–519.

Turner, D. C. and Meister, O. (1988) Hunting behaviour of the domestic cat. In: *The Domestic Cat: The Biology of its Behaviour*, Turner, D. and Bateson, P. (eds). pp. 111–121, Cambridge University Press: Cambridge.

12

Stereotypic and Compulsive Disorders

Introduction

In this chapter we review some of the abnormal behaviours of pets. Abnormal behaviours fall into two major categories: pathophysiological and experiential. Pathophysiological (i.e. resulting from a physical or medical problem) examples have been dealt with in numerous sections throughout this book. These might include genetic physical problems (such as hip dysplasia, deafness or hydrocephalus), or genetic behavioural or physiological problems (such as narcolepsy, or nervousness in Pointers) or acquired problems (such as rabies, nutritional deficiencies or toxins).

Experiential abnormal behaviour might arise during development (e.g. inadequate socialisation), may be reactive (resulting from factors in the environment or management of the pet) or may be conditioned (e.g. owner rewards behaviour). Reactive abnormal behaviour generally results from conflict brought about by the pet's level of arousal and the inability to perform an appropriate behaviour to reduce arousal. The motivation to perform a particular behaviour is brought about by any combination of intrinsic or extrinsic factors. When there are no appropriate behaviours to achieve de-arousal the pet may redirect its behaviour toward a less suitable target, may engage in vacuum activities, or may display displacement activities (normal behaviours out of context) or neurotic behaviour (behaviour which does not seem to be derived from normal).

Because of genetic, medical, hormonal, nutritional and physical differences, and the effects of early learning and experience, two pets exposed to the same external stimuli may achieve different levels of motivation or varying levels of arousal. How an animal copes or responds to this arousal is also dependent on these internal factors and mechanisms. Situations that might lead to stress or arousal include the pet's physical or social environment, the availablity of resources, and the availablity of appropriate releasing stimuli for species-typical behaviours (e.g. chew toys, scratching posts). De-arousal is achieved by satisfying the pet's desires through the performance of normal species-typical behaviours.

Redirected Behaviours

When an animal is motivated to perform an activity toward an appropriate target (e.g. territorial aggression, fear aggression) but is frustrated or in some other way interrupted from reaching the principal target, the pet directs its behaviour towards a less appropriate target or third party. In contrast to displacement activity, an activity is not performed out of context, rather the interrupted or frustrated behaviour is directed towards another target.

Displacement or Conflict Behaviours

In some situations, an animal may be motivated to perform two behaviours that are in conflict with each other (e.g. approach and withdrawal, greeting and fear of being punished). The inability to perform both of the strongly motivated behaviours can lead to conflict that often results in the performance of a displacement behaviour. This is usually a normal behaviour shown at an inappropriate time, appearing out of context for the occasion. The behaviour may be performed in order to decrease arousal and help the animal cope with the conflict. Grooming, yawning, eating and vocalisations may be performed in stressful situations as displacement behaviours.

Neurotic Behaviour

When the animal is highly motivated to perform a behaviour and there are insufficient outlets to achieve de-arousal, neurotic behaviour may develop. These are behaviours which do not appear to be derived from normal behaviour, such as self-mutilation or tail chasing.

Vacuum Activity

An instinctive or unconscious behaviour that is performed in the absence of the stimulus to which it would normally be performed is a vacuum activity. These activities have no apparent useful purpose. Behaviours that are highly motivated but for which there is no outlet (sucking, licking, masturbation) may constitute these activities.

Stereotypies

Stereotypies are generally defined as unvarying, repetitive or constant behaviour patterns that have no obvious goal or apparent function. Stereotypic behaviours may be performed as components of displacement behaviours or compulsive disorders, such as acral lick dermatitis, tail chasing or flank-sucking. They may also be due to physiological changes such as might be seen with a neurological disorder (circling, head bobbing).

Compulsive Behaviours

When an animal is repeatedly placed in a state of conflict, the threshold for performance of a displacement behaviour decreases so that it may be manifested during any state of stress or arousal. Eventually, the behaviour becomes compulsive as the pet loses control over initiating or terminating it. In some cases, the compulsive behaviour may even begin to be seen in non-conflict situations. Compulsive behaviours are often derived from normal behaviour patterns (such as grooming or locomotion) but appear to be abnormal because they are excessive, exceedingly intense, or performed out of context. Compulsive behaviour may extract certain costs from the individual by way of wasting energy, interfering with the maintenance of normal body weight, hindering integral behaviour patterns and restricting normal social interactions. They may also be directly injurious when non-food items are ingested (feline wool-eating) or when the behaviour is directed toward the animal (acral lick dermatitis, feline psychogenic alopecia, tail chasing/biting).

Although some compulsive disorders are repetitive and may therefore be referred to as stereotypic (wool-sucking, pacing, floor scratching, self-mutilation), other compulsive disorders such as standing completely still (freezing) or staring would not be referred to as repetitive or ritualistic.

In human medicine, these compulsive disorders are referred to as obsessive–compulsive disorders. In fact, it has been suggested that the term be used in animal behaviour as well. However, the term obsessive refers to thought processes such as concern with cleanliness or safety, while compulsive refers to repetitive rituals or actions. Thus, the term compulsive (and not obsessive) might be better suited to describing the problems seen in dogs and cats. Some of the drugs used to treat people with obsessive–compulsive disorders may also be used for treating compulsive behaviours in animals.

As certain behaviours are more commonly seen in certain breeds, it is likely that there is a genetic predisposition to specific stereotypies or compulsive behaviours. For example, flank-sucking is most commonly seen in Doberman Pinschers, while whirling and spinning has been observed in Bull Terriers, and fly chasing or star gazing in Miniature Schnauzers. In cats, wool-sucking is recognised as a common stereotypy in the oriental breeds.

There is some blurring of the lines of causality for some compulsive behaviours. For example, the ultimate cause of acral lick dermatitis might be viewed quite differently by behaviourists, dermatologists and neurologists. The same may also be true for excessive grooming, psychogenic alopecia and feline hyperaesthesia.

Although many compulsive or stereotypic behaviours arise spontaneously as a response to conflict or anxiety, it is also possible for behaviours to become compulsive or stereotypic because they have been conditioned. For example, the owner who repeatedly gives the young pet attention when it playfully chases its tail may reinforce the performance of the behaviour.

General Approach to Treatment

Regarding treatment, all compulsive and stereotypic behaviours must be evaluated individually since not all require treatment. In fact, treatment may only be necessary if the behaviour poses health risks to the animal or annoys the owner. For some pets, the compulsive behaviour may be the most practical and acceptable outlet for reducing stress or resolving conflict in their home environment.

Reducing stress or finding methods of decreasing the sources of arousal and conflict are the first aspects of treatment that should be explored for compulsive behaviours. In some cases, the source of conflict, anxiety or arousal is easily identified, while in others it is not. Inconsistencies in the relationship between the pet and the owner may lead to problems, especially when it comes to inconsistent training. The environment should be closely examined to ensure that the pet has sufficient stimulation, particularly when the owners are frequently absent or otherwise occupied. This must include sufficient exercise, play, and social attention, as well as appropriate toys. Obedience training may be helpful and the owner should be cautioned that inappropriate punishment could actually intensify the problem rather than correct it. The owner must also be notified that some stressors in the pet's life may not be easily eliminated or avoided. Also, since some stereotypic or compulsive behaviours may be initiated by underlying medical problems, a complete medical work-up is critical in all cases.

It has also been suggested that if the compulsive, stereotypic or displacement behaviours are causing no apparent physical or behavioural 'harm', that they may, in fact, be an acceptable way for the animal to cope with stress or conflict in the environment. For example, if flank-sucking causes no physical harm and occupies, relaxes and calms the dog, is this not preferable to the use of calming drugs, or the development of other physical (e.g. gastrointestinal disorders or acral lick dermatitis) or behavioural disorders (e.g. wholesale destruction of the household or constant vocalisation) associated with stress and anxiety?

Sources of stress that cannot easily be eliminated include:

- New home
- Owner departures
- Change in owner's daily schedule
- Renovations
- Vacation
- New additions to household (spouse, baby)
- Family strife.

In some cases, owners can contribute to the pet's problem by inadvertently rewarding the behaviours. This happens when owners try to divert the pet's attention by offering food and social rewards or when the owners give social attention to a pet performing a behaviour that initially seems 'cute', such as tail chasing, shadow chasing or barking.

Behavioural modification is most appropriate when owners can identify and predict those situations and times when compulsive behaviours are likely to arise. They can then initiate an alternative activity (before the compulsive behaviour is overt) that is incompatible with the problem behaviour, such as play, training or feeding, or provide a chew toy. Although extreme, remote punishment techniques (e.g. remote shock collars) have also been used successfully to treat some cases of obsessive disorders such as acral lick dermatitis. Counterconditioning and desensitisation techniques may also be helpful at reducing the frequency or intensity of the stereotypy. Distraction devices (ultrasonics, water gun, siren, or leash and halter) may help when the owner is unable to interrupt the stereotypic behaviour and re-establish normal or alternative behaviour with simple commands.

Denying the pet access to the focus of its obsession has often been tried, but with mixed results. For example, a bandage or an Elizabethan collar may allow acral lick dermatitis (granuloma) to heal, but once the collar is removed most cases relapse. In many cases, restricting access might actually potentiate the problem by increasing anxiety or arousal.

Drug therapy is gaining popularity for use in pets with stereotypies just as it is in humans with obsessive–compulsive disorders. There are many theories for why different drugs are effective, but the exact mechanism is unknown. There are also many apparent contradictions with drug therapies. For example, acral lick dermatitis responds to therapy with some narcotics (e.g. hydrocodone) as well as narcotic antagonists such as naltrexone. Since endogenous endorphin (opioid) release is believed to be a factor in some compulsive disorders, supplying exogenous sources of opioids or utilising opiate antagonists may both be effective. This same condition also responds sometimes to antidepressants, corticosteroids, flunixin meglumide, cryosurgery, antibiotics, occlusion therapy, radiation therapy and cobra antivenom. Since lowered serotonin and increased dopamine levels may be associated with some compulsive disorders, drugs that bring about a normalisation of one or both of these neurotransmitters (tricyclic antidepressants, fluoxetine, pimozide, lithium) may also be effective in the treatment of these disorders. A short course of therapy with antianxiety drugs (clorazepate, diazepam, buspirone)

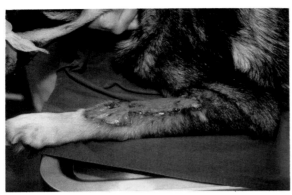

Fig. 12.1 Acral lick dermatitis: self-trauma to the foreleg of a dog. Reprinted with permission from Ackerman, L. *Practical Canine Dermatology.* American Veterinary Publications, 1989.

may also be useful when the pet must be exposed to a potentially stressful or anxiety-producing situation (new home, dramatic change in schedule, new baby).

Acral Lick Dermatitis (Lick Granuloma)

Acral lick dermatitis is a distinct clinical entity in which dogs lick at one or more of their limbs, often causing significant damage (Fig. 12.1). It is not unusual to find the area denuded of skin and it may be raw and weeping, or thickened and granulomatous. The exact cause is not yet known but dermatological, behavioural and neurological theories have all been promulgated. Large breeds such as Doberman Pinschers, Great Danes, German Shepherd Dogs, Labrador Retrievers, Golden Retrievers and Irish Setters are most commonly affected. Males are affected twice as often as females. Dogs with acral lick dermatitis may have mild sensory polyneuropathy. Lack of stimulation is frequently cited as an underlying cause, but underlying anatomical abnormalities (e.g. arthritis, fracture, neural entrapment,) may be contributory. Also, acral lick dermatitis may be a compulsive disorder with a fundamental problem of conflict between the pet and its environment. The condition arises when the pet is repeatedly stressed or anxious, and this leads to excessive licking.

Damage is then done to the skin, which potentiates the sensation and persistent licking. Affected dogs begin licking at a site, removing hair, causing inflammation and finally removing layers of the skin,

sometimes down to the bone. The area becomes raw and weeping, and the chronic trauma itself becomes irritating, further stimulating the dog to lick and chew.

Diagnosis and Prognosis

The underlying aetiology cannot always be confirmed by clinical signs alone. Differential diagnoses include: stress or conflict, neoplasia (e.g. mast-cell tumour), parasitism (e.g. demodicosis), mycotic dermatitis, trauma (e.g. fracture, neural injury, prior wound, foreign body), focal allergic manifestation (e.g. id reaction, contact eruption, adverse food reaction, atopy), and acral mutilation syndrome. Bacterial and fungal cultures, skin scrapings, cytological examination and biopsies must be performed to rule out organic causes. Radiography of the affected limb is recommended and periosteal reactions of underlying bone are commonly seen.

In most cases, a fair to guarded prognosis is given to dogs with acral lick dermatitis. If the underlying cause can be determined and eliminated, the prognosis improves dramatically.

Management

With true acral lick dermatitis, treatment must be directed at both the psychological impairment and the skin disorder. Therefore, even if an underlying psychological problem can be diagnosed and treated with behavioural management and drug therapy, concurrent treatment of the skin condition is essential. Medical therapy might consist of treatment with long-term antibiotics, anti-inflammatory agents and denying access to the area until the lesion begins to heal. Behavioural management might include the diagnosis and treatment of those situations and stimuli that lead to stress or anxiety, as well as drug therapy with tricyclic antidepressants or fluoxetine. In general, several months of therapy are likely to be needed before the lesions (and the compulsive licking) are resolved. At that point, if the underlying problems have been resolved, the lesions may not recur if the drug is withdrawn.

Any situation leading to conflict may be an inciting factor for acral lick dermatitis in dogs that are genetically predisposed to developing these problems. In time, as with other compulsive disorders, the problem may become generalised to other situations, even those in which the pet's level of stress, anxiety or conflict is relatively low. When the licking occurs in the owner's presence, those stimuli that directly precede the licking should be identified. These stimuli might then be eliminated, reduced or modified, or desensitisation and counterconditioning techniques can be used to teach the pet to perform an alternative competing behaviour in these situations. Distraction or aversive devices (including audible and ultrasonic alarms, water rifles or a halter and long leash) may also be successful at interrupting the behaviour; however, these techniques do not help to resolve the problem if it occurs in the owner's absence. For these cases, increasing play and exercise before departures and increased environmental stimulation (objects to chew and tear apart, toys and boxes with food hidden inside, providing food in a variety of locations or with a timed feeder, getting another pet, day care) may be useful for keeping the pet occupied and distracted (*see separation anxiety and destructive chewing in Chapter 7*). Although aversive techniques are seldom practical or effective, treatment with remote control shock collars and bandaging the area and applying 'hot' or 'bitter' sprays have been successful. The key to therapy is that the aversion must be strong enough to deter the behaviour, and that the pet receives the aversive stimulus continuously (every time) until the behaviour ceases. Whenever the aversive treatment cannot be effectively applied, an Elizabethan collar should be used to prevent access to the area. Care should be taken when considering the use of aversive stimuli in treating this condition because some cases may take a turn for the worse with this approach.

Pharmacological intervention is often required as an adjunct to most treatment programmes for compulsive disorders (Fig. 12.2). Medication such as tricyclic antidepressants, narcotic antagonists, fluoxetine and hydrocodone are the primary considerations. Other treatments that have also been used with variable success include cryosurgery, radiation therapy, excisional therapy, acupuncture and injections of cobra antivenin. Corticosteroids injected into the lesion or applied topically with a penetrating agent, such as dimethyl sulphoxide (DMSO), have been quite successful, but the potential dangers of long-term corticosteroid use must be considered. One of the most popular topical remedies has been adding 3 ml of flunixin meglumide to an 8 ml container of fluocinolone and DMSO; the mixture is applied once to twice daily.

In a recent study using radiation therapy, a successful clinical response was seen in 6 of 17 cases

DRUG THERAPIES FOR ACRAL LICK DERMATITIS		
Drug	**Dose**	**Comments**
Naltrexone	2.2 mg/kg PO sid–bid	Narcotic antagonist.
	1 mg/kg SC	Successful about 65% of time.
Nalmefene	1–4 mg/kg SC	Successful about 70% of time.
Hydrocodone	5 mg/20 kg PO tid	Supplies exogenous source of opioid? Mood altering? Successful about 65% of time.
Doxepin	0.5–1.0 mg/kg bid	Tricyclic antidepressant; moderately sedating; strongly antihistaminic, moderate anticholinergic.
Amitriptyline	1.0–4.4 mg/kg PO sid–bid	Tricyclic antidepressant; moderately sedating; potent anticholinergic; strongly antihistaminic.
Clomipramine	1–3 mg/kg PO bid	Tricyclic antidepressant. Serotonergic; moderately sedating; moderately anticholinergic. Successful about 65% of time. (See Chapter 4 for further details.)
Fluoxetine	1 mg/kg PO sid	Antidepressant. Potent serotonergic agent. (See Chapter 4 for further details.)
Pentazocine + Naltrexone	50 mg + 0.5 mg PO bid	Combination narcotic and narcotic antagonist.
Orgotein	5–10 mg every 7–10 days or two or three times intralesionally	Success rate not determined, but presumed low.
Pimozide	1–10 mg daily	Used in humans with antidepressants for refractory obsessive–compulsive disorders.

Fig. 12.2 Drug treatment for the behavioural component of acral lick dermatitis.

(35%). In another 24% (4 cases), there was resolution but with eventual recurrence. Total radiation dosage was within the range of 625–4500 cGy, delivered in fractions of 261–1000 cGy, and administered at 3-, 4-, or 7-day intervals. Thus, radiation therapy might be considered in cases that do not respond to other treatment modalities.

It is sometimes necessary to use bandaging or Elizabethan collars to deny access to the lesions for the first few weeks of therapy. On the other hand these techniques could lead to increased anxiety, thereby compounding the problem. Concurrent use of bactericidal antibiotics (such as cephalosporins, potentiated penicillins, and trimethoprim–sulphonamides) are recommended for a minimum of 6 weeks to treat secondary infection which can contribute to perpetuation or recurrence of lesions.

Prevention

Acral lick dermatitis is almost impossible to prevent because it can arise from so many different underlying causes, both behavioural and medical. The best approach to preventing a chronic ingrained behaviour is to recognise the compulsive nature early and initiate behavioural modification at that time.

Owners of dogs that have been treated for acral lick dermatitis should be counselled about controlling stress in the pet's life. Consideration should be given to the prophylactic use of psychoactive medication, exercise and environmental stimulation when highly stressful situations cannot be avoided.

Case examples

Case 1

Midnight, a 4-year-old, spayed female Labrador Retriever cross, was presented for a 2 cm thickened ulcerated lesion on the left foreleg. The owner reported that the pet had started intermittently licking the area 4 months ago. There was no history of trauma. During the past month the licking had been constant. Yelling at the pet was only successful in distracting it temporarily. The owner had had a baby 2 months previously. Prior to the middle of the pregnancy, the owner and the dog often jogged together and spent a lot of time in the park. The pet had had little training and had always been a bit unruly. Since the baby was born, the unruliness had

been a major problem and the owner frequently found herself scolding the pet. A thorough medical work-up uncovered no other problems. The underlying problem was conflict due to major changes in the dog's daily life and a change in the relationship with the owner.

The wife and husband were encouraged to alternate in taking the pet on at least one long walk each day and to hire a dog walking service to provide a second long daily walk. The owners were taught how to teach the dog to sit, lie down and stay on command so that it could be given commands that would keep it out of the way when needed and prevent unruly behaviour. Food lure training using an upbeat tone was stressed. This gave the owners a way of controlling the pet and preventing undesirable behaviour so that scoldings decreased. The owners were told to develop a set of rules for how they expected the pet to behave and to reinforce desired behaviour consistently and avoid reinforcing undesired behaviour. Cephalexin was prescribed for 6 weeks and the lesion was bandaged lightly and sprayed with a bitter spray when the owners were not available to supervise.

Six weeks later the dog was re-examined: the lesions were well on their way to healing. The owners felt that there was considerable improvement but that the dog still licked the area occasionally, although not as often as before. A solution of topical fluocinolone and DMSO was dispensed to be applied to the area as 5 drops bid for the next 10 days. It was suggested that a bitter topical solution be applied to the area for another 3 weeks after that. The rationale was that the behaviour may have been ingrained enough that the dog was licking out of habit. A re-evaluation one month later revealed a dog that was essentially normal and all therapy was discontinued. A follow-up 6 months later showed the condition was still in remission.

Case 2

Darcy, a 2-year-old Doberman Pinscher, was presented with a 6-month history of licking and chewing at his right forelimb. The area was ulcerated and the owner was sure she could see all the way to the bone. They had tried punishing him whenever they caught him chewing and he would stop temporarily. However, they could not police him day and night and the condition continued to get worse. Careful history-gathering failed to reveal evidence of boredom or change in the dog's life. He jogged with his owner 2 miles each day, just as he had always done. They did not believe he was 'stressed' and were sure there had to be another reason for the problem.

Clinical evaluation revealed a normal healthy happy dog with no evidence of any medical problems. Radiographs of the limb revealed a periosteal inflammatory reaction but no evidence of foreign bodies. Biopsies were done to rule out organic causes such as dermatophytosis, demodicosis, subcutaneous mycoses and mast cell tumour. Findings included marked ulceration, dermal hyperplasia and a mixed-cell inflammatory infiltrate, consistent with self-induced acral lick dermatitis.

The leg was treated with a mild antiseptic solution and bandaged to prevent further access. A 6-week course of amoxicillin-clavulanate was prescribed. The owners telephoned 2 weeks later to report that Darcy was now busy licking at the other forearm and causing similar damage. Re-examination confirmed the owner's fear; he had left the bandaged leg alone and now was destructively chewing his left foreleg. A solution of fluocinolone and DMSO combined with flunixin meglumide was dispensed with instructions for the owner to apply 5 drops of the mixture BID for 10 days.

Re-evaluation 14 days later was not promising. Although there had been some improvement, it was evident that Darcy was still busy chewing his leg. The owners consented to an experimental therapy, using the human drug pimozide. They were cautioned about possible side effects but were still anxious to give it a try. A pre-therapy electrocardiogram was done with plans to repeat ECGs once weekly while on therapy.

The owners phoned 4 days later to say that Darcy was not chewing his leg but that he was acting 'funny'. He bared his teeth at them (while still wagging his tail), began barking at the neighbour's cat (which he had never done before) and once they found him sleeping in a hall cupboard. It was not known whether these behaviours were drug-related, but it was recommended that the dosage be decreased by 25%. Darcy was seen weekly for his ECG but without evidence of any cardiac problems. His lesions continued to regress and were completely gone by about 10 weeks into therapy. However, when we attempted to discontinue therapy altogether, the behaviour resurfaced. Before he could do any harm, treatment was reinstituted. After some manipulation of drug dosage, it was determined that Darcy could be controlled with a relatively small alternate-day dose.

If medication was not administered for 72 hours, the behaviour resumed.

In this case, control required long-term use of pimozide on an alternate-day basis. Darcy was re-examined every 3 months for cardiac evaluation, haematology, urinalysis and serum biochemistry.

Feline Psychogenic Alopecia

Alopecia can result when cats overgroom and remove fur, usually over their topline. The diagnosis of psychogenic alopecia is reserved for those cases in which no underlying medical problem is evident. Obviously, a cat with fleas that removes fur by chewing is not a candidate for the diagnosis. Cats are normally fastidious groomers and as much as 30–50% of their time awake is spent performing some type of grooming behaviour.

It is thought that feline psychogenic alopecia may be a displacement activity resulting from anxiety or frustration, which in time might become compulsive. Nervousness, lack of stimulation and the desire for human contact can result in excessive grooming. Changes in the owner's schedule resulting in separation anxiety, inappropriate punishment, and new people or animals in the environment may all be potential causes of this type of problem.

Recently, a study was completed which examined grooming time in relation to stress and drugs that increase or decrease dopamine levels. Grooming was significantly increased after an injection of apomorphine and decreased following an injection of haloperidol. The results support the concept that stress is able to induce excessive grooming and emphasises the role of dopamine in relation to stress.

Diagnosis and Prognosis

The first diagnostic step is to confirm that the fur is being removed by excessive grooming and that the hairs are not being shed. This can be quickly and effectively confirmed by a trichogram in which hairs are plucked, placed on a microscope slide, and viewed microscopically. Whereas endocrine conditions have hairs with telogen bulbs predominating, fur that has been removed by licking shows evidence of shear. This confirms only that the alopecia is due to excessive grooming, not the ultimate cause. This alone can be valuable, because many cats are

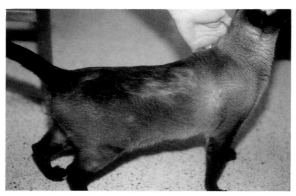

FIG. 12.3 Patchy hair loss on the dorsum of a cat with psychogenic alopecia.

secretive groomers and owners may report that they never see their cat lick or chew. The other clinical clue is that a cat with psychogenic alopecia will only have hair loss on those parts of the body that can be reached with the tongue. In contradistinction to conditions such as dermatophytosis and allergy, in cats with psychogenic alopecia the top of the head and back of the neck are always spared from hair loss (Fig. 12.3).

It is essential that a thorough medical examination be conducted before a diagnosis of psychogenic alopecia is given. Many cats with presumed psychogenic tendencies have been shown to have inhalant allergies (atopy). This finding is also supported by the breed predisposition towards Siamese, Abyssinians and Himalayans. Thus, apparent overgrooming can result from the pruritus of an allergic skin condition and there need not be concurrent primary dermatological lesions. Feline inhalant allergies are most appropriately diagnosed by intradermal allergy testing; blood tests are not accurate. Complete remission with corticosteroid therapy, while not diagnostic of any specific medical condition may help to rule out a behavioural cause. Referral to a dermatologist is often warranted. Therapy often includes antihistamines (especially chlorpheniramine and clemastine), fatty acids (combinations of cis-linoleic acid, gamma-linolenic acid, and eicosapentaenoic acid) and immunotherapy.

The cat with alopecia must also be evaluated for internal and external parasites, dermatophytes and adverse food reactions. Fleas are not always evident immediately and several minutes should be spent with a flea comb concentrating on several areas, particularly the base of the tail, shoulders, perineum, axillae and

behind the ears. Skin scrapings should also be taken from several representative sites (cheyletiellosis can closely mimic psychogenic alopecia) as well as dermatophyte cultures. Whenever possible, a hypoallergenic diet trial should be conducted for a minimum of 8 weeks using, for example, lamb-based baby food or fresh-cooked lamb. Commercial hypoallergenic diets are less reliable for diagnostic testing because they will miss the diagnosis approximately 20% of the time. A word of caution: these diets are suitable only for the diagnostic process, they are not nutritionally balanced for long-term feeding. Blood tests designed to identify cats with food allergies are extremely unreliable and are of little practical value. Additional laboratory tests that should be performed include: complete blood count, thyroxine, serum alanine transaminase, urinalysis and faecal evaluation.

Important historical information should include a description of events, schedule changes or environmental changes that occurred prior to or at the time of the initiation of the grooming behaviour, as well as how the cat responded to these changes. The occurrence of other concurrent anxiety-associated behaviours such as hiding, anorexia, avoidance and nervousness might suggest that the problem has a behavioural rather than a medical aetiology.

Management

The diagnosis of feline psychogenic alopecia is reserved for those cases for which an underlying medical cause cannot be found. Whenever possible, treatment should include eliminating the cause of the cat's stress. Although it is questionable whether cats suffer from true separation anxiety, the techniques used for reducing destructive behaviour and increasing environmental stimulation (play centres, chew toys, food- or catnip-packed toys, videos, increased interactive play) can all be tried if the behaviour tends to occur in the owner's absence. (*See feline destructive behaviour in Chapter 7.*) Gradually helping the cat adapt to long owner absences by providing a number of short departures of varying lengths may help. Reducing access to any stimuli that might cause anxiety and perhaps even obtaining a second compatible cat may improve (or perhaps aggravate) the condition. If behavioural therapy alone is not successful, drug treatment is often initiated, using diazepam, amitriptyline, clomipramine, fluoxetine, chlorpheniramine maleate, phenobarbital or progestins (Fig. 12.4).

DRUG TREATMENT FOR FELINE PSYCHOGENIC ALOPECIA		
Drug	**Dosage**	**Comments**
Diazepam	0.25–2.2 mg/cat sid–tid	Potential hepatic toxicity. (*See Chapter 4 for details.*)
Amitriptyline	5.0–10.0 mg/day or 1–2 mg/kg sid	May take 2 weeks to see effect. (*See Chapter 4 for details.*)
Clomipramine	0.5–1.5 mg sid	May take 2 weeks to see effect. (*See Chapter 4 for details.*)
Chlorpheniramine maleate	1–2 mg PO bid–tid	*See Chapter 4.*
Phenobarbital	2–3 mg/kg PO sid–bid or as needed	*See Chapter 4.*
Fluoxetine	0.5–1.0 mg/kg every 24 h	SSRI
Megoestrol acetate	2.5–10 mg/cat sid for 2 weeks, then half dose every 2 weeks	Numerous potential toxic effects. (*See Chapter 4 for details.*)

Fig. 12.4 Drug therapies used to treat feline psychogenic alopecia.

Response to medication varies greatly between individuals and some cats will not respond to any of these drugs. The owner should be counselled to avoid inadvertently reinforcing the behaviour by giving the cat attention when it is grooming. Well timed distractions, unassociated with the owner, are more beneficial than aversive stimuli in stopping the performance of the behaviour.

Prevention

Reducing stress in the cat's life and using anxiolytic medication prior to and during stressful situations for the cat with a history of psychogenic alopecia may prevent further problems. Owners of cats that have been treated for psychogenic alopecia should be counselled about controlling stress in the cat's life. Consideration should be given to prophylactic use of psychoactive medication, exercise and environmental stimulation when highly stressful situations cannot be avoided.

For those cases that are actually due to allergies, a familial nature is likely. Affected individuals should not be used for breeding. There is also some hypothetical information that supplementing allergy-prone kittens with oils containing eicosapentaenoic acid (EPA), docosahexaenoic acid (DHA) and gamma-linolenic acid may lessen the impact of allergies when they are more fully mature.

Case Example

Thai, a 9-year-old neutered female Siamese cat, was presented for alopecia along the sides and dorsum of the lumbar area. The owner had noticed little change in the cat's grooming behaviour, but it had been hiding quite a lot since a new roommate and his dog moved into the apartment 2 weeks ago. A complete medical/dermatological work-up (including intradermal allergy testing following an 8-week hypoallergenic diet trial) revealed no underlying medical aetiology.

The cat received 5 mg amitriptyline sid and was confined to a quiet area of the apartment for the initial 2 weeks. During that time, the owner set about doing a number of things with the cat that would distract it from the dog. New toys were purchased, a 'kitty garden' of sprouting wheat was provided and a chair was moved to a window so the cat could look outside. The owner had daily play sessions with the cat and used food rewards to teach it to come when he whistled. Obedience training was recommended for the dog so that sit–stays could be used to control its behaviour when the cat was present. After 2 weeks, a baby gate was placed in the doorway to the cat's confinement room. This allowed the cat to see the dog and move about in its room without being bothered by the dog. It also allowed the dog to habituate to the cat, so it didn't get excited every time it saw it. After 4 more weeks, the owner held exercises during which the dog would be on a leash responding to sit–stays for its owner, 6 metres (20 feet) away from the door to the cat's room. While standing next to the gate, the cat's owner would whistle and call the cat for a treat. Gradually, the cat was called through the gate into the main room. High resting areas were provided for the cat, so that when it started spending more time in the main room, it could rest in a safe area. As the cat showed less anxiety, hair regrowth was noted. Once the cat started spending an appreciable amount of time in the living areas of the apartment, it was gradually weaned off the amitriptyline.

Feline Hyperaesthesia

Feline hyperaesthesia is a poorly understood condition that has also been referred to as rippling skin syndrome, rolling skin syndrome, twitchy skin syndrome, atypical neurodermatitis, neuritis and feline neurodermatitis. The onset of clinical signs may be spontaneous and intermittent and the manifestations vary considerably between different cats. The normal response of many cats to scratching of the dorsal area can include rippling of the skin, an arched back and varying degrees of vocalisation. In hyperaesthesia, the affected cat may have a more exaggerated response to touching, rubbing or scratching of the back. This behaviour may then become a compulsive disorder as the frequency increases, the response becomes more intense and the signs begin to appear with little or no apparent stimuli. In addition to rolling skin over the dorsum, muscle spasms and vocalisation, the cat may have dilated pupils and may seem to startle, hallucinate and dash away. Some cats will defecate as they run away, leaving stool deposited in a linear pattern. There may also be some displacement grooming or self-directed biting at the flank, tail or back displayed along with the above behaviours.

Diagnosis and Prognosis

The term 'hyperaesthesia' was coined because these cats are extremely sensitive to touch along the back, especially the dorsal lumbar area. Being touched in these areas can result in rippling of the skin, biting or licking of the area, and displacement grooming or licking directed into the air. This behaviour may be a normal response to physical stimulation and arousal in some cats or may be a conflict or displacement behaviour in response to high levels of arousal or anxiety. The problem may also become a compulsive disorder as the frequency and intensity increase, and the stimuli that initiate the behaviour become milder or generalised to out-of-context (non-contact) situations. Medical conditions that might cause or contribute to the problem include any condition that might irritate or cause discomfort of the skin, lumbar or perineal regions. Differential diagnosis of those problems that might cause or contribute to hyperaesthesia include flea bite dermatitis, food allergy, toxins, anal sacculitis, intervertebral disc disease, Feline lower urinary tract disease (FLUTD), trauma, infection and neoplasia. The prognosis is extremely variable from one individual to the next.

Management

At present it is not known whether hyperaesthesia represents a distinct syndrome or the common endpoint of many different conditions. Any medical problems that cause or contribute to pain, discomfort or irritation must be diagnosed and treated. Behavioural management requires the identification and control of those stimuli that lead to the behaviour. Avoiding or minimising these stimuli or desensitising and counterconditioning techniques so that the cat learns to 'tolerate' these stimuli, may be successful at reducing the cat's level of arousal. Hyperaesthesia may also represent a form of epilepsy. This can be

DRUG THERAPY FOR FELINE HYPERAESTHESIA SYNDROME		
Drug	**Dosage**	**Comments**
Amitriptyline	5–10 mg/cat/day	May take up to 2 weeks to see effect.
Clomipramine	0.5–1.5 mg/kg	May take up to 2 weeks to see effect.
Phenobarbital	2–3 mg/kg PO sid–bid or as needed	(See Chapter 4.)
Diazepam	1–3 mg bid	(See Chapter 4.)
Prednisone	1–2 mg/kg per day for 5 days then alternate days (concurrent flea treatment if needed)	
Buspirone	0.5–1.0 mg/kg sid-tid	Anxiolytic with wide margin of safety
Fluoxetine	0.5–1.0 mg/kg q24h	SSRI
Megoestrol acetate	0.5–10 mg/cat sid for 2 weeks, the ½ dose q2wks	Numerous potential risks. (See Chapter 4 for details.)

Fig. 12.5 Drug treatment for feline hyperaesthesia syndrome.

partially validated by the response to antiepileptic therapy although these drugs may also serve to reduce the cat's level of arousal. Treatment with cortico-steroids and progestins may also be occasionally successful (Fig. 12.5).

Prevention

Until more is known about feline hypaeresthesia, it is unlikely that we can effectively prevent the condition, except to avoid or desensitise the cat to those stimuli that cause arousal.

Case Example

Rip was a 3-year-old neutered male Burmese cross that the owners claimed had always been sensitive about being stroked or groomed along his hind end. From the time he was obtained at 4 months of age, any time Rip was petted or brushed over his dorsal lumbar region, his skin would ripple, he would vocalise, and within a minute or two he would run away and begin to groom himself. However, over the past few months, any time the owners would attempt any grooming or physical contact distal to his shoulders, Rip would immediately howl, his skin would ripple, his pupils would dilate, and he would run away and begin to lick around the perineal region. This behaviour also was observed a few times each week when there was no approach or contact by the owners.

On examination, Rip was physically restrained by being wrapped in a large blanket. With his head covered he allowed visual examination of the skin but as soon as his lumbar region was touched, he howled, the skin rippled and he made frantic attempts to escape. There were no physical abnormalities noted except for a small amount of hair loss in the perineal region. A basic blood profile was drawn and revealed no abnormalities. Rip was then admitted for examina-tion under anaesthesia. No fleas or flea dirt were noted and there were no physical abnormalities except for moderately enlarged and impacted anal sacs, which were thoroughly flushed. Rip was sent home with 2 weeks of a trimethoprim–sulphoamide combi-nation, but there was no apparent improvement in signs. It was suspected that Rip had always had a mild displacement behaviour but the pain and irritability associated with the anal sacculitis had aggravated the condition and he had now developed a conditioned response with both medical and behavioural compo-

nents. Rip was placed on 2 mg diazepam twice daily, and the owners were given a desensitisation and counterconditioning programme which incorporated hand-feeding of all food and treats, and increasing levels of contact during these feeding times. At first, contact was limited to touching the back just distal to the shoulder region but in time the owner moved farther back and increased to a slightly stronger level of petting. After 2 weeks the diazepam dose was decreased to 1 mg twice daily and the owner was gently stroking the hind end successfully (with mild skin rippling and vocalisation). However, when the diazepam dose was further reduced the vocalisation and rippling dramatically increased. The cat was re-admitted for examination and although the anal sacs were only minimally distended, they were removed prophylactically. The cat was subsequently main-tained on 1 mg of diazepam twice daily. Whether the diazepam helped to reduce the cat's level of arousal and sensitivity to touch or whether there was a neurological component to the problem was never determined.

Flank-Sucking

Flank-sucking represents a poorly understood con-dition in which a dog nurses a patch of skin on its flank. The dog will hold a section of flank skin in its mouth and hold the position, resulting in changes as simple as a dampened, ruffled haircoat to more severe changes including raw, open sores. The Doberman Pinscher is the breed most commonly affected and the trait has been followed through certain bloodlines, suggesting a hereditary component. The cause has not been determined but the problem may occur more frequently when the dog is under stress. In time the condition often becomes compulsive (to a point where some dogs perform the behaviour whenever they are sleeping or engaged in some other activity). Psycho-motor epilepsy is another possible underlying cause.

Diagnosis and Prognosis

Flank-sucking is an exclusion diagnosis so a thorough medical evaluation is warranted before this label is applied. A minimum database should include multiple skin scrapings, fungal culture, faecal evalu-ation and impression cytology. Biopsies of affected areas and radiographic studies are extremely helpful

MANAGEMENT OF FLANK-SUCKING IN DOGS	
Approach	**Comments**
Reduce stress	Remove underlying stressful situations that may lead to the behaviour. Providing mental stimulation (training, activities) and exercise may also help
Avoid reinforcing	Owner attention during the behaviour (consoling or scolding) may contribute to an increased frequency of the behaviour
Deny access	Use an Elizabethan collar or similar device so that the dog cannot access the area and cause further damage
Aversion therapy	Apply bitter-tasting medicaments to the area so that taste aversion deters the dog from licking at the site
Provide alternatives	Food-laden toys, alternative devices or objects for chewing, and activities (find the food), must be offered, especially if aversion therapy or denying access is being used. (*See canine destructive chewing and separation anxiety in Chapter 7.*)
Behavioural modification	Use counterconditioning so that the dog has to respond in a manner that does not allow it to lick
Drug therapy	Progestin therapy has been advocated in the past but newer drugs such as the tricyclic antidepressants (clomipramine) and fluoxetine are likely to be more useful in compulsive disorders and may actually be more effective (*see acral lick dermatitis*). If anxiety is a component of the arousal, antianxiety drugs may also be effective. In addition, if flank-sucking is actually a manifestation of psychomotor epilepsy, phenobarbital may very well be effective. Studies have been lacking to date

FIG. 12.6 The management of canine flank-sucking

at eliminating the possibility of other contributing medical causes. Flank-sucking becomes the operative diagnosis when no physiological reasons can be found for the behaviour.

Management

Too few reports of cases of flank-sucking have been published to be able to make generalisations about treatment. In many cases the sucking does not cause significant lesions or damage and does not interfere with the apparent health or behavioural welfare of the pet. In these cases, the flank-sucking, although compulsive, may be an acceptable 'coping' mechanism. When the behaviour does cause physical damage or becomes so compulsive as to contribute to other behaviour problems (decreased eating, poorly responsive or aggressive towards owners when approached during sucking) then treatment is necessary (Fig. 12.6). In these cases behavioural modification and medical intervention may be useful.

Prevention

Until more is known about the causes of flank-sucking, prevention remains an elusive goal. Since the condition is most commonly reported in Doberman Pinschers, affected dogs should not be used in breeding programmes.

Case Example

Bart, a 2-year-old intact male Doberman Pinscher, was presented for sucking on the skin in the flank area. The problem had started 6 months previously and occurred most frequently in the early evening. The owner was concerned that some local discomfort was causing the behaviour and would gently talk to the pet as she inspected the skin in the area that was being sucked. Differential diagnoses included flank-sucking, demodicosis, dermatophytosis and foreign body reaction (including injection site granuloma). Skin scrapings and fungal culture were both negative, although a contaminant growth of *Alternaria* was found on the dermatophyte test medium. Foreign body reaction could not be eliminated from our considerations without a biopsy, which the owner was reluctant to permit. It was decided that the problem would be pursued on a behavioural basis and that further diagnostic work would be done if this failed to resolve the situation

Bart was fitted with an Elizabethan collar to prevent sucking when the owner was not able to observe and correct it. Each time she had to leave the dog alone, he was provided with a dental rope toy coated with a small amount of peanut butter, and rubber toy with a piece of meat tucked inside. The owner started a vigorous exercise programme with the dog just prior to the time at which the sucking usually occurred. She was told not to say anything to Bart when she noticed him sucking. Whenever the dog started sucking, the owner was instructed to blow a whistle to distract him, wait 10 seconds or longer (but before the sucking resumed) and then play with him, review obedience or take him for a long walk.

Bart improved markedly but the owner reported that whenever she was lax in the exercise programme, the problem started to recur. Given the options of additional testing and drug therapies, she elected to perservere and see that Bart received the exercise he apparently needed.

Tail Chasing

Compulsive tail chasing is not an uncommon behaviour in dogs, the cause of which is unknown. It has variably been described as a subepileptic episodic behaviour, a neuropathological disorder, a psychosis, an opioid-mediated compulsive disorder and a displacement behaviour. It has also been reported subsequent to physical trauma, surgery or medical illness. Some cases such as those seen in Bull Terriers may exhibit a more intense spinning or whirling behaviour which may be refractory to behaviour modification techniques. Other concurrent behaviour problems, such as aggression, have been reported in 'spinning' Bull Terriers. In some cases, the problem may have started as play behaviour that was conditioned by the owner.

Diagnosis and Prognosis

The diagnosis is based on the findings of a dog with tail chasing behaviour and no evidence of a medical problem. The minimum database should consist of a complete blood count, biochemical profile, urinalysis, faecal evaluation and, when possible, an electroencephalogram (EEG). The tail should be carefully evaluated for any evidence of foreign body penetration, trauma or inflammation. Any deviations to the tail or pain on palpation are good reasons to consider radiographic studies. The prognosis is good for those behaviours that have been reinforced and conditioned but will otherwise be guarded to poor, unless an effective drug can be found to resolve the condition.

Management

Management of this problem must be based on treatment of the potential causes and contributing factors to the problem. Tail chasing behaviour that has been inadvertently reinforced can be treated by removing all attention and rewards when the behaviour begins. Interrupting the behaviour with distraction, aversive devices, or a halter and leash might also be successful. Identifying those stimuli that initiate the behaviour and either avoiding these stimuli or desensitising and counterconditioning the dog to these stimuli might also be effective (*See treatment for acral lick dermatitis for more details*). When the behaviour cannot be interrupted, when the behaviour occurs independent of specific stimuli, or when the specific stimuli cannot be avoided or controlled through desensitisation and counterconditioning, drug therapy is likely to be required (Fig. 12.7). If the condition is responsive to narcotic antagonists (e.g. naltrexone), then endogenous opioid release is likely to be at least one of the mechanisms involved. Since narcotic antagonists are inconvenient to administer long term, and also expensive, combinations of pentazocine and naloxone may be used instead. It is

DRUG TREATMENT FOR TAIL CHASING		
Drug	**Dosage**	**Comments**
Clomipramine	1–3 mg/kg bid	*See Chapter 4*
Doxepin	5–10 mg/kg bid	*See Chapter 4*
Carbamazepine	4–10 mg/kg divided tid	*See Chapter 4*
Amitriptyline	1–4 mg/kg PO sid – bid	*See Chapter 4*
Phenobarbital	2–3 mg/kg PO bid or as needed	*See Chapter 4*
Fluoxetine	0.5–1.0 mg/kg sid	*See Chapter 4*
Naltrexone	2.2 mg/kg PO sid	*See Chapter 4*
Naloxone	11–22 μg/kg Sc/IM/IV	*See Chapter 4*
Pentazocine plus naloxone	50 mg pentazocine + 0.5 mg naloxone bid	*See Chapter 4*

FIG. 12.7 Drug treatment for tail chasing.

also possible that narcotic therapy (hydrocodone) may be useful in these cases. Subepileptic conditions may respond to phenobarbital or potassium bromide therapy. Compulsive disorders may be responsive to treatment with clomipramine, fluoxetine, amitriptyline, or doxepin, combined with behavioural modification techniques.

Tail amputation rarely results in resolution of the problem. For most of the idiopathic cases, it seems that any of the treatment regimens will result in success in some cases and failure in others. Each case must be evaluated and treated individually.

Prevention

Until the cause of compulsive tail chasing is better understood, there are no clear-cut ways of preventing it. Owners must be advised as to how attention and rewards contribute to behaviour problems, so that these factors can be prevented. Appropriate selection and use of distraction and agents to interrupt the problem might also be successful. Since there seems to be some breed predilection, at least for Bull Terriers, there may be a genetic component to the problem. Thus, affected dogs and their siblings should not be used in breeding programmes.

Case Example

Rocky was a 3-year-old male neutered Lhasa Apso who barked incessantly and chased his tail whenever the owner entered the home. The problem began about one year ago during a time when Rocky had a lapse in housetraining and for several weeks in a row, the owner frequently punished Rocky upon arriving home and finding a mess in the house. The pet would start to approach the owner, then, back away and run in circles while barking. The owners admitted that at the start they had found the tail chasing 'funny' and 'cute' and had encouraged the behaviour. When the behaviour became incessant, the owner then attempted to calm Rocky down by patting or lifting him, but recently had resorted to stopping the behaviour by feeding Rocky as soon as the behaviour started.

The barking and tail chasing initially developed as a result of anxiety. The pet was caught in an approach-avoidance conflict, wanting to greet the owner, but fearful of being punished. The owners' attention rewarded the behaviour and it became a conditioned response. A reinforcement of basic obedience com-

mands and a session at obedience school was recommended to gain more control over Rocky. Interruption of the behaviour with a startle device was suggested and, provided the dog responded by stopping his barking and circling, the owner could reward Rocky with a favourite treat such as a piece of freeze-dried liver. In the interim the owners were advised to ignore Rocky completely at homecomings until he calmed down. After a few weeks of success with obedience training the owners began to apply the retraining techniques. At first a shake can was thrown on the floor when they entered but although Rocky was deterred for a few seconds he would not respond to the command and reward cue so that he soon habituated to the shake can. The owners were therefore advised to try entering the home through their side door (which would provide a slightly different set of cues), and Rocky was fitted with a citronella spray anti-bark collar. As soon as the owner entered and barking began, the citronella collar was activated and Rocky would shake his head and retreat. Although the collar did not have any direct effect on the circling, it effectively interrupted both behaviours. The owner would then call Rocky to come and sit and provide the food reward, and the conditioned circling and barking behaviours were permanently subdued. The owners decided to leave the citronella collar on whenever they were out, and were aware that all barking was eliminated (the type that disturbed the neighbours as well as the territorial barking) while Rocky was wearing the collar.

Miscellaneous Compulsive and Stereotypic Disorders

There are a number of additional problems that have been described in dogs and cats that might arise in situations of conflict, anxiety or stress. These behaviours may then become more frequent or repetitive and be initiated by numerous other stimuli, which were not associated with the original conflict or displacement behaviour.

In dogs these might include pacing, circling, digging, phantom chewing, incessant or rhythmic barking, fly snapping or chasing unseen objects, freezing and staring, polydypsia, sucking, licking, or chewing on objects (or owners), and other forms of self-mutilation. In cats, excessive sucking and chewing, hunting and pouncing at unseen prey, running and

MANAGEMENT OF MISCELLANEOUS COMPULSIVE DISORDERS

Approach	Comments
Rule out medical problems that may cause or contribute to the problem	Neurological, ophthalmic, otic, hormonal and other medical conditions may be responsible for numerous behaviour changes
Treat medical conditions	Whether the medical problem is causing the problem or whether the behaviour problem has led to a medical condition, these must be treated in order to resolve the problem
Is there a normal explanation for the behaviour?	Digging, pouncing, chasing, swatting or freezing and staring at imaginary objects may be an actual response to a stimulus (underground, in a wall, in the air) that the owner is unable to see, hear or otherwise detect. Exuberant play, digging, and incessant barking may also be normal behaviours that appear abnormal to the owners
Change the owner's response to the behaviour	Some behaviours persist and progress due to the owner's response to the behaviour. Punishment can lead to an increase in anxiety while any attention given to the pet (positive or negative) during the behaviour can act as a reinforcer. All attention and reinforcement must be removed
Are the consequences of the behaviour serious enough to deal with?	Even though a behaviour is unusual or excessive, if it is not detrimental to the pet, the owner or the environment it may be an acceptable 'coping' mechanism, and attempts to change the behaviour may than lead to more dire consequences
Identify the causes of conflict, anxiety and arousal and reduce if possible	Provide more attention, increased exercise, providing distractions in the form of play toys, food treats, activity centres, chew toys or additional pets
Identify stimuli – minimise, modify, reduce or avoid	Identify those stimuli that initiate the behaviour and try to avoid, reduce or change these stimuli
Restrain or prevent pet from performing the undesirable behaviour	Elizabethan collars, bandaging, bark collars, booby-traps or cages might be used to prevent the pet from performing the undesirable behaviour but caution must be taken that these techniques do not aggravate the problem (or cause new problems) by increasing anxiety
Aversion or distraction	Distraction or aversive devices can be used to interrupt or deter the behaviour in the owner's presence. Alarms, water pistols and a harness or halter with a remote leash can be used
Aversive conditioning by remote or booby-trap techniques	For problems that occur in the owner's absence, it may be occasionally possible to deter behaviour through consistent and properly timed application of remote punishment techniques or the use of booby-traps in problem areas (e.g. remote shock, taste deterrents, shock mats)
Desensitise and countercondition	If the stimuli that initiates the behavioural response can be identified, it may be possible to desensitise and countercondition the pet to these stimuli
Drug therapy – medical	Treat medical conditions that might cause or contribute to the problem as well as those conditions that have arisen as a result of the problem. If a possible seizure focus is suspected phenobarbital, carbamazepine or diazepam (cats) therapy might be effective
Drug therapy – antianxiety	Antianxiety agents such as benzodiazepines, buspirone or propranolol might be useful at reducing anxiety and arousal if these are the cause of the problem
Drug therapy – narcotic antagonists	Previously discussed
Drug therapy – narcotics	Previously discussed
Drug therapy – antidepressants	Tricyclic antidepressants and fluoxetine alone or in combination with other agents (*See chapter 4 for details*)
Drugs – miscellaneous agents	A variety of other drugs have been used in human medicine or infrequently in veterinary medicine and should be reserved for specific applications or refractory cases, either alone, or in combination with some of the other drugs mentioned above (*see Chapter 4 for details*). Examples are clozapine, haloperidol, thoridiazine, pimozide and lithium

Fig. 12.8 Steps in the management of miscellaneous compulsive disorders.

chasing, paw shaking, freezing, excessive vocalisation and self-directed aggression such as tail chasing or foot chewing, may all be manifestations of displacement or compulsive disorders.

In each case it is essential to diagnose, rule out or treat any medical condition that might contribute to the problem. In addition, medical problems might arise as a result of the chewing, digging, or licking and these have to be treated as part of the therapy (as in acral lick dermatitis, tail chewing or gum chewing). If the problem persists after all medical problems are diagnosed, treated or ruled out, behavioural modification, environmental manipulation and drug therapy may also be indicated (Fig. 12.8).

Further Reading

Ackerman, L. (1989) *Practical Canine Dermatology*, 3rd Edition. American Veterinary Publications: Goleta, CA.

Ackerman, L. (1989) *Practical Feline Dermatology*, 2nd Edition. American Veterinary Publications: Goleta, CA.

Beaver, B. V. (1989) Disorders of behaviour. In: *The Cat: Diseases and Clinical Management*, pp. 163–184. Sherding, RG (ed.) Churchill Livingstone: New York.

Blackshaw, J. K. Sutton, R. H. and Boyhan, M. A. (1994) Tail chasing or circling behaviour in dogs. *Canine Practice*, **19**(3), 7–11.

Brignac, M. M. Hydrocodone treatment of acral lick dermatitis. *Proceedings of the 2nd Annual World Congress of Veterinary Dermatology, Montreal, 1992.*

Brown, S. A., Crowell-Davis, S., Malcolm, T. and Edwards, P. (1987) Naloxone-responsive compulsive tail chasing in a dog. *Journal of the American Veterinary Medical Association*, **190**(7), 884–886.

Dodman, N. H., Bronson, R. and Gliatto, J. (1993) Tail chasing in a bull terrier. *Journal of the American Veterinary Medical Association* **202**(5), 758–760.

Dodman, N. H., Shuster, L., White, S. D. *et al.* (1988) Use of narcotic antagonists to modify stereotypic self-licking, self-chewing, and scratching behaviour in dogs. *Journal of the American Veterinary Medical Association*, **193**(7), 815–819.

Eckstein, R. A. and Hart, B. L. (1996) Treatment of acral lick dermatitis by behavior modification using electronic stimulation. *J Am Anim Hosp Assoc*, **32**, 225–230.

Fox, M. W. (1965) Environmental factors influencing stereotyped and allelomimetic behaviour in animals. *Laboratory Animal Care*, **15**, 66–67.

Goldberger, E. and Rapoport, J. L. (1991) Canine acral lick dermatitis: response to the anti-obsessional drug clomipramine. *Journal of the American Animal Hospital Association*, **27**, 179–182.

Hart, B. L. (1976) The role of grooming activity. *Feline Practice*, **6**, 14.

Hawkins, J. (1992) Gum-chewer syndrome: self-inflicted sublingual and self-inflicted buccal trauma. *Compendium for Continuing Education for Practicing Veterinarians*, **14**(2), 219–222.

Hewson, C. J. and Luescher, U. A. (1996) Compulsive disorders in dogs. In: *Readings in Companion Animal Behavior* Voith, V. L. and Borchelt, P. L. (eds) pp. 153–158. Veterinary Learning Systems: Trenton, NJ.

Luescher, U. A., McKeown, D. B. and Halip, J. (1991) Stereotypic or obsessive–compulsive disorders in dogs and cats. *Veterinary Clinics of North America, Small Animal Practice*, **65**(2), 401–413.

Manteca, X. (1994) Fly snapping syndrome in dogs. *Veterinary Quarterly*, **16**(Suppl. 1), S49.

Mason, J. D. (1991) Stereotypies: a critical review. *Animal Behaviour*, **41**, 1015–1037.

McKeown, D., Luescher, A. and Machum, M. (1988) Coprophagia: food for thought. *Canadian Veterinary Journal*, **29**(10), 849–850.

McKeown, D. B., Luescher, U. A. and Halip J. Stereotypies in companion animals and obsessive compulsive disorder. In: *Behavioural Problems in Small Animals*, pp. 30–35. Ralston Purina Company.

Nesbitt, G. H. and Ackerman, L. J. (1991) *Dermatology for the Small Animal Practitioner*. Veterinary Learning Systems: Trenton, NJ.

Overall, K. L. (1992) Recognition, diagnosis, and management of obsessive–compulsive disorders. *Canine Practice*, **17**(2), 40–41; **17**(3), 25–27; **17**(4), 39–43.

Overall, K. L. (1994) Use of clomipramine to treat ritualistic stereotypic motor behaviour in three dogs. *Journal of the American Veterinary Medical Association*, **205**(12), 1733–1741.

Rivers, B., Walter, P. A. and McKeever, P. J. (1993) Treatment of canine acral lick dermatitis with radiation therapy: 17 cases (1979–1991). *Journal of the American Animal Hospital Association*, **29**, 541–546.

Schwartz, S. (1993) Naltrexone-induced pruritus in a dog with tail-chasing behaviour. *Journal of the American Veterinary Medical Association*, **202**(2), 278–280.

Shell, L. G. (1994) Feline hyperesthesia syndrome. *Feline Practice*, **6**, 10.

Stein, D. J. and Hollander, E. (1992) Dermatology and conditions related to obsessive–compulsive disorder. *Journal of the American Academy of Dermatology*, **26**, 237–242.

Tuttle, J. (1980) Feline hyperesthesia syndrome. *Journal of the American Veterinary Medical Association*, **176**, 47.

Tuttle, J. L. and Parker, A. J. (1980) Diagnosing, treating feline hyperesthesia syndrome. *D. V. M.*, **11**, 72.

Voith, V. L. and Marder, A. R. (1988) Feline behavioural disorders. In: *Handbook of Small Animal Practice*. Morgan, R. (ed.) pp. 1045–1051. Churchill Livingstone: New York.

Walton, D. K. (1986) Psychodermatoses. In: *Current Veterinary Therapy. IX. Small Animal Practice*, Kirk R. W. (ed). WB Saunders: Philadelphia, PA.

Willemse, T. and Spruijt, B. M. (1995) Preliminary evidence for dopaminergic involvement in stress-induced excessive grooming in cats. *Neuroscience Research Communications*, **17**(3), 203–208.

Young, M. S. and Manning, T. O. (1984) Psychogenic dermatoses. *Dermatological Reports*, **3**, 1.

13

Behaviour Problems in Geriatric Pets

Distribution of Behaviour Cases

Studies of canine cases at behaviour referral practices indicate that aggression is the primary reason for referral, followed by housesoiling, destructiveness, excitability, phobias, separation anxiety, vocalisation and submission (Fig. 13.1). Approximately 6% of referred cases in those studies were over the age of 9 years. Although aggression cases were not uncommon in older dogs, there was a relative increase in cases referred for phobias and separation anxiety (including vocalisation, destructiveness and housesoiling).

In cats, the most common reasons for referral are inappropriate elimination (including spraying), followed by aggression, destructiveness, overactivity, vocalisation, fears and ingestive behaviours. In one study of 130 cats (unpublished data, G. M. Landsberg), 15% of all referred cases were over the age of 9. Inappropriate elimination was the most common reason for referral, followed by aggression, hyper-

activity, excessive vocalisation and destructive scratching.

It is important to note that the number of cases seen in older pets is relatively small. In dogs, only 62 of 1094 referred cases, or approximately 6% of all referred cases, were over the age of 9 years (Fig. 13.1). In contrast, it has been estimated that in North America 13.9% of all dogs are over the age of 11. In cats, approximately 11% of 420 cases were over the age of 9 years, while approximately 11% of all cats are over 11. The relatively small numbers of behaviour cases in older dogs may reflect the decrease in aggressive cases (particularly dominance aggression), while in cats, inappropriate elimination still represents the primary reason for referral.

Since behaviour problems are due to genetic influences, combined with the effects of training, environment and early socialisation, it is not surprising that most canine behaviour problems emerge within the first few years. By the time pets are behaviourally mature (2 to 3 years of age), it is likely

CANINE BEHAVIOUR CASES IN DIFFERENT AGE GROUPS				
Age at referral:	Under 9 years (Landsberg, 1991)	Over 9 years (Landsberg, 1991)	Over 9 years Additional cases*	Over 9 Years All cases
Total cases:	421	28	34	62
Aggression (people)	225 (53%)	11 (39%)	6 (23%)	17 (27%)
(intraspecies)	30 (7%)	2 (7%)	1 (3%)	3 (5%)
Housesoiling	78 (19%)	3 (11%)	11 (32%)	14 (23%)
Destructive	59 (14%)	5 (18%)	13 (38%)	18 (29%)
Excitable/unruly	29 (7%)	0	0	0
Phobias	23 (5%)	4 (14%)	6 (23%)	10 (16%)
Separation anxiety	22 (5%)	2 (7%)	16 (47%)	18 (29%)
Vocalisation	22 (5%)	4 (14%)	9 (26%)	13 (21%)
Submission	11 (3%)	0	0	0
Compulsive/stereotypic	8 (2%)	1 (4%)	2 (6%)	3 (5%)
Waking/restless	0	3 (11%)	2 (6%)	5 (8%)

* Additional cases include those at the Veterinary Hospital of the University of Pennsylrania 1984–1987, and those in Toronto between 1992 and 1994

Fig. 13.1 Distribution of behaviour cases by age (from Landsberg, 1995). Some cases were referred for more than one problem.

that most owners would have recognised and dealt with significant problems by treating, resolving, or learning to live with the problem, or have removed the pet from the home. Problems that emerge at an older age can also be due to environmental changes, but when there has been little or no change in the pet's environment, age-related medical conditions and cognitive decline should be strongly considered.

Aggression toward People

Canine dominance aggression is most commonly exhibited by 2 to 3 years of age so that a decrease in dominance aggression referrals (the most common reason for canine aggression referrals overall) is to be expected. Therefore, it is somewhat surprising that a considerable number of dominance aggression cases are still seen in older dogs. A number of these dogs showed possessive aspects of aggression, so that if the problem is newly emerging and there is no recognisable change in the household, medical conditions affecting appetite, mobility, cognition, sensory function, or hormonal status, and conditions leading to increased pain or irritability might contribute to an increase in aggression. A number of aggressive cases in older dogs were referred because of fear or anxiety associated with a toddler or new baby in the household.

Intraspecies Aggression

Introduction of a new dog or cat, changes in the household, and physical or behavioural changes associated with the ageing pet may lead to intraspecies aggression. Changes such as sensory dysfunction, decreased mobility, increased pain and irritability, and cognitive decline may affect the manner in which the pet interacts with its conspecifics. In dogs, the younger dog may begin to challenge the dominant older dog as it becomes unable to maintain its dominant position. Owners may then make the situation worse by supporting or coming to the aid of the older dog, and reprimanding the younger dog, rather than allowing the new hierarchy to develop.

Excessive Vocalisation

Elderly pets may be particularly susceptible to stress, so that either environmental changes or medical problems that lead to increased anxiety can

trigger a variety of behaviour problems such as destructiveness, distress vocalisation, housesoiling and compulsive disorders. Some of the cases of excessive vocalisation in older dogs are a component of separation anxiety, while others are related to an increase in night-time restlessness and vocalization. Sensory dysfunction (particularly auditory dysfunction), age-related cognitive dysfunction, CNS pathology, and age-related medical conditions may contribute to increased vocalisation in older dogs and cats.

Separation Anxiety

Older dogs may be more resistant than younger dogs to changes in their schedule or their household. Sensory deficits can lead to numerous behaviour changes and may affect the pet's level of anxiety, particularly when left alone. Noise-related phobias may also contribute to departure anxiety.

Housesoiling

In older dogs, some of the housesoiling problems are due to separation anxiety. Elimination during the owner's absence, followed by owner punishment on arrival home would further aggravate the dog's anxiety. Any change to a dog or cat's environment or schedule may also contribute to housesoiling or marking behaviours. Medical conditions that increase the frequency of elimination or cause a decrease in control may also be contributing factors. Sensory dysfunction, conditions that affect mobility, age-related cognitive decline, and some forms of neurological pathology may also lead to housesoiling.

Destructive Behaviour

Most cases of canine destructiveness are seen as a component of separation anxiety.

Restlessness/Waking at Nights

Dogs and cats that are restless or do not sleep through the night should be closely evaluated for medical problems that might lead to an increased frequency of elimination, restlessness, or discomfort. Sensory changes can affect the pet's depth of sleep. With age there may also be altered sleep–wake cycles and decreased REM sleep.

Noise Phobias

A number of medical and age-related conditions might cause or contribute to canine noise phobias such as sensory dysfunction, medical conditions leading to increased irritability and restlessness, cognitive dysfunction and other ageing or pathological effects on the brain or its neurotransmitters. In time these very same changes (e.g. marked loss of hearing or sight) might help to ameliorate these problems. The locus ceruleus and its neurotransmitter noradrenaline are vital in the genesis of fear and panic (Schull, 1991), so that age-related changes that affect the limbic system, the locus ceruleus and its noradrenaline levels can either ameliorate or aggravate fearful and phobic responses. Another consideration is that some loud noises are extremely intermittent (e.g. thunder and fireworks) so that there may be a lengthy learning component to the behaviour. In other words, over the years the owners intermittently give attention to the fearful pet and reward the fearful behaviour so that the problem is gradually accentuated.

Submissive and Overly Excitable Behaviours

Since these behaviours would generally develop at a much younger age, it is likely that owners would have corrected or learned to live with them (or given up the pet) well before the pet reached 9 years old.

Compulsive and Stereotypic Behaviours

Compulsive and stereotypic behaviours encompass a wide spectrum of behaviours with numerous causative factors. Although there is often a genetic component to these problems, conflict, stress, or anxiety-producing stimuli or situations are required to trigger the problems. It may take varying lengths of time and multiple exposures to the stimuli for the behaviours to become compulsive. Medical conditions, pathology of the CNS, and changes in neurotransmitters may further contribute to the problem in the ageing pet.

Diagnostic Considerations

Even though a behaviour case may be presented to the veterinarian at an older age, the age of onset of the problem may be much earlier. In some cases, perhaps due to changes in intensity or frequency of the problem, or changes in the household that preclude living with the problem any longer, the behaviour problem may have begun at a relatively young age. Therefore, a critical part of history-taking is to determine the age at which the problem began to emerge and, if it is of long standing, why the owners have waited until this time to seek assistance.

Clinical History

History-taking is one of the most important aspects of behaviour problem diagnostics. In older pets with a problem of recent onset, the behavioural and medical history beginning just before and at the time of onset is often the key to separating a primary behaviour problem from those associated with medical conditions.

● Search for situations/changes that might indicate a behavioural cause associated with environmental changes around the time of onset of the problem.
● Search for situations/responses that might be maintaining or reinforcing the problem.
● Identify potential genetic and medical conditions associated with the age of onset of the problem.
● Identify any changes in elimination, behaviour, appetite, mobility, etc. that might be associated with potential medical causes.

Physical Examination

Although a standard physical examination is required for every behaviour case, neurological examination and sensory evaluation may also be necessary in the older pet. This is of particular importance when the pet was previously well behaved and there is no clearly identifiable environmental cause of the problem. For each behaviour problem, it is essential to determine which body systems might be affected so that, where indicated, a more in-depth assessment can be carried out.

Laboratory/Radiographic Assessment

A purely behavioural diagnosis can only be made after ruling out all possible medical factors.

- Identify the problem (i.e. owner complaint, clinical signs) and determine potential medical problems that could cause or contribute to the problem.
- Run appropriate diagnostic tests for those medical problems considered.
- The minimum tests for an older pet with behaviour problems, would included a basic biochemical profile, complete blood count, and urinalysis. These tests are also essential if drug therapy is to be considered. Specific tests might also be required depending on the clinical signs and behaviour problem (e.g. faecal, endocrine assessment, water intake, radiography, additional blood testing, or specialised tests such as endoscopy, ECG, ultrasonography, CSF evaluation, or even CT or MRI scans).

Effects of Age on Behaviour

Ageing can have an effect on virtually every body system, which may in turn have a direct or indirect affect on the behaviour of a pet (Fig. 13.2). Ageing changes are generally progressive and irreversible. Disease, stress, nutrition, exercise, genetics and environment all play a role in the ageing process. Older animals seldom have disease or dysfunction of a single organ system. Rather, it is the combined or interactive effect of multiple organ disease that affects the overall health and behaviour of the geriatric pet.

Cognitive Dysfunction and Senile Dementia in Dogs

It is generally believed that, as in people, a dog's cognitive ability tends to decline with age. The diagnosis of cognitive dysfunction generally requires the presence of one or more of the following behavioural changes in the absence of any physical causes: decreased reaction to stimuli, confusion, disorientation, incontinence, decreased interaction with the owners, increased irritability, slowness in obeying commands, alterations in sleep–wake cycle, decreased responsiveness to sensory input, and problems performing previously learned behaviours such as housetraining. Should these changes advance to a point where the dog is no longer able to function as a pet, the condition may be consistent with senile dementia. Senility in dogs is often associated with some of the same neuropathological lesions and changes in neurotransmitters seen in people with Alzheimer's disease and dementia. One of these changes is a decrease in dopamine levels due to an increase in monoamine oxidase B (MAO B) activity. The drug L-deprenyl, a selective MAO B inhibitor, may therefore, be of use in ameliorating or slowing the onset of some of the signs of age-related cognitive dysfunction. An initial clinical trial was conducted in which elderly dogs, with signs of behavioural or cognitive problems, were placed on L-deprenyl (provided there was no concurrent neurological or systemic disease). Some improvement was seen in dogs that showed disinterest in food, housesoiling, decreased ability to recognise commands, places, people or other animals, weakness, stiffness or difficulty navigating stairs, disruption of the sleep–wake cycle, stereotypic behaviours, and tremors or shaking. (Available in U.S. and Canada as Anipryl.)

Another drug that might be considered is nicergoline (available in the UK as Fitergol®, Rhone Merieux). It is an alpha-1 and alpha-2 adrenoceptor antagonist which acts on the vascular system and cells of the brain. The manufacturer claims that it increases cerebral blood flow, increases oxygen supply to the brain, and that it has a neuro-protective action on the neural cells which limits damage caused by chronic hypoxia or anoxic attacks. Drug trials suggest that the drug may help older dogs that have problems such as: loss of activity; sleep disorders; episodes of collapse/fits/'stroke'-like symptoms; loss of house training or incontinence; loss of appetite; and decreasing awareness. Literature from the manufacturer reports a success rate of over 80 per cent in dogs with age-related disorders, a safety margin in excess of 90 times the recommended dose and once-daily administration. No independent studies are currently available.

Management of Behaviour Problems of Geriatric Onset

The guidelines for management are:

- Diagnosis: determine if any underlying pathology exists and treat where possible.

EFFECTS OF AGEING ON BEHAVIOUR

Effects of Ageing	Behavioural Implications
METABOLIC EFFECTS	
Decreased metabolic rate – increased obesity	Decreased activity; obesity may affect locomotion, elimination, and other systems
Decreased immune competence	May affect any organ system
Increase in autoimmune diseases	
Thermoregulation capacity reduced	Decreased tolerance of temperature changes, seeks warmth, avoids cold
Less sensitive to thirst – tissue dehydration	
Decreased ability to metabolise or excrete drugs	Caution with all forms of drug therapy!
Increase in metabolic disorders affecting nervous system: hypothyroid, hypoglycaemia (insulinoma), hepatic disorders, hyperlipidaemia (Schnauzers)	Pacing, seizures, restlessness, decreased mental system – alertness, geriatric-onset behaviour changes
Decrease REM sleep, intermittent sleep	Increased waking, appearance of restlessness
GASTROINTESTINAL SYSTEM	
Increase in dental disease; can increase incidence of disease of other internal organs	Pain, increased irritability, aggression?
Decreased nutrient absorption	Nutritional effects on behaviour? Changes in stool consistency leading to housesoiling?
Decreased colonic motility	Constipation – stool housesoiling
Liver function decreases	Hepatic encephalopathy and associated behaviour
RESPIRATORY SYSTEM	
Decreased respiratory capacity, reduced efficiency	Hypoxaemia: nocturnal confusion?, signs of senility?
Decreased oxygen at the cellular level	Decreased ability to do work
URINARY SYSTEM	
Decreased renal function – decreased blood flow	Polyuria–decreased control. Housesoiling
	Behaviour changes associated with uraemia
Anaemia due to erythropoietin decrease and uraemia – hypertension	CNS hypoxia? – confusion – restlessness
Prostatic hypertrophy	Pollakiuria/incontinence
Incontinence due to urethral incompetence, urinary tract infections and conditions leading to polyuria/polydypsia	Housesoiling due to decreased control or incontinence
ENDOCRINE SYSTEM	
Decreased hormone production by thyroid, testis, ovary, and pituitary – may also be overproduction due to functional tumours (*see below*)	Decreased activity level – increased irritability or aggression
	Decreased tolerance to cold
Testicular tumours (60% of older dogs): Sertoli cell – oestrogen increase/androgen decrease Interstitial cell tumours – increased androgens Prostatic hypertrophy	Medical/behavioural effects of increased oestrogens Medical/behavioural effects of testosterone increase Pollakiuria/Incontinence
Dysregulation of hypothalamic–pituitary–adrenal axis	Polyuria/polydypsia/panting/polyphagia/increased restlessness/housesoiling?
MUSCULOSKELETAL SYSTEM	
Loss of bone and muscle mass	Weakness – decreased mobility – housesoiling?
Neuromuscular function deteriorates	Decreased mobility/activity – incontinence – housesoiling?
Cartilage degenerates/arthritis	Increased pain/irritability

Fig 13.2 – continued

EFFECTS OF AGEING ON BEHAVIOUR	
Effects of Ageing	**Behavioural implications**
CARDIOVASCULAR SYSTEM AND BLOOD	
Heart disease in 33% of dogs over 13 years old	Decreased exercise tolerance
Tissue and cellular anoxia leading to dysfunction or deterioration of other organs	Brain hypoxia leading to signs of senility?
Propensity toward anaemia	Brain hypoxia – signs of senility?
NERVOUS SYSTEM	
Increasing hypoxia due to anaemia, cardiovascular disease, respiratory deterioration	Senility? – cognitive decline?
	Effects on memory and previous learning
Tumour formation – primary or secondary	Cerebral: abnormal sleep, change in eating, loss of housetraining, aggression, docility, visual deficits, circling, weakness
	Cerebellar: ataxia, tremor, head tilt, circling
	Brainstem: state of consciousness, cranial nerve deficits
Neurotransmitter changes:	
Increase in MAO B – decrease in dopamine	Cognitive dysfunction, tremors?, pituitary-dependent Cushing's syndrome?
Decrease in cholinergic system, decreased serotonin	Depression, sleep, and neuromuscular disorders
Cell numbers decrease: neurons of the locus ceruleus and substantia nigra most affected	Reduced reaction to stimuli
Thickening of meninges	Irritable when disturbed, slow to obey commands, problems with orientation and learned behaviour
Amyloidosis – lipofuschinosis – gliosis – meningial fibrosis – Alzheimer-like and other age-related pathology	Cognitive decline? Senility? – Urinary incontinence, disorientation – alteration of sleep–wake cycles – geriatric-onset behavioural problems
	Decreased performance in recognition/memory
SPECIAL SENSES	
Decreased sight, smell, hearing	Hypersensitive to stimuli with less affected senses (e.g. sensitive to noise if blind)
	Less responsive and alert to stimuli with affected senses
	Increased irritability? – Increased fear? Changes in sleep–wake cycle – aggression – decreased appetite
	Increased vocalisation

Fig. 13.2 The effects of ageing on the body and consequent possible changes in behaviour.

- Determine stimuli that incite or reinforce the problem and remove or modify where applicable.
- Environmental modification may be required to the environment due to changes in the pet's medical health, mobility, and level of cognitive dysfunction (e.g. dog doors, confinement).
- Behaviour modification: rewards, punishment, counterconditioning, desensitisation, flooding. Techniques and applications may have to be modified.
- Drug/medical therapy: although drugs may be needed or indicated for a variety of medical and behavioural problems in older dogs, extra caution

should be taken before administering drugs to older dogs. Drug metabolism, excretion, and level of toxicity may be markedly affected by the dog's medical health.

Housesoiling

In many cases, the older dog will require access to the outdoors more frequently. A decrease in bladder capacity may occur due to obesity, reduced elasticity or prostate enlargement. This can increase the need to void more frequently. Polyuria due to a variety of medical problems seen in older dogs or cats may increase the volume of urine produced and increase the need to void more frequently. If the litterbox is not changed more frequently, the cat may avoid the constantly wet box. The frequency of defecation may increase when the overweight pet is changed to a high-fibre diet. If the owners are unable to change their schedule to accommodate the pet dog's need to go outdoors more frequently, a dog door or paper training may be necessary.

Musculoskeletal problems, such as weakness, muscular atrophy and arthritis, can make it difficult for the dog to get outdoors to eliminate or for the cat to navigate stairs to get to its litterbox. When it is painful for the pet to get up or down stairs to eliminate, it may choose to avoid the discomfort and eliminate in convenient but inappropriate areas. Adjusting the height, size or location of the litterbox may increase a cat's ability or desire to use its litterbox. Medication to control pain, carpet runners on stairs for traction, and control of obesity should help.

Specific behavioural treatment for the house-soiling dog involves accompanying the pet outdoors as often as possible so that elimination in a desired location may be reinforced, consistent supervision/confinement, and a regular feeding schedule. Punishment must be discussed since owners often punish too harshly or too long after the behaviour. A light scolding given only during the misbehaviour is all that is acceptable. Harsh or delayed punishment may make the problem worse. The approach to treatment of feline housesoiling is the same for geriatrics as it is for young adults and has been described in chapter 6. Some older cats will stop using the box due to the mental confusion associated with cognitive dysfunction. The only solution for these pets is to confine them to a small room that can be easily cleaned.

Environmental/Social Stress

The elderly pet is less able to handle stress. Any major, stressful situation has the potential to trigger anorexia, destructive behaviours, excessive vocalisation, housesoiling, displacement behaviours and stereotypical behaviour. Changes in the amount of time the owner spends with the pet or changes in the owner's schedule can be very unsettling. In Chapman and Voith's (1990) study of older dogs referred for behaviour problems, separation anxiety was the most common cause of destructive behaviour and excessive vocalisation. Treatment for separation anxiety has been described and involves changing the way the owner interacts with the pet so that it is not always getting attention on demand, gradually accustoming the pet to absences by the owner and, in some cases, medication. Once the underlying cause has been addressed, it is helpful to reward play with toys when the owner is present and to provide food-laced toys at departure. Taste-aversive sprays can be used on objects around the house to teach the pet to avoid chewing them.

Long trips and boarding should probably be limited or carefully thought out. If major changes in the pet's life are anticipated, some care should be taken gradually to introduce the pet to these. If sudden, major changes are unavoidable and the pet responds very anxiously, medication may be helpful. Tricyclic antidepressants such as amitriptyline or anxiolytics such as clorazepate or buspirone may be effective. Appropriate precautions should be taken based on the physical health of the pet.

Aggression

Emerging medical, physical and neurological problems can contribute to behaviour problems such as aggression. Seldom do these conditions directly cause abnormal or undesirable behaviour. However, they often serve to push the pet beyond a certain threshold so that aggression is exhibited in situations where it did not formerly appear. It is important to rule out underlying painful disease for all aggressive pets. Arthritis and dental disease commonly occur in older pets and should be considered when aggression problems develop. The appearance of an aggression problem can also be associated with the development of sensory deficits. Pets that are fearful of humans usually learn to avoid them by simply moving away. The pet that loses its ability to hear or see someone approaching is more likely to be startled and display defensive or fearful aggression.

Once the owner notices that the pet is losing its hearing, hand signals can be taught by repeatedly associating specific hand movements with obedience commands. Visitors should always be advised about approaching the pet with sensory deficits. In some cases it may be prudent simply to confine the pet to a safe, quiet area when visitors are in the home.

CNS diseases (such as brain tumours), cognitive decline, and the effects of age and disease on the endocrine system and the resultant hormonal changes may also contribute to an increase in aggression. Cerebral vascular disorders are frequently blamed for apparent sudden onset of aggression, but they are relatively rare in dogs and cats. A good medical and behavioural work-up will usually uncover more common aetiologies such as pain-elicited aggression or dominance aggression.

The importance of ruling out or treating medical problems cannot be stressed enough. Failure to treat these will probably prevent successful resolution of the aggression problem. The treatment for fear aggression involves desensitisation and counterconditioning. The owners of dominant dogs need to establish a dominant role for themselves in respect to their pet. This involves obedience training, control of resources, counterconditioning and desensitisation exercises.

Intraspecies Social Problems

As the family dog gets older, two types of social problems with other dogs in the family may occur. These include problems associated with the addition of a puppy to the home and hierarchy problems involving other adult dogs in the home.

Most puppies are full of energy and engage in a considerable amount of assertive play that involves chasing, attacking and biting. If the older dog is strong enough and has had adequate intercanine socialisation, it will usually use threats and inhibited bites to control the puppy. If the adult dog is weak, passive or fearful it may retreat and hide. Some dogs will become exceptionally anxious about having an active young puppy in the home. This may lead to anorexia, housesoiling, excessive vocalising or destructive problems. When the older dog appears to be overwhelmed by the young puppy, the two should be separated whenever the owner is not around to supervise. Before allowing the puppy and older dog to interact, the owner should provide enough exercise or play to fatigue the puppy. This will help ensure desirable interactions. The owner should reward all gentle play. The noise of a squeak toy may help distract the puppy from engaging in play attacks. A long lead on the puppy can be used for control and to apply a light correction. A head halter and lead can be very helpful for control. Occasionally, a timely squirt from a water gun or a toy tossed near the puppy will provide the distraction necessary to stop or prevent rough play.

Sometimes, aggression develops between two adult dogs who have lived together for years when the older, dominant dog becomes weaker and less assertive. The younger dog may challenge the older dog in competitive or social situations. These may include soliciting attention from the owner, greeting visitors, exhibiting territorial displays, and guarding food or toys. The owners may make the situation worse by trying to protect and maintain the older pet's dominant position. Theoretically, the owner should support a dominant role for the younger pet by allowing it to have what it wants, such as receiving treats and attention first from the owner, desired sleeping areas, etc. But, in reality, it is very difficult for most owners to force the older dog to defer to a younger pet who has been a member of the family for a shorter period of time. Another solution is for the owners to reaffirm the family's dominant role in respect to both dogs. Obedience commands should be taught or reviewed. Both dogs should then be taught that the owners have complete control over anything that the pets desire. The owner can do this by requiring a response to a command before either pet receives anything (food, treats, play, a walk outdoors, and, especially, social attention). Whenever the dogs start to approach the owner, a guest, doorway or food bowl, they should both be commanded to stay and, then, released, one at a time. The order in which the pets are released should vary each time. Establishing a strong dominant role for the owners tends to reduce aggressive tension between the pets. In some cases, muzzles or head halters may be necessary for control and for safety.

The main social problem between cats occurs when another cat is introduced into the home. The older cat, especially if it has lived alone for a long period, may be particularly resistant to accepting another member of the same species into the home. An initial separation period, gradual exposure and counterconditioning exercises may help. A quiet kitten (7–9 weeks old) of the opposite sex is most likely to be accepted, although some older cats will not accept another cat into the home, no matter what choice is made or what the owner does to try to facilitate the introduction.

Waking at Night – Excessive Vocalisation

Dogs and cats normally sleep through short cycles day and night, so that even those pets that remain quiet through the night are not necessarily sleeping the entire time. Age-related cognitive decline, sensory decline and a variety of medical conditions (especially those that affect frequency and control of elimination) may contribute to sleep restlessness, increased discomfort, increased vocalisation, and overly demanding behaviours (rather than a decrease in sleep). Endocrine dysfunction, such as hyperadrenocorticism, diabetes mellitus, hypothyroidism and hyperthyroidism, may cause increased night-time restlessness and increased vocalisation for a variety of reasons including polyuria and polydypsia, polyphagia, an increase in panting, or changes in thermoregulatory ability. Diagnosing and treating the underlying medical problem, altering the pet's elimination schedule, providing sufficient daytime and evening exercise and attention periods, and behavioural drug therapy with benzodiazepines, tricyclic antidepressants or L-deprenyl (if cognitive dysfunction is suspected) may be useful.

Cognitive Dysfunction

Problems due to deteriorating mental function, such as difficulty recognising familiar places or people, excessive vocalisation, spatial disorientation, confusion, pacing, changes in the sleep–wake cycle and housesoiling that is refractory to conventional treatment techniques are very frustrating for the owner. In most cases, management is the only way to decrease the impact of these problems, although L-deprenyl and perhaps nicergoline hold some promise, as was mentioned earlier. Treatment for cognitive dysfunction has traditionally been palliative involving changes in management, changing the pet's environment and nursing care.

Preventive measures such as providing a consistent, moderate amount of mental stimulation and exercise for the older pet may help. Owners should review obedience commands and tricks with the pet as well as frequently engaging it in simple games.

Case Examples

Case 1

Tony, an 11-year-old orange male tabby cat, began to spray on the patio doors. Neighbourhood cats often frequented the patio but until recently Tony had exhibited no indoor spraying. A complete behavioural assessment revealed no obvious changes to Tony's household or environment, and there were no obvious changes on physical examination. Before behaviour therapy was instituted, a complete laboratory work-up was performed, including complete blood counts, serum biochemistry, a thyroid profile and urinalysis. Tony's thyroxine (T_4) level was markedly elevated and a diagnosis of hyperthyroidism was confirmed with further imaging studies. Thryoidectomy was performed and Tony's spraying immediately ceased.

Approximately 6 months later Tony began to spray again near the patio door. A cause could not be found. Tony was on thyroxine supplementation but laboratory testing revealed that levels were in the normal range. The owners were able to prevent further spraying by confining Tony away from the patio doors when they were out and installing vertical blinds and supervising him when they were at home.

Case 2

Jody was a 13-year-old, 6 kg, spayed female Beagle cross who had begun to wake the owners every night by pacing and vocalising. Jody traditionally slept on the bedroom floor and when the problem first began the owners attempted to leave Jody outside the bedroom with the door closed. This only led to louder vocalisation as well as digging and scratching at the door. The owners would attempt to put Jody outdoors to eliminate but she merely waited outside the door to be allowed back in.

Medical evaluation, routine laboratory testing and physical examination revealed no significant abnormalities, except for a moderate increase in serum alkaline phosphatase. Further studies were conducted in consideration of a possible diagnosis of hyperadrenocorticism. Results of a low-dose dexamethasone suppression test were equivocal but there was no measurable increase in water intake. A diagnosis of hyperadrenocorticism could not be confirmed at this time. During the daytime there was no apparent increased frequency of elimination and the owners noted no other apparent, although changes except a decreased responsiveness to previously trained commands. The owners also felt there was a decrease in hearing ability although the dog could be successfully distracted with an ultrasonic device.

Although specific causes for the night waking and increased restlessness could not be identified, the decrease in hearing ability and, perhaps, age-related cognitive decline were presumed to play a role in the problem. The owners were instructed to provide additional play, attention, and exercise during the late afternoon and evening, and to attempt to keep Jody awake with play, and chew toys for the few hours prior to bedtime. They were also instructed to review obedience training including extended 'down–stays'. When this was unsuccessful, the owners attempted to move the feeding schedule from morning only to half at 8 a.m. and half at 8 p.m. If Jody did wake at night, the owners were instructed to ignore her or to utilise a 'down–stay' command. If she did not respond, she was to be locked into the basement until she quietened down.

Although every attempt was made to avoid drug therapy, behavioural techniques did not successfully ameliorate the problem. Alprazolam was then dispensed at 0.25 mg to be given each night prior to bedtime (and appropriate drug releases were drawn up and signed). An ultrasonic device was kept under the owner's pillow to deter the behaviour if it recurred. Evening exercise, feeding, chew toys and obedience training were continued. The first few nights Jody slept through the night and on the third night when Jody awoke and approached the bed, the owner used the ultrasonic device to deter the behaviour. Jody backed away and after another attempt (and response to the device) she lay down and returned to sleep. After another week the medication was reduced by 50% and after the second week it was withdrawn completely. The owner reported no recurrences.

References

Chapman, B. L. and Voith, V. L. (1990) Behavioural problems in old dogs: 26 cases (1984–1987). *Journal of the American Veterinary Medical Association*, **196**, 944.

Landsberg, G. M. (1991) The distribution of canine behavior cases at three referral practices. *Veterinary Medicine*, **86** (11), 1011.

Schull, E. (1991) Advances in the understanding and treatment of noise phobia. *Veterinary Clinics of North America, Small Animal Practice*, **21**(2), 353–367.

Further Reading

Beaver, B. (1994) Owner complaints about canine behavior. *Journal of the American Veterinary Medical Association*, **204**, 1953–1955.

Borchelt, P. L. and Voith, V. L. (1986) Elimination behaviour problems in cats. *Compend Contin Educ*, **8**, 197–205.

Chapman, B. L. and Voith, V. L. (1990) Cat aggression redirected to people: 14 Cases (1981–1987). *J Am Vet Med Assoc*, **196**(6), 947–950.

Chapman, B. L. and Voith, V. L. (1990) Behavioral problems in old dogs: 26 cases (1984–1987). *Am Vet Med Assoc*, **196**(6), 944–946.

Chapman, B. L. (1995) Behavioural disorders. In: *Geriatrics and Gerontology of the Dog and Cat*, Goldston, R. T. and Hoskins, J. D. (eds). pp. 51–62, W. B. Saunders Co.: Philadelphia, PA.

Chapman, B. L. (1993) Geriatric behaviour. In: *Animal Behaviour. Proceedings of the T. G. Hungerford Refresher Course, Sydney*, **133**, 133–143. Postgraduate Committee in Vetinary Science, University of Sydney: Sydney.

Fenner, W. R. Neurology of the geriatric patient. *Veterinary Clinics of North American, Small Animal Practice*, **18**(3), 711–724.

Goldston, R. T. Introduction and overview of geriatrics. In: *Geriatrics and Gerontology of the Dog and Cat*, Goldston, R. T. and Hoskins, J. D. (eds). pp. 1–9, W. B. Saunders Co.: Philadelphia, PA.

Hunthausen, W. (1994) Identifying and treating behaviour problems in geriatric dogs. *Veterinary Medicine*, **89**(9), 688–700.

Hunthausen, W. (1995) Housesoiling and the geriatric dog. *Geriatric Medicine*. Supplement to *Vetinary Medicine*, August, 4–15.

Landsberg, G. M. (1995) The most common behavior problems of older dogs. *Veterinary Medicine*, August, Supplement, 18–24.

Milgram, N. W., Ivy, GO., Head, E., Murphy, M. P. *et al.* (1993) The effect of L-deprenyl on behavior, cognitive function and biogenic amines in the dog. *Neurochemical Research*, **18**(12), 1211–1219.

Mosier, J. E. (1989) Effect of aging on body systems of the dog. *Veterinary Clinics of North America, Small Animal Practice*, **19**(1), 1–12.

Neer, T. M. The nervous system. In: *Geriatrics and Gerontology of the Dog and Cat*, Goldston, R. T. and Hoskins, J. D. (eds). pp. 325–346, W. B. Saunders Co.: Philadelphia, PA.

Ruehl, W. W., Bruyette, D. S., DePaoli, A., Cotman, C. W., Head, E., Milgram, N. W. and Cummings, B. L. (1995) Canine cognitive dysfunction as a model for human age-related cognitive decline, dementia and Alzheimer's disease: clinical presentation, cognitive testing, pathology and response to l-deprenyl therapy. In: *Progress in Brain Research*, Yu, P. M., Tipton, K. F. and Boulton, A. A. Vol. 106, pp. 217–225. Elsevier: Netherlands.

Appendix: Drug Dosages

Before using any of the following drugs please refer to chapter 4 for treatment suggestions, contraindications, and potential adverse effects. Where more than 1 dose is listed, it is because a variety of doses have been published, and the lowest effective dose should be utilised. Most of the drugs listed below are not licensed for veterinary use, and few controlled studies have been performed. It is therefore the practitioner's responsibility to know the local regulations regarding off-label dispensing and to have appropriate consent or release forms signed.

The authors have made every effort to ensure the accuracy of the information with regards to drug dosages. However, appropriate information sources should be consulted, especially when new or unfamiliar drugs are first being utilised. It is the responsibility of every veterinarian to evaluate the appropriateness of a particular opinion in the context of actual clinical situations and with due consideration to new developments.

All drugs are per os unless otherwise indicated. prn = as needed, sid = once per day.

DRUG DOSAGES				
Class	Drug	Indications/Comments	Dosage (Dog)	Dosage (Cat)
CNS stimulants		• Hyperkinesis • Narcolepsy		
	Methylphenidate	• Paradoxical calming effect in hyperkinesis • Narcolepsy	narcolepsy: 0.05–0.25 mg/kg bid **or** hyperkinesis: 2–4 mg/kg bid-tid	
	Dextroamphetamine	• Test for hyperkinesis • Narcolepsy	0.2–1.3 mg/kg prn narcolepsy: 5–10 mg sid	Narcolepsy: 1.25 mg prn
	Levoamphetamine	Test for hyperkinesis	1.0–4.0 mg/kg prn	
Anticonvulsants	Phenobarbital	• Tranquillisation • Epileptic seizures • Cats: Excessive vocalisation	1–4 mg/kg bid **or** prn – (up to 16 mg/kg/day)	1–4 mg/kg sid–bid **or** prn
	Carbamazepine	• Psychomotor epilepsy • Compulsive disorders • Aggression – cats • Antianxiety	4–10 mg/kg divided q8h **or** 5–10 mg/kg bid	Approximately 25 mg bid – adjust to serum levels **or** 4–8 mg/kg q12h
Benzodiazepines		• Urine marking in cats • Noise Phobias • Feline aggression • Anxiety		
	Clorazepate	• Antianxiety • Noise phobias • Thunderstorm phobia (peak serum levels within 1–2 h)	0.55–2.2 mg/kg sid–bid or prn	0.55–2.20 mg/kg sid–bid **or** prn
	Alprazolam	• Refractory feline housesoiling • Acute fears and fear aggression • Night waking	0.02–0.10 mg/kg **or** 0.25–2.0 mg/dog bid–tid	0.125–0.25 mg/cat bid **or** prn **or** 0.1 mg/kg tid **or** prn

		DRUG DOSAGES continued		
Class	**Drug**	**Indications/Comments**	**Dosage (Dog)**	**Dosage (Cat)**
	Diazepam (half-life of 2.5 hours in dogs and 5.5 hours in cats)	• Antianxiety • Appetite stimulant • Urine marking • Noise phobias • Seizures	0.5–2.2 mg/kg tid **or** prn	0.2–0.4 mg/kg sid–bid **or** Appetite stimulant: 0.5–1.0 mg/kg
	Diazepam (sustained release)	As above	0.5–1.0 mg/kg sid to bid	0.5–1.0 mg/kg sid to bid
	Flurazepam	• Appetite stimulant • Altered sleep cycles	0.2–0.4 mg/kg for 4–7 d	0.2–0.4 mg/kg for 4–7 d
	Oxazepam	• Appetite stimulant • Antianxiety • Urine marking	0.2–1.0 mg/kg sid–bid	0.2–0.5 mg/kg sid–bid **or** 1–2 mg/cat bid
	Triazolam	• Aggression in cats • Altered sleep cycles		0.03 mg/cat bid
	Clonazepam	• Sleep disorders • Seizures • Psychomotor epilepsy	0.1–0.5 mg/kg bid–tid	0.016 mg/kg sid–qid
	Chlordiazepoxide	• Anxiety • Appetite stimulant • Urine spraying	2–20 mg prn	0.2–1.0 mg/kg sid–bid
	Chlordiazepoxide/clinidium	• Stress colitis	1–2 tabs bid	
Neuroleptics		• Decrease vocalisation • Travelling • Noise phobias • Sedation		
	Acepromazine	• Restraint/sedation • Reduce activity • Reduce response to stimuli • Car travelling	0.1–2.2 mg/kg sid–qid	0.5–2.2 mg/kg prn
	Chlorpromazine	• Reduce response to stimuli • Reduce activity • Sedation	0.5–3.3 mg/kg sid–qid	0.5–3.3 mg/kg sid–qid
	Promazine	• Reduce activity • Reduce response to stimuli • Sedation	1.0–4.4 mg/kg prn	2.0–4.0 mg/kg prn
	Thoridiazine	• Aggression • Anxiety • Phobias • Compulsive disorders	1.1–2.2 mg/kg sid–bid	
	Perphenazine	• Anxiety • Fears • Phobias	0.88 mg/kg bid to tid	0.88 mg/kg bid to tid
	Pimozide	Compulsive disorders	1–10 mg sid	
	Haloperidol	• Compulsive disorders • Aggression	1–4 mg bid	
Tricyclic Antidepressants		• Depression • Anxiety • Aggression • Feline urine spraying • Narcolepsy • Enuresis • Compulsive behaviours • Mood stabilising		
	Amtriptyline	As above (peak levels 2–12 h)	1.0–6.0 mg/kg sid–bid	0.5–1.0 mg/kg/d

DRUG DOSAGES continued				
Class	**Drug**	**Indications/Comments**	**Dosage (Dog)**	**Dosage (Cat)**
	Doxepin	• Acral lick dermatitis • Compulsive behaviours	3–5 mg/kg bid **or** 0.5–1.0 mg/kg bid	
	Clomipramine	• Compulsive behaviours • Anxiety, including separation anxiety • Refractory urine marking	1–3 mg/kg/bid	0.5 mg/kg sid

	Imipramine	• Separation anxiety
		• Anxiety
		• Enuresis
		• Narcolepsy/Cataplexy (peak effects 1–2 h)
			2.2–4.4 mg/kg sid–bid
			Stereotypy:
			  1.0–2.0 mg/kg bid–tid
			Narcolepsy or cataplexy:
			  0.5–1.0 mg/kg tid
			Enuresis: 10 mg bid
				1–2 mg/kg bid–tid
				Enuresis – 2.5–5 mg bid

	Protriptyline	Narcoleptic hypersomnia (e.g. Labrador Retrievers) • Cataplexy	10 mg before bedtime **or** 0.2–0.5 mg/kg sid–bid	
Selective serotonin reuptake inhibitors (SSRIs)		• Depression/panic • Compulsive disorders • Aggression • Mood stabilising • Refractory urine marking		
	Fluoxetine	• Compulsive behaviours • Aggression • Mood stabilizing (half-life of fluoxetine in dogs – 1 day and half-life of norfluoxetine 5 days)	1.0 mg/kg sid	0.5–1.0 mg/kg q24 h
	Sertraline	See SSRI's above	1–3 mg/kg prn	
	Paroxetine	See SSRI's above		1 mg/kg sid
Hormones		• Aggression • Inappropriate elimination • Suppress male behaviour • Calming effect • Appetite stimulant		
	Megoestrol acetate	As above	1.1–4.4 mg/kg sid, then half dose q2wks to lowest effective dose	2.5–10 mg sid for 1 to 2 weeks then half dose q2wks to lowest effective dose
	Medroxyprogesterone acetate	As above	5–11 mg/kg sq/im 3X/yr	5–20 mg/kg sq/im 3X/yr
	Diethylstilboestrol	Oestrogen-responsive incontinence	0.1–1.0 mg/dog/day for 3–5 days then reduce to once or twice weekly	
	Testosterone cypionate	Urinary incontinence in neutered males	2.2 mg/kg im monthly	5–10 mg im
Ergot alkaloids	Bromocriptine	• Feline urine marking • False pregnancy – dogs • Pituitary dependent hyperadrenocorticism	0.01–0.10 mg/kg once or divided twice per day	

<div align="center">**DRUG DOSAGES continued**</div>				
Class	**Drug**	**Indications/Comments**	**Dosage (Dog)**	**Dosage (Cat)**
Antihistamines		• Compulsive scratching • Self trauma • Mild sedation • Car travelling • Waking at night		
	Hydroxyzine	As above	2.2 mg/kg bid–tid	2.2 mg/kg bid–tid
	Chlorpheniramine	As above	2–8 mg bid–tid **or** 0.2–0.8 mg/kg tid (maximum 1 mg/kg/24 hours)	1–2 mg bid–tid **or** 0.4–0.7 mg/kg sid to bid
	Diphenhydramine	As above	2–4 mg/kg bid–tid	2–4 mg/kg bid–tid
	Trimeprazine	As above	0.5–5.0 mg/dog tid	
	Cyproheptadine	• Serotonin antagonist • Antihistaminic • Appetite stimulant	Antihistamine: 0.3–2.0 mg/kg bid	2.0–4.0 mg/cat bid-tid
Opiate agonists/ antagonists		• Compulsive – stereotypic behaviours • Self mutilation		
	Naltrexone	As above	2.2 mg/kg sid–bid	2–4 mg/kg sid (up to 25–50 mg/cat)
	Pentazocine/Naloxone	As above	50 mg pentazocine/ 0.5 mg naloxone bid	
	Hydrocodone	Compulsive dermatologic disorders	0.22 mg/kg bid–tid	0.25–1.0 mg/kg bid–tid
Beta-blockers		Decrease somatic components of anxiety		
	Propranolol	Mild fears and anxiety	0.5–3.0 mg/kg bid **or** prn	0.2–1.0 mg/kg tid
	Pindolol	Mild fears and anxiety	0.125–0.25 mg/kg bid	
Alpha–adrenergics and sympathomimetics		• Urinary incontinence • Excitement urination • Submissive urination • Nocturnal urination		
	Phenylpropanalamine	As above	1.1–4.4 mg/kg bid–tid	12.5 mg tid
	Ephedrine	As above	15–50 mg bid–tid **or** 5–15 mg tid	2–4 mg/cat bid–tid
Alpha-adrenergic antagonists	Nicergoline	• Cognitive dysfunction • Diminished vigor • Sleep disorders • Psychomotor disturbances	0.25–0.50 mg/kg/day × 30 days. Tablets should not be broken for small dogs. A solution can be concocted with manufacturer's directions	
Antipsychotics	Lithium	• Unpredictable severe aggression	6–12 mg/kg q12–24 h – titrate dose by blood levels	
Miscellaneous antianxiety	Buspirone	• Chronic fears/anxiety • Phobias • Feline urine marking • Aggression • Stereotypy–obsessive	1.0–2.0 mg/kg sid–tid	0.5–1.0 mg/kg sid–tid
	Meprobamate	• Antianxiety • Aggression	20–40 mg/kg bid–qid	50 mg/kg prn
MAO inhibitors	Deprenyl	• Cognitive dysfunction • Neurodegenerative disease • Pituitary-dependent hyperadrenocorticism	Cognitive: 0.5 mg/kg sid Cushing's: 1–2 mg/kg sid	
For indications, contraindications, adverse effects and references see chapter 4.				

Index